HEMOSTASIS

A Case Oriented Approach

HEMOSTASIS

A Case Oriented Approach

Douglas A. Triplett, M.D.
Professor of Pathology and
Assistant Dean
Indiana University School of Medicine

Director, Muncie Center for Medical Education

Director of Hematology
Ball Memorial Hospital
Muncie, Indiana

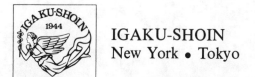

IGAKU-SHOIN
New York • Tokyo

Interior Design by Hudson River Studio
Typesetting by Ampersand Publisher Services, Inc.
  in Times Roman
Printing and Binding by Edwards Brothers, Incorporated
Cover Design by Paul Agule Design

Published and distributed by

IGAKU-SHOIN Ltd.,
5-24-3 Hongo, Bunkyo-ku, Tokyo

IGAKU-SHOIN Medical Publishers, Inc.,
1140 Avenue of the Americas, New York, N.Y. 10036

Library of Congress Cataloging in Publication Data

Triplett, Douglas A.
  Hemostasis : a case oriented approach.

  Includes index.
1. Blood—Coagulation, Disorders of—Case studies.
2. Blood—Coagulation. 3. Hemostasis. I. Title.
[DNLM: 1. Hemostasis. 2. Blood coagulation
  disorders.
WH 310 T835h]
RC647.C55T736   1985   616.1'57   83-2654

ISBN: 0-89640-099-9 (New York)
ISBN: 4-260-14099-X (Tokyo)

Printed and bound in U.S.A.

10 9 8 7 6 5 4 3 2 1

Preface

In the last several years, a number of comprehensive reference books have appeared in the field of thrombosis and hemostasis. The number of new publications reflects an increased interest in the pathogenesis of thrombotic disease and various treatment modalities. This interest is appropriate in view of the frequency of vascular thrombotic disease in the western world. However, these encyclopedic texts are difficult for clinical or laboratory physicians to utilize in the diagnosis and management of patients with thrombotic or hemorrhagic disorders. Therefore, there is a real need for a text that presents the information required for the care and diagnosis of such patients in a logic case oriented format.

The idea for this book came from a number of workshops and symposia that have been presented at the annual meetings of the American Society of Clinical Pathologists. Without exception, the most popular format for presentation of new concepts in the complex area of hemostasis has been the case oriented programs. The participants' critiques always request additional case material. This has also been the situation in teaching house officers, medical students, and medical technologists.

The cases utilized in this book have been gathered from the files of the Hematology section of the Department of Pathology at Ball Memorial Hospital. Without the cooperation and active support of the clinicians and the clinical staff, this book would not have been possible. I am also deeply indebted to the indulgence and support of my associates in the Department of Pathology, Drs. Willman, Branam, Baldwin, Kocoshis, Pearson and House. The medical technologists in the Hematology section also deserve credit for their outstanding technical support and frequent thoughtful comments in individual cases. Also, the residents in pathology and hematopathology fellows have been a source of inspiration and provocative insights.

A special acknowledgement is necessary for my secretary, Linda Glaze. She has cheerfully worked on the manuscript despite my frequent revisions and seemingly endless deadlines. This book represents "our efforts." We hope that the reader will find it stimulating and useful.

Douglas A. Triplett, M.D.

Contents

HEMOSTASIS

A Case Oriented Approach

PART

ONE

FUNDAMENTALS
OF HEMOSTASIS

Chapter
ONE

Biochemistry of Blood Coagulation

The hemostatic mechanism has two primary functions: confining circulating blood to the vascular bed and arresting bleeding at the site of an injured vessel. These dual functions are readily appreciated by clinical states in which there is an abnormality of the hemostatic process. Patients may bleed spontaneously (e.g., classical hemophilia A and B) or after damage to a vascular wall due to trauma. The hemostatic process depends on delicate and complex interactions among at least five components: blood vessels, plasma coagulation proteins, physiologic protease inhibitors, platelets and the fibrinolytic system.

The hemostatic response may be conveniently divided into two steps: primary and secondary hemostasis. The primary response involves interaction between a blood vessel and circulating platelets. With exposure of various components of the vascular wall after endothelial injury, platelets adhere and undergo a complex sequence of reactions that culminates in the formation of a primary platelet plug. Secondary hemostasis involves interactions of coagulation proteins which result ultimately in the generation of cross-linked fibrin which stabilizes the platelet plug.

This chapter will focus on coagulation proteins and on physiologic inhibitors of the coagulation process.

Historical Perspectives

Although a hemorrhagic tendency found in males of certain families was described in the Jewish Talmud in the second century (1), disorders of coagulation received little attention until the appearance of hemophilia in members of the royal families of Europe (2,3). In 1853, Queen Victoria, a carrier of hemophilia, gave birth to her fifth son, Leopold, who suffered from the disease. After receiving a minor blow to the head, Leopold died of a cerebral hemorrhage at the age of 31. Two of Queen Victoria's daughters were identified as carriers of hemophilia after they gave birth to affected sons. One of Queen Victoria's granddaughters, Alexandra, became the Czarina of Russia and gave birth to a son, Alexis, who suffered from hemophilia. The role of hemophilia in the Russian revolution has been the subject of a number of popular histories (4).

In 1905, Paul Morawitz (5) proposed a theory of coagulation that has become widely accepted. This theory can be summarized as follows:

$$\text{Prothrombin} \xrightarrow[\text{Ca}^{2+}]{\text{Thrombokinase}} \text{Thrombin}$$

$$\text{Fibrinogen} \xrightarrow{\text{Thrombin}} \text{Fibrin}$$

Morawitz proposed that coagulation takes place in two stages. In the first stage, prothrombin is converted to its active form by thrombokinase, a poorly defined factor that requires the presence of calcium. In the second stage, thrombin acts on fibrinogen to yield fibrin. Thus, Morawitz recognized four essential components: thrombokinase, prothrombin, calcium and fibrinogen.

Following Morawitz's theory, Addis, in 1911 (6), demonstrated that normal plasma would correct the prolonged clotting time of hemophilic plasma. Subsequently, in 1935, Armand J. Quick, a young physician biochemist in New York City, and his colleagues (7) devised a test for measuring "prothrombin". In this test, a potent tissue factor, thromboplastin, is added to oxalated plasma and then calcium is added. This test (prothrombin time) has found wide spread popularity and is currently the most commonly performed procedure in coagulation laboratories.

As a result of the development of this test, a number of important advances in the field of coagulation were made. They include the elucidation of hemorrhagic disease of the newborn and the identification of a substance, 3' methylene bis[4-hydroxycourmarin], in spoiled sweet clover that is responsible for a hemorrhagic disease noted in cattle feeding on the clover (8). With the discovery of dicumarol, the first oral anticoagulant in the clinical armamentarium was identified. Measurement of the prothrombin time also led to the discovery of additional coagulation factors, including labile factor (factor V) (9,10), serum prothrombin conversion accelerator (factor VII) (11–13) and Stuart-Prower factor (factor X) (14).

In 1953, Langdell and coworkers at the University of North Carolina (15) described the partial thromboplastin time as a measure of the "intrinsic system" of coagulation. In contrast to the "extrinsic system" of coagulation, which involves the participation of a "tissue factor," all components of the intrinsic system are found in the circulating blood. The concept of intrinsic and extrinsic systems of coagulation is useful in the evaluation of patients with abnormalities of hemostasis. Nevertheless, in vivo, after vascular injury, there are a number of interactions between the two systems.

The partial thromboplastin time was further refined by Proctor and Rapaport (16), who proposed the addition of a substance (kaolin) to accelerate the contact phase of coagulation thus giving rise to the activated partial thromboplastin time. Thus, two relatively simple tests, the prothrombin time and the activated partial

Table 1

Nomenclature of Coagulation Factors

Factor	Synonyms
I	Fibrinogen
II	Prothrombin
III	Tissue thromboplastin, tissue factor
IV	Calcium
V	Proaccelerin, labile factor, Ac globulin
VI	Not used
VII	Proconvertin, Serum Prothrombin Conversion Accelerator, stable factor, autoprothrombin I
VIII	Antihemophilic factor A (AHF), antihemophilic globulin (AHG)
IX	Christmas factor, plasma thromboplastin component (PTC), antihemophilic factor B
X	Stuart-Prower factor, autoprothrombin III
XI	Plasma thromboplastin antecedent (PTA), antihemophilic factor C
XII	Hageman factor
XIII	Fibrin-stabilizing factor, Laki-Lorand factor
●	Fletcher factor (prekallikrein)
●	Fitzgerald factor (high-molecular-weight kininogen)
●	Protein C
●	Protein S

thromboplastin time became the mainstays of the modern coagulation laboratory.

In the 1950s, investigators using these two procedures identified additional coagulation factors (factors IX, XI and XII) (17–19). To reduce the confusion created by the existence of various names for many coagulation factors, the International Committee on Nomenclature of Blood Coagulation Factors assigned Roman numerals to define the recognized coagulation proteins (Table 1).

In 1964, the "cascade" (MacFarlane) (20) and "waterfall" (Davie and Ratnoff) (21) mechanisms of blood coagulation were proposed. These two theories likened blood coagulation to a linear sequence of proteolytic reactions. It soon became clear that the

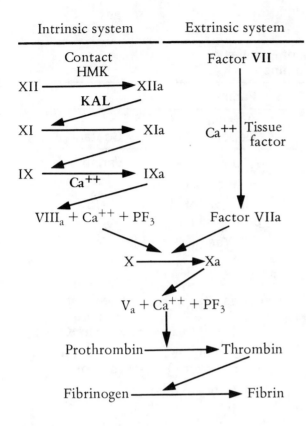

HMK = High molecular weight kininogen
KAL = Kallikrein
PF₃ = Platelet phospholipide

Figure 1. Intrinsic and extrinsic systems of coagulation. Both Factors VIII and V are converted from procofactors to *active* cofactors.

zymogens involved in the coagulation process have extensive sequence homology with zymogens of the pancreatic serine proteases. Two separate pathways of coagulation, intrinsic and extrinsic, which were defined by the activated partial thromboplastin time and the prothrombin time, were recognized. More recent work, however, has emphasized the interdependence of the classical intrinsic and extrinsic systems as well as the complexity of the coagulation reactions (22–27). In addition to the enzymes that participate actively in the coagulation process, it is now appreciated that several steps involve membrane phospholipid surfaces and protein cofactors and have a requirement for calcium ions. Current concepts of the coagulation process are illustrated in Figure 1.

Properties of Coagulation Proteins

Rather than discuss the coagulation proteins in numerical sequence, it is convenient to divide them into three groups on the basis of biochemical properties. The three groups are vitamin K dependent, contact and thrombin sensitive factors (Table 2). Table 3 lists the physical properties of all the coagulation proteins.

Vitamin K-Dependent Coagulation Factors

Vitamin K-dependent coagulation factors include prothrombin and factors VII, IX and X. Four additional vitamin K-dependent plasma proteins have recently been discovered. They include protein C, which was initially identified by Seegers and associates (28,29), protein S, protein Z and protein M (Table 4). The characteristic chemical feature of these proteins is a unique amino acid residue referred to as γ carboxyglutamic acid (30). γ Carboxyglutamic acid results from a vitamin K-dependent postribrosomal modification. Carboxylation of glutamic acid in the γ position results in the formation of this amino acid (Figure 2).

The γ carboxyglutamic acid residues enable the vitamin K-dependent proteins to bind calcium ions. As a result, these proteins can bind to vesicles composed of acidic phospholipids. The ability to bind calcium and form "calcium bridges" with acidic phospholipids is essential for the enzyme and substrate functions of the vitamin K-dependent proteins in the coagulation mechanism. Use of oral anticoagulants or dietary vitamin K deficiency results in inhibition of the vitamin K-dependent carboxylation reactions. As a consequence, nonfunctional vitamin K-dependent proteins are secreted into the circulation causing a reduction in the efficiency of the coagulation mechanism (Figure 3) (31–33).

Four vitamin K-dependent proteins have been recognized since the discovery of factor X in 1956. During the past decade, further studies on the structure and function of these proteins have led to elucidation of the primary structure of three of these factors. Of the newly characterized vitamin K-dependent proteins, protein C is of greatest interest. Seegers and associates (29) initially termed this protein autoprotrhombin IIa and correctly identified it as an inhibitor of coagulation. Protein C also appears to play a role in fibrinolysis (34). Hereditary and acquired deficiencies of protein C have been described (35,36).

Figure 2. γ-Carboxyglutamic acid.

Table 2

Biochemical Properties of Families of Coagulation Proteins*

| | Family | | |
Property	Thrombin Sensitive	Vitamin K Dependent	Contact
Molecular weight	300,000+	57,000–69,000	Variable
Stability	Heat labile	Heat stabile	—
Consumed during coagulation	Yes	No (except prothrombin)	No
Adsorbed by $BaSO_4$, $Al(OH)_3$, etc.	No	Yes	No
Destroyed by plasmin	Yes	No	No
Synthesis	Does not require vitamin K	Requires vitamin K	Does not require vitamin K
Reagent for correction studies	Plasma	Serum (except factor II)	Plasma or serum
Present in platelets	α granules and cytoplasm	No	No
Acute-phase reactant	Yes	No	No

*For a more complete summary of the physical properties, see Table 3. Thrombin-sensitive proteins are present in platelets. Fibrinogen, factor VIII R:Ag and factor V are located in the α granules, whereas factor XIII is located in the cytoplasm. Note that factor VIII:C activity does not occur in platelets. The factor XIII found in platelet cytoplasm is composed of a chains only.

Table 3

Properties of Coagulation Proteins

Factor	Molecular Weight	Migration in Electrophoresis	Structure of Zymogen	Structure of Active Enzyme	Functional Activity
Fibrinogen	340,000	β Globulin	Symmetric with six subunits		
Prothrombin	72,000	α- or β-Globulin	Single polypeptide chain	Two subunits linked by disulfide bond	Serine protease
Factor V	330,000	β-Globulin	Single chain	Several fragments	Cofactor
Factor VII	48,000	α-Globulin	Single polypeptide chain	Two-chain form	Serine protease

(A) Normal Liver Cell

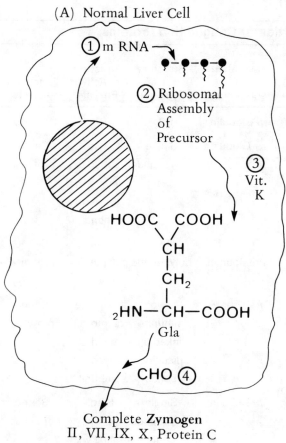

(B) Liver Cell in Vitamin K **Deficiency**

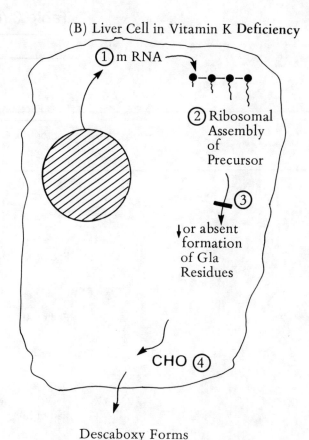

Figure 3. Synthesis of vitamin K-dependent proteins is similar in many respects to synthesis of other proteins. Nuclear DNA "instructs" (1) messenger RNA, which regulates (2) ribosomal assembly of polypeptide chains. After ribosomal assembly, (3) vitamin K partici- pates in the conversion of amino-terminal glutamic acid residues into γ-carboxyglutamic acid (Gla). The final step (4) is addition of carbohydrate and secretion of the completed zymogen into the circulation. In Proteins C and S, as well as Factors IX and X, an additional post-ribosomal step involves the hydroxylation of aspartic acid to B-hydroxyaspartic acid.

Biologic Half-life	Carbohydrate Content	Site of Production	Dependent on Vitamin K	Concentration in Plasma	Presence in $BaSO_4 =$ Adsorbed Plasma	Presence in Serum
90 hours	4.5%	Liver	No	300–400 mg/dl	Yes	No
60 hours	8.2%	Liver	Yes	10–15 mg/dl	No	No
12–36 hours	13%	Liver	No	0.5–1.0% mg/dl	Yes	No
4–6 hours	—	Liver	Yes	0.1 mg/dl	No	Yes

Table 3 *(continued)*

Properties of Coagulation Proteins

Factor	Molecular Weight	Migration in Electrophoresis	Structure of Zymogen	Structure of Active Enzyme	Functional Activity
Factor VIII: C	70–240,000	β-Globulin	?	?	Cofactor
Factor IX	57,000	α_1-Globulin	Single polypeptide chain	Two subunits linked by disulfide bond	Serine protease
Factor X	58,900	From α to prealbumin	Two polypeptide chains	Two polypeptide chains	Serine protease
Factor XI	160,000	As β- or γ- Globulin	Two subunits linked by disulfide bonds	Cleavage of internal bond of each subunit	Serine protease
Factor XII	80,000	β-Globulin	Single polypeptide chain	Single chain, mol. wt 28,000	Serine protease
Prekallikrein (Fletcher factor)	85,000	Fast γ-globulin	Single polypeptide chain	Two chains linked by disulfide bond	Serine protease
High-molecular-weight kininogen	110,000	α-Globulin	Single chain		Cofactor
Factor XIII (fibrin stabilizing factor)	320,000	α_2-Globulin	2a (75,000) and 2b (88,000) chains	Two a chains	Trans-Amidase
Plasminogen	90,000	β-Globulin	Single polypeptide chain		Serine protease
Protein C	62,000	—	Two chains linked by disulfide bonds	Two chains linked by disulfide bonds	Serine protease (anti-coagulant)
Protein S	69,000	—	One chain	—	—

Biologic Half-life	Carbohydrate Content	Site of Production	Dependent on Vitamin K	Concentration in Plasma	Presence in BaSO₄= Adsorbed Plasma	Presence in Serum
12 hours	17.1%		No	—	Yes	No
24 hours	15%	Liver	Yes	0.75 mg/dl	No	Yes
40 hours	5%	Liver	Yes	1.2 mg/dl	No	Yes
48–52 hours	16.8%	Liver	No	0.4 mg/dl	Yes decreased one-third	Yes
48–52 hours	15%	Liver	No	0.29 mg/dl	Yes	Yes
		Liver	No	0.15–0.45 mg/dl	Yes	Yes
6.5 days	12.6%	Liver	No	0.70 mg/dl	Yes	Yes
3–5 days	4.9%	Liver	No	2.5 mg/dl	Yes	No
		Liver	No	10–15 mg/dl	Yes	
6 hours	23%	Liver	Yes	0.5 mg/dl	No	Yes
—	7.8%	Liver	Yes	—	No	Yes

Table 4

Additional Vitamin K-Dependent Proteins*			
	Protein C	Protein S	Protein M	Protein Z
Molecular weight	62,000	69,000	50,000	44,000
Plasma concentration (μg/ml)	3.5	1	<1	<1
Number of chains	2	1	1	1
Number of glutamic acid residues	11	10	(+)	6
Carbohydrate (%)	(+)	(+)	(+)	(+)
Function	Anticoagulant and fibrinolytic	Complement C4b, Cofactor for Protein C	Procoagulant	Platelet function(?)

The physical properties of other vitamin K-dependent plasma proteins are summarized in Table 4. Protein C is currently the most important of these proteins. Patients with a hereditary or an acquired deficiency of protein C have been described.

In addition to vitamin K-dependent plasma proteins, various tissue proteins with γ-carboxyglutamic acid residues have been discovered. They include osteocalcin in bone, atherocalcin in atherosclerotic plaques and an unnamed protein in the kidneys.

Prothrombin

Prothrombin was the first coagulation factor to be highly purified. Following purification, sequencing studies led to the discovery of γ carboxyglutamic acid residues on the amino-terminal end of the molecule. The molecular weight of prothrombin in 72,000 (Figure 4). The conversion of this coagulation factor to thrombin involves a series of enzymatic steps (37). Factor Xa first cleaves prothrombin at position #2 and then at position #3 yielding the amino-terminal "pro" fragment and active alpha-thrombin. Alpha-thrombin is composed of an A chain of 5,700 daltons and a B chain of 31,000 daltons which are linked by disulfide bonds. The active serine containing enzymatic pocket of thrombin is located in the heavy (B) chain. Unlike the other vitamin K-dependent coagulation proteins, thrombin does not

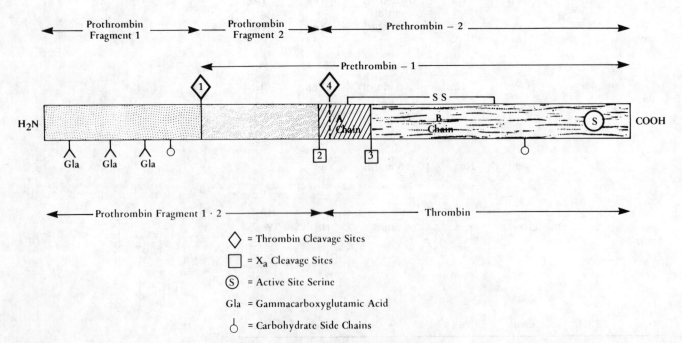

Figure 4. Prothrombin activation.

remain bound to phospholipid surfaces by the calcium bridges formed by the carboxyglutamic acid residues on the amino-terminal end of the molecule. In addition to the peptide bonds that are cleaved by Factor Xa, prothrombin is also cleaved by thrombin.

Thrombin can cleave prothrombin at two sites. Cleavage at the first site, position #1, yields prothrombin fragment one (23,000 daltons) from the amino terminal of the molecule (38). The remaining portion of the prothrombin molecule is called prethrombin 1. Prethrombin 1 has a molecular weight of 55,000. The second thrombin cleavage site is position #4. This site is located 13 amino acid residues from the cleavage site that gives rise to the A chain of thrombin. This cleavage is autocatalytic, consequently, isolated human thrombin always lacks these 13 residues. The physiologic importance of this thrombin cleavage site is unknown.

Factor VII

Factor VII was initially thought to be unique to the extrinsic system of coagulation. However, recent data indicate that factor VII is capable of activating factor IX (22–27, 39, 40). As a result the clear compartmentalization of coagulation into intrinsic and extrinsic systems is now obsolete. Nevertheless, for a laboratory approach to coagulation, it is still useful to think in terms of an intrinsic and extrinsic system. Recently the possible role of factor VII as the initial enzyme in the coagulation process has been suggested. The single chain form of factor VII is unique among the coagulation factors because it is biologically active and does not require proteolytic activation. The zymogen or single chain form of factor VII can incorporate diisopropylfluorophosphate (DFP) into the active site serine. Depending on the experimental conditions, the molecular weight of factor VII has been reported as varying from 45,000 to 54,000 (Figure 5). The single-chain form of factor VII can be

cleaved by a number of serine proteases with further enhancement of its activity. The enzymes that further activate factor VII include: factors XIIa, IXa, Xa and thrombin. Plasmin will also activate factor VII. Cleavage at site #1 by factor Xa or thrombin will yield a 100-fold increase in the activity of factor VII. As a result of this cleavage, a two-chain molecule linked by disulfide bonds is formed. There is no activation peptide. The active site is located in the carboxy-terminal peptide. The two-chain form called VIIa may be cleaved at site #2 by factor Xa and/or thrombin to yield B VIIa. The cleavage at site #2 occurs at a slow rate and will divide the heavy-chain into two peptides. Beta VIIa does not possess coagulant activity.

Factor IX

The zymogen form of factor IX is a single chain molecule with a molecular weight of 55,000 (Figure 6). The activation of the zymogen can be mediated by either factor XIa or factor VIIa. As previously discussed, the active form of factor IX can activate factor VII. Thus, there is a reciprocal relationship in the activation of factors IX and VII. The activation of factors IX involves two proteolytic cleavages and requires calcium. The first reaction, which appears to be rate limiting, involves the cleavage of site #1 an arginine-valine bond, resulting in a disulfide linked two-chain intermediate that lacks enzymatic activity. The second reaction is slower and occurs at site #2. With this reaction there is a liberation of an activation peptide (9000 daltons) from the heavy chain of the inactive intermediate. The resulting two-chain form of factor IX is the active enzyme having a molecular weight of 46,500. An enzyme from the venom of Russell's viper also activates Factor IX, but the mechanism of activation involves a single cleavage at site #2 (41). Thus, no activation peptide is released. This form of IXa has approximately 50% of the activity of

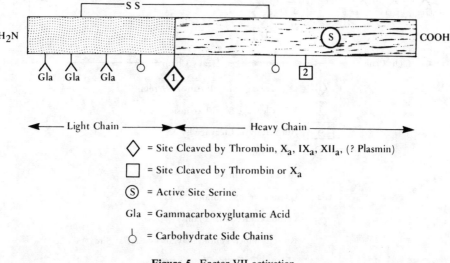

Figure 5. Factor VII activation.

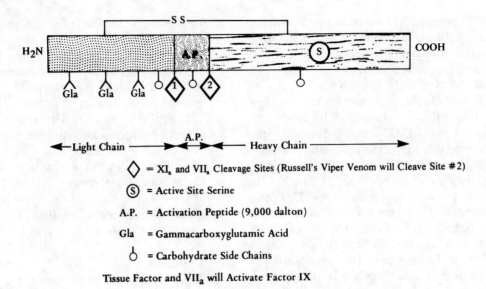

$\Diamond$ = XI$_a$ and VII$_a$ Cleavage Sites (Russell's Viper Venom will Cleave Site #2)

$\circledS$ = Active Site Serine

A.P. = Activation Peptide (9,000 dalton)

Gla = Gammacarboxyglutamic Acid

ϕ = Carbohydrate Side Chains

Tissue Factor and VII$_a$ will Activate Factor IX

Figure 6. Factor IX activation.

factor IXa produced by the actions of factors XIa and VIIa.

Factor X
Factor X may be thought of as the crossroads of the coagulation system. Both the intrinsic and extrinsic systems of blood coagulation will activate factor X. Macromolecular complexes are involved in both systems (intrinsic: IXa, VIII, calcium, and phospholipid; extrinsic: VIIa, tissue factor, calcium, and phospholipid). Factor X is a two-chain molecule with a heavy chain of 37,000 daltons and a light chain of 17,000 daltons (Figure 7). The two chains are linked by disulfide bonds. The light chain contains 12 γ carboxyglutamic acid residues and is analogous to the amino-terminal portion of other vitamin K-dependent proteins. The zymogen form of factor X is activated by the cleavage of site #1 by either VIIa or IXa to yield factor Xa α. Subsequent autocatalytic cleavage of the enzyme at site #2 will produce XaB. In addition, factor Xa α also cleaves the factor X molecule at site #3. This cleavage at site #3 is slow and is presumably of no physiologic importance.

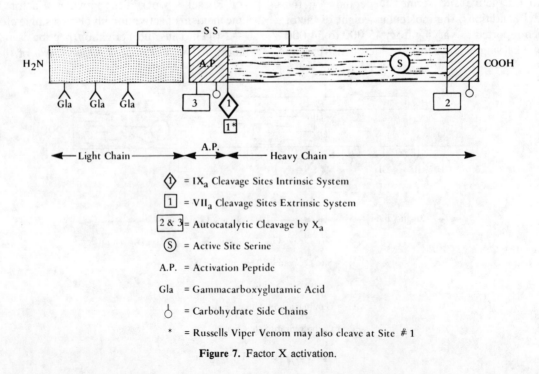

$\Diamond$ = IX$_a$ Cleavage Sites Intrinsic System

$\boxed{1}$ = VII$_a$ Cleavage Sites Extrinsic System

$\boxed{2\ \&\ 3}$ = Autocatalytic Cleavage by X$_a$

$\circledS$ = Active Site Serine

A.P. = Activation Peptide

Gla = Gammacarboxyglutamic Acid

ϕ = Carbohydrate Side Chains

* = Russells Viper Venom may also cleave at Site #1

Figure 7. Factor X activation.

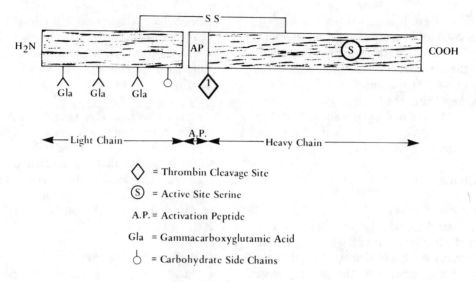

Figure 8. Protein C activation.

Protein C

Protein C was initially identified in 1960 by Seegers and associates (28). In 1976, Stenflo purified and partially characterized protein C (42). During his isolation procedure, Stenflo obtained four peaks in his chromatographic elution steps. These peaks were labeled sequentially A through D; the third peak contained a "new" protein that was arbitrarily given the name protein C. Protein C is a glycoprotein with a heavy and light chain linked by disulfide bonds (43). The heavy chain has a molecular weight of approximately 41,000 and the light chain 21,000. The human protein C molecular appears to be more glycosylated than bovine protein C and contains approximately 23% carbohydrate. The γ carboxyglutamic acid residues are located on the light chain while the active site serine is found on the heavy chain. Recently, a new amino acid, beta hydroxyaspartic acid, has been found in protein C. In contrast to the other vitamin K-dependent coagulation proteins, activated protein C is a potent anticoagulant. Physiologically protein C is thought to be activated by thrombin which has complexed with a cofactor, thrombomodulin, on the surface of endothelial cells. Thrombin will cleave protein C in the amino terminal region of the heavy chain at position #1 (Figure 8). As a result, a 14 chain activation peptide is released and activated protein C is formed. In the laboratory protein C is also activated by trypsin and Russell's viper venom. Normal plasma contains a protein that inhibits activated protein C (ie, a physiologic inhibitor), which has only recently been isolated (44,45). Protein C functions in plasma by inactivating the activated cofactors Va and VIIIa (Figure 9) (46,47). Activated protein C will inactivate the activated forms of these cofactors more rapidly than the native forms.

Other Vitamin K-Dependent Plasma Proteins

With the discovery of γ carboxyglutamic acid, a number of additional vitamin K-dependent proteins have been discovered. Of these, proteins S, Z, and M are plasma proteins. Protein S has a molecular weight of 69,000 (48). It has an association with complement component

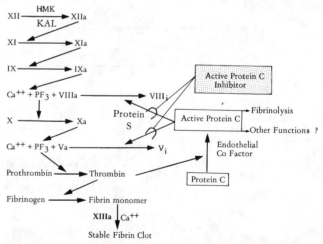

Figure 9. Active protein C inactivates two cofactors: VIIIa and Va. This anticoagulant activity is of clinical importance because patients with a hereditary deficiency of protein C have a thrombotic tendency. Protein C is activated by thrombin. Thrombin in the form of a complex thrombomodulin on surfaces of endothelial cells rapidly converts protein C into its active form. The role of another vitamin K-dependent protein, protein S, has yet to be fully characterized.

Plasma contains a physiologic inhibitor of activated protein C. The rare hereditary disorder of combined factors V and VIII deficiency was thought to be due to an absence of this inhibitor. However, recent experiments have suggested that this is not the case. (With permission from Dr. John Griffin, Scripps Clinic and Research Foundation, La Jolla, California.)

C4b (49). In addition, there is some evidence to suggest that protein S is a cofactor in accelerating the activity of activated protein C. Presumably this reaction takes place on the surface of the activated platelet. Protein Z has a molecular weight of 44,000 and contains six γ carboxyglutamic acid residues (50). The function of this protein is unknown. Protein M has a molecular weight of 50,000 and appears to be a procoagulant involved in the activation of prothrombin to thrombin (51).

Contact Factors

Factor XII (Hageman Factor)

Factor XII is a single chain glycoprotein with a molecular weight of 80,000 (Figure 10). Surface bound (factor XII) is more susceptible to cleavage by kallikrein and by undergoing configurational change may also manifest evidence of an active site (52). Cleavage within the disulfide loop (site 1) gives rise to α factor XIIa which can activate factor XI. Alpha-factor XIIa remains bound to the surface. If the cleavage occurs outside the disulfide loop (site 2), β factor XIIa is generated. Beta XIIa has a molecular weight of 28,000 and possesses both esterase and amidolytic activity. Beta XIIa is not bound to the activating surface and will only poor activate factor XI; however, it will activate prekallikrein.

As noted above, it appears that cleavage of factor XII may not be necessary for expression of α XIIa activity (53,54). For instance, exposure of factor XII to immobilized ellagic acid will impart most of the α XIIa activities to the surface bound molecule without enzymatic cleavage (55). Similarly, reactions with kaolin, sulfatides, gangliosides and stearic acid potentiate the activity of factor XII without altering its structure (56).

The interaction between factor XII and the cofactor of the contact phase of coagulation, high molecular weight kininogen (Fitzgerald factor) is still the subject of study. It appears that high molecular weight kininogen is involved in orienting the binding of Factor XII to negatively charged foreign surfaces. This "directed" binding facilitates the surface interactions of factor XII.

Prekallikrein (Fletcher Factor)

Prekallikrein is a single-chain glycoprotein with a molecular weight of approximately 85,000 (Figure 11). A single cleavage (site 1) of the zymogen yields the disulfide-linked active enzyme kallikrein. In its zymogen form, prekallikrein appears to incorporate DFP into its active site serine. Thus, in a manner similar to factor VII, prekallikrein may possess a low level of intrinsic activity. Prekallikrein circulates as a 1:1 molar complex with high molecular weight kininogen. Prekallikrein is involved in the surface activation of factor XII. The kallikrein that is generated by α XIIa is relatively rapidly released from the surface upon which the contact factors are assembled. In contrast, factor XIa will remain associated with the surface. Beta XIIa will also activate prekallikrein in

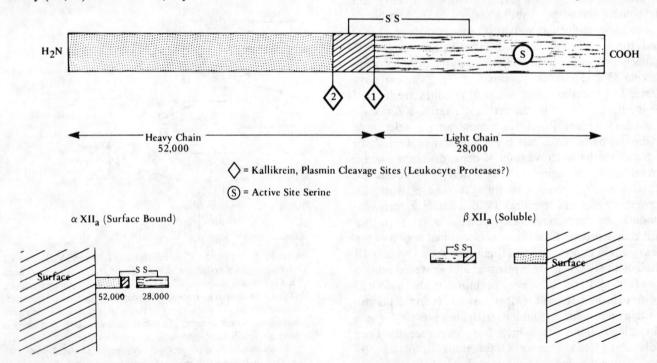

Figure 10. Factor XII has a molecular weight of approximately 80,000. When it is exposed to a negatively charged surface, it attaches to the surface. This attachment is mediated through the heavy chain. After becoming attached, factor XII undergoes a conformational change that makes it more readily cleaved by kallikrein. Cleavage at site 1 results in surface-bound alpha-factor XIIa. Cleavage at site 2 gives rise to soluble beta-factor XIIa. Beta-factor XIIa activates prekallikrein but activates factor XI only poorly.

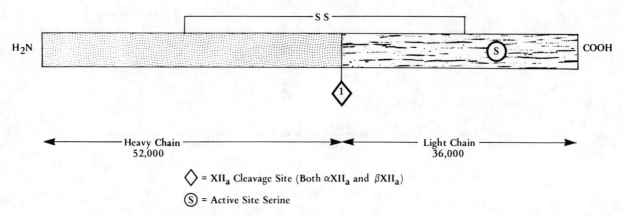

Figure 11. Prekallikrein activation.

solution. The physiologic substrates for kallikrein include plasminogen, factors IX, and XII and high molecular weight kininogen. Recently, it has been discovered that kallikrein will activate prorenin. The fluid phase activation of prekallikrein by β XIIa has been implicated in the hypotensive episodes that follows administration of albumin preparations.

Factor XI

Factor XI is a symmetric two chain molecule with each of the constituent chains having a molecular weight of 80,000 (Figure 12). Activation of factor XI by factor XIIa follows cleavage of both chains (site 1) yielding two 50,000 dalton and two 30,000 dalton chains covalently linked by disulfide bridges. The active site of factor XIa is similar to other serine proteases.

The native factor XI circulates in plasma bound to high molecular weight kininogen in a 1:1 molar complex. The surface bound or α XIIa will activate factor XI. After activation, XIa will remain bound to the surface.

The physiologic substrates for XIa are factors XII and IX. The activation of IX is of greatest importance.

High-Molecular-Weight Kininogen (Fitzgerald Factor)

High-molecular-weight kininogen has a molecular weight of approximately 110,000 (Figure 13). This protein is a substrate for plasma kallikrein giving rise to bradykinin. After release of bradykinin, the molecule consists of a heavy chain of 66,000 daltons and a light chain of 44,000 daltons linked by disulfide bonds. The coagulant activity of the molecule resides in the light chain. As has been previously noted, high-molecular-weight kininogen circulates in plasma as a complex with factor XI or prekallikrein. Thus, high-molecular-weight kininogen serves as a carrier protein for two of the contact components and, in addition, serves to orient the various components of the contact phase of coagulation on foreign surfaces to maximize productive surface interactions.

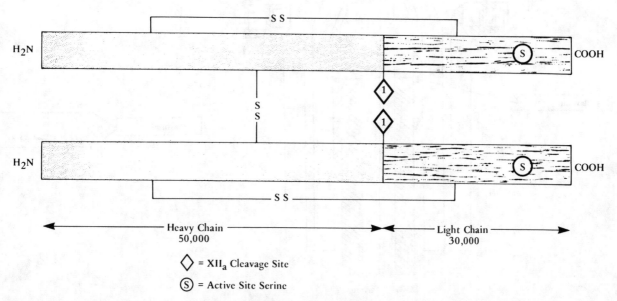

Figure 12. Factor XI activation.

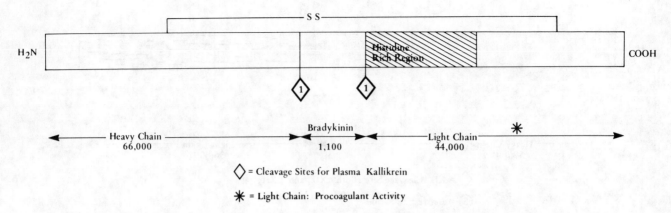

Figure 13. Cleavage of high-molecular-weight kininogen.

Thrombin-Sensitive Coagulation Factors

Fibrinogen

Fibrinogen is a symmetrical dimer that contains three pairs of different polypeptide chains linked by disulfide bonds (Figure 14). The constituent polypeptide chains are called alpha, beta and gamma. The molecular weight of fibrinogen is 340,000. The primary structure of fibrinogen is known. Therefore, the study of abnormal or dysfibrinogen molecules has advanced rapidly. By identi-

fying single amino acid substitutions in certain dysfibrinogens (eg, fibrinogen Detroit) the physiologic importance of certain regions of the molecule has been appreciated. The conversion of fibrinogen to fibrin results from the thrombin mediated cleavage of specific arginine-glycine bonds with the release of fibrinopeptides A and B. These fibrinopeptides are released from the amino-terminal ends of the alpha and beta chains. Fibrinogen is also substrate for plasmin. Plasmin will progressively digest fibrinogen ultimately yielding the plasmin-resistant fragments D and E (for further discussion, see section on fibrinolysis).

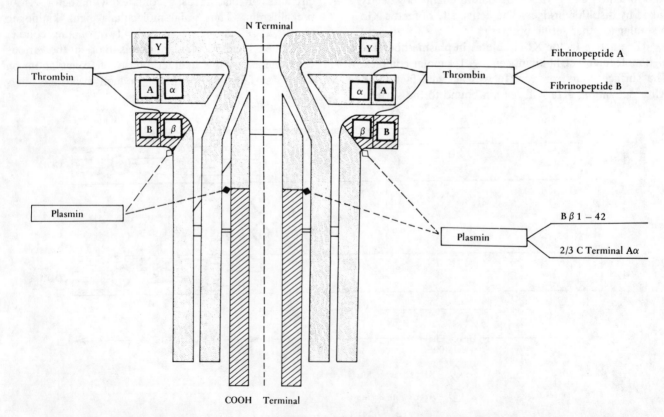

Figure 14. Proteolytic digestion of fibrinogen. (Modified from Blömback B, Blomback M: *Ann NY Acad Sci* 202:77–97, 1972.)

Factor V

Factor V is a single chain glycoprotein with a molecular weight of 330,000. Factor V is found in plasma as well as the alpha granules of the platelet. Of all the coagulation proteins, factor V is the most labile. The native factor V in plasma is a procofactor that must be proteolytically cleaved in order to express its cofactor activity in the conversion of prothrombin to thrombin. Thrombin will proteolytically activate factor V by attacking specific sites in the molecule giving rise to the active cofactor Va. The activation of factor V is depicted in Figure 15. Generation of factor V activity is associated with the cleavage producing component D (not to be confused with the fibrinogen breakdown product D)(58). Inactivation of factor V by activated protein C involves cleavage of component D (94,000 dalton peptides). It appears that the minimum species that displays factor Va activity is a complex of components D and E. Association of these two components is dependent on the presence of a tightly bound calcium ion. Platelet factor V may play a more important role in vivo than plasma factor V (59,60).

Factor VIII

Factor VIII is a complex protein that consists of at least two components: factor VIII:C which is deficient or abnormal in patients with hemophilia A, and the von Willebrand factor, which is deficient or abnormal in patients with von Willebrand's disease (61–65). Von Willebrand factor plays no part in blood coagulation but is essential for primary hemostasis. The function of von Willebrand factor in primary hemostasis is dependent upon its ability to mediate platelet adhesion to components of damaged vessel walls. The components of the complex circulate in plasma linked noncovalently. Both components are acute phase proteins; consequently their levels increase in a parallel fashion in response to varying non-specific stimuli (eg, exercise, surgery, stress, etc.)(66–69). Current nomenclature of the various properties of factor VIII is summarized in Table 5.

Presently, there is no consensus regarding the molecular weight of factor VIII:C. Molecular weights ranging from 35,000 to 310,000 have been reported (70–73). Although there is disagreement regarding the unactivated factor VIII:C, there is general agreement

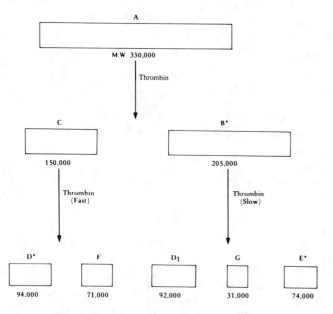

Figure 15. Activation of factor V to Va involves proteolytic cleavage of the molecule by thrombin. In the diagram, the asterisks indicate the peptide fragments that are involved in expression of factor Va activity. Components C and B are intermediates in the conversion of factor V to Va. Factor Va activity is expressed when peptide D* is formed. Factor Va may be inactivated by protein C. Activated protein C cleaves peptide D*. (Mann KG, Fass DM: The molecular biology of blood coagulation in VF Fairbanks (ed). *Current Hematology*. New York: John Wiley & Sons 1983, vol 2, p 359.)

Table 5

Nomenclature of Factor VIII/von Willebrand Factor		
Factor	VIII:C	Procoagulant activity; measured with factor VIII assay
Factor	VIII:C:Ag	Factor VIII:C antigen; measured with homologous or monoclonal antibodies by immunoradiometric assay or radioimmunoassay
Factor	VIII R:RCo	Ristocetin cofactor; activity necessary for ristocetin-induced platelet agglutination *Invitro*
Factor	VIII R:Ag	Factor VIII-related antigen; reacts with heterologous antisera to factor VIII*; measured by rocket immunoelectrophoresis, radio immunoassay or immunoradiometric assay
Factor	VIII R:WF	von Willebrand factor; bleeding time factor; activity necessary for formation of in vivo platelet plug

Recently, the use of hydridoma monoclonal antibodies has permitted the identification of a number of antigenic determinants on the factor VIII R:Ag portion of the molecule.

that proteolysis by thrombin yields a digest of polypeptide chains with molecular weights that are between 50,000 and 80,000 (74,75). The lability of factor VIII:C when it is separated from other plasma proteins has prevented accurate measurements of its activity. Recent calculations suggest that its plasma concentration is less than 100 ng/ml. The site of production of factor VIII:C is also unknown, although experimental evidence points to the liver. In the porcine model of von Willebrand's disease, synthesis of factor VIII:C is stimulated by the von Willebrand portion of the factor VIII molecule. An alternative hypothesis suggests that the von Willebrand component of the factor VIII molecule merely stabilizes factor VIII:C.

Factor VIII-WF (von Willebrand Factor) is present in plasma, platelets, megakaryocytes and endothelial cells and is synthesized by the latter two cell types (61,62). In platelets, factor VIII-WF is located in the alpha granules and in cultured endothelial cells, it is located in the perinuclear region and in a meshwork of filaments between cells. In vivo, factor VIII-WF is also found in the subendothelium. The plasma concentration of factor VIII-WF is 5 to 10 ug/ml.

Purified Factor VIII-WF is large, having a molecular weight in excess of 1,000,000. Complete reduction of the protein with mercaptolethanol or dithiothreitol leads to a single detectable subunit with a molecular weight of 200,000 to 230,000 (76–79). Recently, the multimeric structure of unreduced factor VIII-WF has been explored by various electrophoretic procedures. The molecular weight of the multimers has been estimated to vary between 800,000 and 12,000,000. The multimers appear to be built from a basic 220,000 dalton subunit or from dimers or tetramers of such subunits. The presence of multiple molecular forms of factor VIII-WF can be demonstrated by crossed immunoelectrophoresis. Crossed immunoelectrophoresis of plasma factor VIII-WF shows an asymmetric pattern due to the differing electrophoretic mobilities of the variably sized multimers. The larger multimers have the least anodal electrophoretic mobilities, whereas the small multimers have the greatest anodal mobilities. The large forms of

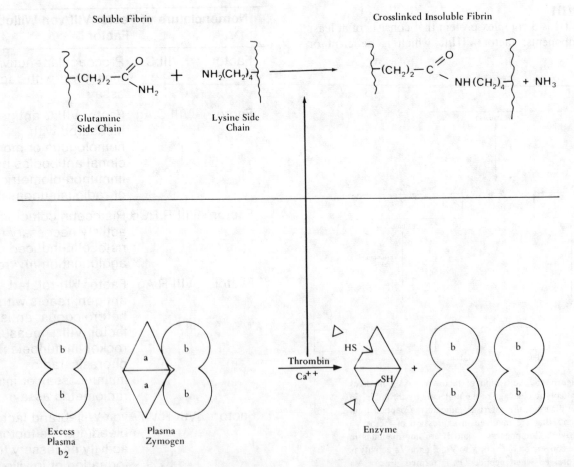

Figure 16. After activation of factor XIII by thrombin, there is cleavage of an activation fragment, which is indicated by △ in the figure. There is also a conformational change to expose the sulfhydryl group of the active cysteine site. Activated factor XIII is a transamidase, in contrast to all other coagulation enzymes, which are serine proteases. (Modified from McDonagh J: Structure and function of Factor XIII in Colman RW, Hirsh J, Marder VJ, Salzman EW (eds): *Hemostasis and Thrombosis*. Philadelphia: J. B. Lippincott Company, 1982, pp 166, 167.)

factor VIII-WF appear to possess von Willebrand factor activity in vivo. Commercially prepared concentrates of factor VIII have a relative lack of the large forms of factor VIII-WF. Von Willebrand's disease may result from an absence of factor VIII-WF or a decrease in its activity or from the presence of an inactive form of this factor.

Factor XIII

Factor XIII is a transamidase that is essential for the formation of covalent bonds between fibrin monomers (80). Deficiency of factor XIII is associated with a hemorrhagic diathesis that is also characterized by poor wound healing (81,82). Fibrin clots that have not been stabilized by factor XIII lack tensile strength and are readily soluble in 5 molar urea or 1% monochloroacetic acid. In addition to forming covalent bonds between fibrin monomers, factor XIII_a links $\alpha 2$ antiplasmin and fibronectin to fibrin.

Plasma factor XIII consists of two dissimilar subunits, a and b chains that form a molecular complex that consists of two a chains and two b chains held together by non-covalent interactions (Figure 16). The molecular weight of factor XIII is approximately 320,000 which each a chain being 75,000 daltons and each b chain being 80,000 daltons. All the catalytic function resides in the a chain, which contains six free sulfhydryl groups, one of which is located in the active center. The a chains contain no disulfide bonds (83). The tetrameric form of factor XIII is designated a_2b_2 and its concentration in plasma is approximately 8 μg/ml. In addition to the tetrameric form, there is an excess of free b chains, which may represent as much as 50% of the total plasma concentration of the b chain. These free b chains circulate as dimers (b_2). The plasma concentration of b_2 is approximately 4 μg/ml.

The platelets also contain factor XIII, which is found in the cytoplasm in contrast to the other members of the thrombin sensitive coagulation proteins that are found in the alpha granules. Platelet factor XIII is composed of a chains only and has a molecular weight of 160,000 (80). About one-half of the total factor XIII activity is localized to the platelets. The platelet a chains are immunologically identical to the plasma a chains.

Other Components of the Blood Coagulation System

In addition to the three families of coagulation proteins discussed above, tissue factor is involved in the extrinsic system of coagulation. It is appropriate to classify tissue factor as a cofactor. The interaction between tissue factor, factor VII and factor X is not yet fully elucidated (84). It is assumed that tissue factor reacts with factor VII to form a complex that will activate factor X. Tissue factor is found in many organs including the brain, lungs,

kidneys, liver, spleen and placenta, and in large vessels such as the aorta and vena cava. Damaged endothelium will also express tissue factor activity.

Tissue factor appears to be a large lipoprotein complex. The apoprotein form has some tissue factor activity, but the addition of the phospholipid component increases its activity approximately 950 fold. The mechanism by which tissue factor interacts with the extrinsic system is a subject of controversy. Tissue factor has been shown to possess peptidase activity that is not sensitive to DFP (85,86). It is not clear whether the interaction with factor VII involves proteolysis.

Physiologic Interactions of the Coagulation Proteins

Intrinsic System

The stimulus that initiates the coagulation mechanism in vivo is unknown, but is thought to be associated with endothelial injury. In vitro, exposure of plasma to various negatively charged surfaces such as silica and kaolin will activate the contact phase of the intrinsic system. The contact activation will also lead to the activation of the fibrinolytic system and complement pathways. In addition there is kinin generation and conversion of prorenin to renin (Figure 17).

The initial step involves binding of factor XII to a negatively charged surface resulting in a confirmational change (Figure 18). This binding is oriented so as to maximize productive interactions by high-molecular-weight kininogen (Fitzgerald factor). After the conformational change has taken place, factor XII is very susceptable to activation by kallikrein. High-molecular-weight kininogen also binds to the exposed surface. Prekallikrein and factor XI are complexed with high-molecular-weight kininogen in a 1:1 molar relationship. Thus, these two components of the contact system are also selectively localized to the exposed foreign surface. Activation of prekallikrein to kallikrein results in further enzymatic conversion of factor XII to XIIa, which, in turn, will convert prekallikrein to kallikrein. This reciprocal proteolysis is thought to be the major pathway of in vivo factor XII activation. This hypothesis, does not, however, explain the initial factor XII activation which may be a result of expression of trace XIIa activity following conformational change without proetolysis. The activated surface bound XIIa will then activate factor XI, which remains bound to the foreign surface.

Factor XI then activates factor IX. This step of the coagulation sequence is dependent on calcium in contrast to the earlier phases of contact activation. Factor IX can also be converted to its activate form by factor VIIa and tissue factor. Activated factor IX will then form

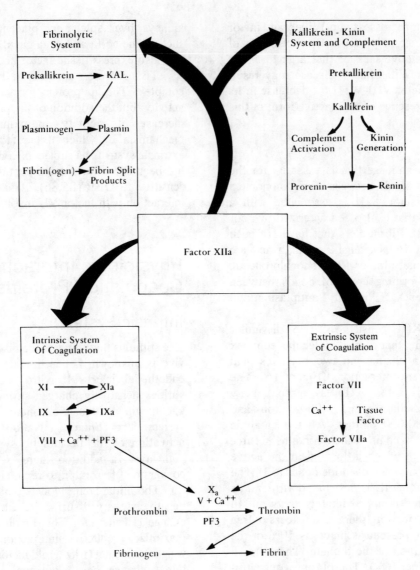

Figure 17. Activation of factor XII is pivotal in a number of physiologic processes. Factor XIIa initiates intrinsic coagulation by activating factor XI. Also, factor XIIa activates the extrinsic system by converting factor VII into VIIa. In addition to its role in coagulation, factor XII activates the fibrinolytic, kallikrein-kinin, complement and renin-angiotensin systems.

a macromolecular complex composed of factor VIII, phospholipids, and calcium which will then activate factor X to Xa. The activation of factor X by IXa is markedly accelerated by factor VIII. It is estimated that factor VIII will accelerate this reaction in excess of 1000 fold. Factor VIII, which participates in this reaction, is the activated form of the procofactor. Activation of factor VIII involves thrombin proteolysis of the procofactor.

Factor Xa will form a complex with Factor V, phospholipid and calcium, which converts prothrombin to thrombin. The macromolecular complex of Xa-V-phospholipid-calcium is analogous to the factor IXa-VIII-phospholipid-calcium complex. In a manner similar to its action of factor VIII, thrombin activates factor V proteolytically.

The activation of prothrombin involves cleavage of two peptide bonds by factor Xa. Conversion of prothrombin to thrombin is illustrated in Figure 4. The calcium binding sites of the prothrombin molecule are located in its amino-terminal end, specifically in fragment 1. Removal of fragment 1 by thrombin proteolysis will impede formation of the prothrombin converting macromolecular complex with resulting slow generation of thrombin. Fragment 1 will also compete with prothrombin for the factor Xa complex, consequently inhibiting thrombin generation. This competition may represent one means of controlling thrombin production.

Thrombin cleaves specific arginine-glycine bonds in fibrinogen giving rise to fibrinopeptides A and B from the alpha and beta chains, respectively. The resulting fibrin monomers then spontaneously polymerize both end-to-end and laterally. Reptilase, an enzyme derived from snake venom will remove fibrinopeptide A. However, removal of fibrinopeptide A is followed by formation of fibrin.

The last step of coagulation involves the conversion of the relatively unstable fibrin gel to a stable fibrin clot. This step is mediated by factor XIIIa. Thrombin in the presence of calcium will convert factor XIII to XIIIa. Factor XIIIa functions as a transamidase by catalyzing formation of E (γ glutamyl) lysine linkages between a glutamine side chain in one fibrin monomer with a lysine side chain in another fibrin monomer. The formation of these convalent bonds primarily involves the γ chains of the fibrin monomer.

Extrinsic System

In the extrinsic system, tissue factor functions as a cofactor. Tissue factor will form a complex wih VIIa that converts factors X to Xa and IX to IXa. This ability of the extrinsic system to activate factor IX essentially bypasses the initial phases of the contact system. This may explain the lack of bleeding associated with hereditary deficiencies of factor XII, prekallikrein and high-molecular-weight kininogen. As mentioned earlier, factor VII may express a low level of activity without proteolytic activation. Thus, factor VII may be the key regulatory protein in the initiation of the coagulation response.

Down Regulation of Blood Coagulation

Clearly coagulation involves an amplification system. Therefore, there must be a balancing mechanism(s) to prevent formation of excess thrombin. Thrombin may in part modulate the coagulation response. The initial trace amounts of thrombin activate the procofactors V and

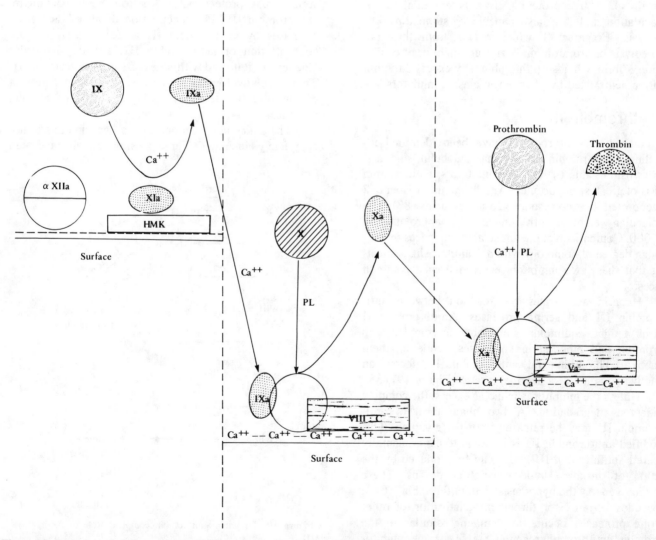

Figure 18. Intrinsic coagulation pathway. (With permission from Dr. John Griffin, Scripps Clinic and Research Foundation, La Jolla, California.)

Table 6

	Physiologic Inhibitors			
Inhibitor	Molecular Weight	Potentiated by Heparin	Rate of Inhibition	Plasma Concentration (mg/dl)
α_1-Antitrypsin	54,000	No	Slow	245–335
Antithrombin III	58,000	Yes	Slow	23–40
α_2-Macroglobulin	820,000	No	Rapid	190–330
C1 inhibitor	140,000	No	Slow	14–30
α_2-Antiplasmin	65,000	No	Rapid	9.6–13.5
Protein C	62,000	No	Slow	0.5

VIII; however, higher concentrations of thrombin will proteolytically degrade these two cofactors. In addition, thrombin, when complexed with thrombomodulin on the endothelial surface will activate protein C to active protein C. Active protein C is a potent inhibitor of coagulation and it is also capable of stimulating fibrinolysis. Fragment 1 which results from thrombin proteolysis of prothrombin is also an inhibitor of coagulation. Fibrin will adsorb thrombin; any excess thrombin will be neutralized by physiologic plasma inhibitors.

Antithrombin III

A number of antithrombins have been identified including: antithrombin III, α_2 macroglobulin, and $\alpha 1$ antitrypsin (Table 6). Of these inhibitors, antithrombin III is of greatest importance. Antithrombin III is an $\alpha 2$ glycoprotein that consists of 425 amino acids (87). The molecular weight of antithrombin III is approximately 58,000. Comparison of the amino acid sequences reveals a high degree of homology with $\alpha 1$ antitrypsin, suggesting that these two inhibitors evolved from a common ancestor.

Heparin accelerates the reaction between antithrombin III and serine proteases. Antithrombin III forms a tight, equimolar, stoichiometric complex with thrombin and other serine proteases, rendering them inactive. Thrombin and antithrombin III forms an inactive complex at a 1:1 molar ratio (Figure 19) (88–89). Unless the inhibitor is in molar excess, the complex undergoes degradation. A two chain form of antithrombin III may be released from the complex. This modified antithrombin III is identical to experimentally altered antithrombin III which can be produced by the action of thrombin under special conditions. These findings support the hypothesis that antithrombin III is a "pseudosubstrate" for thrombin. Inactivation of other serine proteases occurs in a manner similar to the thrombin-antithrombin reaction. Stable enzyme-inhibitor

complexes are formed. Antithrombin III inactivates factors Xa, IXa, XIa and XIIa at slow rates (Figure 20). By contrast factor VIIa is not inhibited by antithrombin III. The binding of factor Xa to the platelet phospholipid surface may protect factor Xa from neutralization by antithrombin III. The inactivation of all of the serine proteases by antithrombin III is dependent upon the concentration of antithrombin III. Pseudo first-order kinetics are followed with an excess of antithrombin III. Thus, a relatively modest decrease in the concentration of antithrombin III may result in a faster clotting response.

The anticoagulant properties of heparin are still not completely elucidated. Three possible models have been

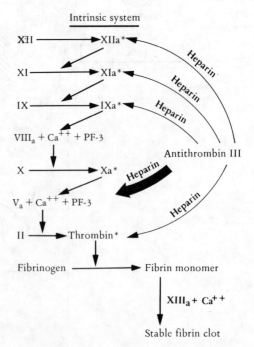

Figure 19. Thrombin-antithrombin complex. Role of Antithrombin III.

(I) Serine Protease — Antithrombin III — Heparin

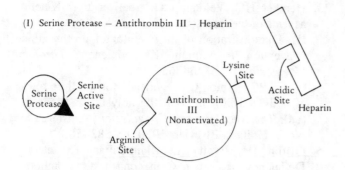

(II) Inactivation of Serine Protease

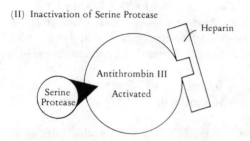

Figure 20. Heparin, an acidic mucopolysaccharide with a high negative charge, reacts with lysine, a positively charged amino acid in the antithrombin III molecule. Antithrombin III then undergoes a conformational change, exposing an arginine site. This arginine site then reacts with the active serine site of the protease. (Triplett DA: Synthetic substrates: A revolution in the diagnostic coagulation laboratory in Homburger HA, Batsakis JG (eds): *Clinical Laboratory Annual: 1982*. New York: Appleton Century Crofts, 1982, pp 243–286.)

proposed: 1) heparin binds to antithrombin and induces a conformational change that promotes the binding of thrombin. On the formation of a stable thrombin-antithrombin III complex, heparin is released and joins another antithrombin III molecule (Figure 19). 2) Heparin binds to thrombin, thereby promoting its reaction with antithrombin III. 3) Heparin binds to antithrombin inducing a conformational change, and also binds to thrombin, approximating the two molecules and accelerating thrombin inhibition. Presently, it is not possible to identify the most important mechanism. Perhaps there are different mechanisms for inactivation of the various enzymes involved in coagulation.

Patients with hereditary or acquired deficiency of antithrombin III are predisposed to thrombotic disease. (90–95). In patients with classical hereditary antithrombin III deficiency, the mean antithrombin III activity is approximately one-half of that found in healthy persons. Many such patients present with thrombotic disease at a young age and the clinical findings are often "atypical." Such patients may have thrombosis in the arms and a fairly frequent finding is mesenteric vein thrombosis. Recently, different types of congenital deficiency of antithrombin III have been described and they have included qualitative as well as quantitative abnormalities (96–98).

References

1. Epstein I: *The Babylonian Talmud, Yebamoth*. Sect 64B. Slotki WI (Trans). London: Soncino Press, 1936, vol 1, p 431.
2. Bulloch W, Fildes P: *Hemophilia. Treasury of Human Inheritance*. Galton Laboratory for National Eugenics, University of London, Parts V and VI, Sect XIVA. London: Cambridge University Press, 1911, pp 169–354.
3. Otto JC: An account of an haemorrhagic disposition existing in certain families. *Med Reposit* 6(1):1802–1803, 1961.
4. McKusick VA: The royal hemophilia. *Sci Amer* 213(2):88–95, 1965.
5. Morawitz P: Die Chemie der Blutgerinnung. *Ergeb Physiol Biol Chem Exp Pharmakol* 4:307, 1905.
6. Addis T: The pathogenesis of hereditary haemophilia. *J Pathol Bacteriol* 15:427–452, 1911.
7. Quick AJ, Stanley-Brown M, Bancroft FW: A study of the coagulation defect in hemophilia and jaundice. *Amer J Med Sci* 190:501–511, 1935.
8. Link KP: The discovery of dicumarol and its sequels. *Circulation* 19:97–107, 1959.
9. Owren PA: The coagulation of blood: Investigations on a new clotting factor. *Acta Med Scand Suppl* 194:1–327, 1947.
10. Owren PA: Parahaemophilia: Hemorrhagic diathesis due to absence of a previously unknown clotting factor. *Lancet* 1:446–448, 1947.
11. Alexander B, Goldstein R, Landwehr G, et al: Congenital SPCA deficiency: A hitherto unrecognized coagulation defect with hemorrhage rectified by serum and serum fractions. *J Clin Invest* 30:596–608, 1951.
12. Alexander B, Goldstein R, Landwehr G: Prothrombin conversion accelerator of serum (SPCA): Its partial purification and its properties compared with acglobulin. *J Clin Invest* 29:881–895, 1950.
13. Owen CA, Jr, Bollman JL: Prothrombin conversion factor of dicumarol plasma. *Proc Soc Exp Biol Med* 67:231–234, 1948.
14. Hougie C, Barrow EM, Graham JB: Stuart clotting defect. I. Segregation of a hereditary hemorrhagic state from the heterogeneous group heretofore called "stable factor" (SPCA proconvertin, factor VII) deficiency. *J Clin Invest* 36:485–496, 1957.
15. Langdell RD, Wagner RH, Brinkhous KM: Effect of antihemophilic factor on one-stage clotting tests: A presumptive test for hemophilia and a simple one-stage antihemophilia factor assay procedure. *J Lab Clin Med* 41:637–647, 1953.
16. Proctor R, Rapaport SI: The partial thromboplastin time with kaolin. *Amer J Clin Pathol* 36:212–219, 1961.
17. Aggeler PM, White SG, Glendening MB, et al:

Plasma thromboplastin component (PTC) deficiency: A new disease resembling hemophilia. *Proc Soc Exp Biol Med* 79:692–694, 1952.

18. Rosenthal RL, Dreskin OH, Rosenthal N: Plasma thromboplastin antecedent (PTA) deficiency. Clinical, coagulation, therapeutic and hereditary aspects of a new hemophilia-like disease. *Blood* 10:120–131, 1955.

19. Ratnoff OD, Colopy JE: A familial hemorrhagic trait associated with a deficiency of a clot promoting fraction of plasma. *J Clin Invest* 34:602–613, 1955.

20. MacFarlane RG: The basis of the cascade hypothesis of blood clotting. *Thromb Diath Haemorrh* 15:591–602, 1966.

21. Davie EW, Ratnoff OD: Waterfall sequence for intrinsic blood clotting. *Science* 145:1310–1312, 1965.

22. Zur M, Nemerson Y: Tissue factor pathways of blood coagulation. In Bloom AL, Thomas DP (eds): *Haemostasis and Thrombosis*. Edinburgh: Churchill Livingstone, 1981, chap 9, pp 124–139.

23. Waaler BA: Simultaneous contribution to the formation of thrombin by the intrinsic and extrinsic blood clotting systems. *Scand J Clin Lab Invest* 9:322–329, 1957.

24. Nemerson Y: The reaction between bovine brain tissue factor and factors VII and X. *Biochemistry* 5:601–608, 1966.

25. Masys DR, Bajaj SP, Rapaport SI: Activation of human factor VII by activated factors IX and X. *Blood* 60:1143–1150, 1982.

26. Jesty J, Nemerson Y: The tissue pathway of coagulation. In Ogston D, Bennett B (eds.): *Haemostasis: Biochemistry, Physiology and Pathology*. London: John Wiley & Sons, 1977, pp. 95–104.

27. Nemerson Y, Pitlick FA: The tissue factor pathway of blood coagulation. In Spaet TH (ed): *Progress in Hemostasis and Thrombosis*. New York: Grune & Stratton, 1972, vol 1, pp 1–37.

28. Seegers WH, McCoy LE, Groben HD, et al: Purification and some properties of autoprothrombin II-A: An anticoagulant perhaps also related to fibrinolysis. *Thromb Res* 1:443–460, 1972.

29. Bruze GJ, Miletich JP: Human Protein Z. (Abstract). *Blood* 62:281a, 1983.

30. Stenflo J: Vitamin K, prothrombin and carboxylglutamic acid. *N Engl J Med* 296:624–626, 1977.

31. Jackson CM, Brenckle GM: Biochemistry of the vitamin K-dependent clotting factors. In Menache D, Surgenor DMacN, Anderson H (eds): *Hemophilia and Hemostasis*. New York: Alan R. Liss, 1981, pp 27–56.

32. Hemker HC, Muller AD, Loeliger EA: Two types of prothrombin in vitamin K deficiency. *Thromb Haemostasis* 23:633–637, 1970.

33. Hemker HC, Veltkamp JJ, Loeliger EA: Kinetic aspects of the interaction of blood clotting enzymes. III. Demonstration of an inhibitor of prothrombin conversion in vitamin K deficiency. *Thromb Haemostasis* 19:346–363, 1968.

34. Comp PC, Esmon CT: Evidence for multiple roles of activated protein C in fibrinolysis. In Mann K (ed): *The Regulation of Coagulation*. Amsterdam: North Holland-Elsevier, 1980, pp 583–588.

35. Griffin JH, Evatt BL, Zimmerman TS, et al: Deficiency of protein C in congenital thrombotic disease. *J Clin Invest* 68:1370–1373, 1981.

36. Bertina RM, Broekmans AW, van der Linden IK, et al: Protein C deficiency in a Dutch family with thrombotic disease. *Thromb Haemostasis* 48:1–5, 1982.

37. Suttie JW, Jackson CM: Prothrombin structure activation and biosynthesis. *Physiol Rev* 57:1–70, 1977.

38. Mann KG, Fass DN: The molecular biology of blood coagulation. In Fairbanks VF (ed): *Current Hematology*. New York: John Wiley & Sons, 1983, Vol. 2, pp 347–374.

39. van den Besselaar AMHP, Ram IE, Bertina RM: Involvement of human factor IX in tissue thromboplastin induced coagulation. (Abstract) *Thromb Haemostasis* 46:34, 1981.

40. Mertens K, Bertina RM: Pathways in the activation of human coagulation factor X. *Biochem J* 185:647–658, 1980.

41. Lindquist PA, Fujikawa K, Davie EW: Activation of bovine factor IX (Christmas factor) by factor XIa (activated plasma thromboplastin antecedent) and a protease from Russell's viper venom. *J Biol Chem* 253:1902–1909, 1978.

42. Stenflo J: A new vitamin K dependent protein: Purification from bovine plasma and preliminary characterization. *J Biol Chem* 251:355–363, 1976.

43. Fernlund P, Stenflo J: Amino acid sequence of protein C. In Suttie JW (ed): *Vitamin K Metabolism and Vitamin K-Dependent Proteins*. Baltimore: University Park Press, 1980, pp 84–88.

44. Marlar RA, Griffin JH: Deficiency of protein C inhibitor in combined factor V/VIII deficiency disease. *J Clin Invest* 66:1186–1189, 1980.

45. Giddings JC, Surgrue A, Bloom AL: Quantitation of coagulant antigens and inhibition of activated protein C in combined factor V/VIII deficiency. *Brit J Haematol* 52:495–502, 1982.

46. Marlar RA, Kleiss AJ, Griffin JH: Human protein C: Interaction of factors V and VIII in plasma by the activated molecule. *Ann NY Acad Sci* 370:303–310, 1981.

47. Marlar RA, Kleiss AJ, Griffin JH: Mechanism of action of human activated protein C, a thrombin-

dependent anticoagulant enzyme. *Blood* 59:1067–1072, 1982.

48. Walker FJ: Regulation of activated protein C by a new protein. *J Biol Chem* 255:5521–5524, 1980.

49. Dahlback B, Stenflo J: High molecular weight complex in human plasma between vitamin K dependent protein S and complement component C4b-binding protein. *Proc Natl Acad Sci USA* 78:2512–2516, 1981.

50. Prowse CV, Esnoug MP: The isolation of a new warfarin-sensitive protein from bovine plasma. *Biochem Soc Trans* 5:255–256, 1977.

51. Seegers WH, Ghosh A, Wu VY: Function of a previously unrecognized plasma protein M in thrombin generation. In Suttie JW (ed): *Vitamin K Metabolism and Vitamin K-Dependent Proteins*. Baltimore: University Park Press, 1980, pp 96–101.

52. Griffin JH: Role of surface in surface-dependent activation of Hageman factor (blood coagulation factor XII). *Proc Natl Acad Sci USA* 75:1998–2002, 1978.

53. Ogston D: Contact activation of blood coagulation. In Poller L (ed): *Recent Advances in Blood Coagulation*. New York: Churchill Livingstone, 1981, vol 3, pp 109–123.

54. Ratnoff OD: The biology and pathology of the initial stages of blood coagulation. In Moore CV, Brown EB (eds): *Progress in Haematology*. New York: Grune & Stratton, 1966, p 204.

55. Silverberg M, Kaplan AP: Enzymatic activities of activated and zymogen forms of human Hageman factor (factor XII). *Blood* 60:64–70, 1982.

56. Tans G, Griffin JH: Properties of sulfatides in factor XII-dependent contact activation. *Blood* 59:69–75, 1982.

57. Katzmann JA, Nesheim ME, Mann KG: Isolation of functional human coagulation factor V using a hybridoma antibody. (Abstract) *Circulation* 62:170, 1980.

58. Katzmann JA, Nesheim ME, Mann KG: The thrombin catalyzed activation of human factor V probed with a hybridoma antibody. (Abstract) *Thromb Haemostasis* 46:88, 1981.

59. Van Zutphen H, Bevers EM, Hemker HC, et al: Contribution of the platelet factor V content to platelet factor 3 activity. *Brit J Haematol* 45:121–131, 1980.

60. Chesney CMcI, Pifer DD, Colman RW: The role of platelet factor V in prothrombin conversion. *Thromb Res* 29:75–84, 1983.

61. Zimmerman TS, Meyer D: Structure and function of factor VIII/von Willebrand factor. In Bloom AL, Thomas DP (eds): *Haemostasis and Thrombosis*. Edinburgh: Churchill Livingstone, 1981, chap 8, pp 111–123.

62. Hoyer LW: The factor VIII complex: Structure and function. In Menache D, Surgenor DMacN, Anderson H (eds): *Hemophilia and Hemostasis*. New York: Alan R. Liss, 1981, pp 1–26.

63. Hoyer L: The factor VIII complex: Structure and function. *Blood* 58:1–13, 1981.

64. Koutts J, Howard MA, Firkin BG: Factor VIII physiology and pathology in man. *Prog Hematol* 11:115–145, 1979.

65. Mannucci PM: Hemophilia diagnosis and management: Progress and problems. In Poller L (ed): *Recent Advances in Blood Coagulation*. New York: Churchill Livingstone, 1981, vol 3, pp 193–226.

66. Jones PK, Ratnoff OD: Sources of variability in antihemophilic factor (factor VIII) procoagulant titers and precipitating antigen levels among obligate carriers of classic hemophilia. *Blood* 57:928–932, 1981.

67. Canale VC, Hilgartner MW, Smith CH, et al: Effect of corticosteroids on factor VIII level. *J Pediatr* 71:878–880, 1967.

68. Lombardi R, Mannucci PM, Seghatchian MJ, et al: Alterations of factor VIII von Willebrand factor in clinical conditions associated with an increase in its plasma concentration. *Brit J Haematol* 49:61–68, 1981.

69. Rizza CR: Effect of exercise on the level of antihaemophilic globulin in human blood. *J Physiol (London)* 156:128–135, 1961.

70. Holmberg L, Borge L, Ljung R, et al: Measurement of antihemophilic factor VIII antigen (VIII:C:Ag) with a solid phase immunoradiometric method based on homologous non-haemophilic antibodies. *Scand J Haematol* 23:17–24, 1979.

71. Fass DN, Knutson GJ, Katzmann JA: Monoclonal antibodies to porcine factor VIII coagulant and their use in the isolation of active coagulation protein. *Blood* 59:594–600, 1982.

72. Knutson GJ, Fass DN: Porcine factor VIII:C prepared by affinity interaction with von Willebrand factor and heterologous antibodies: Sodium dodecyl sulfate polyacrylamide gel analysis. *Blood* 59:615–624, 1982.

73. Muller HP, van Tilburg NH, Derks J, et al: A monoclonal antibody to VIII:C produced by a mouse hybridoma. *Blood* 58:1000–1006, 1981.

74. Lian EC-Y, Nunez RL, Rarkness DR: In vivo and in vitro effects of thrombin and plasmin on human factor VIII (AHF). *Amer J Hematol* 1:481–491, 1976.

75. Cockburn LG, deBeaufre-Apps RJ, Wilson J, et al: Parallel destruction of factor VIII procoagulant activity and an 85,000 dalton protein in highly purified factor VIII/VWF. *Thromb Res* 21:295–309, 1981.

76. Gralnick HR, Williams SB, Morisato DK: Effect of

the multimeric structure of the factor VIII von Willebrand factor protein on binding to platelets. *Blood* 58:387–397, 1981.

77. Meyer D, Obert B, Pietu G, et al: Multimeric structure of factor VIII/von Willebrand factor in von Willebrand's disease. *J Lab Clin Med* 95:590–602, 1980.

78. Ruggeri ZM, Zimmerman TS: Multimeric composition of factor VIII. *Ann NY Acad Sci* 370:205–209, 1981.

79. Zimmerman TS, Voss R, Edgington TS: Carbohydrate of the factor VIII von Willebrand's factor in von Willebrand's disease. *J Clin Invest* 64:1298–1302, 1979.

80. McDonagh JM: Structure and function of factor XIII. In Colman RW, Hirsh J, Marder VJ, et al (eds): *Hemostasis and Thrombosis*. Philadelphia: JB Lippincott, 1982, pp 164–173.

81. Kitchens CS, Newcomb TG: Factor XIII. *Medicine (Baltimore)* 58:413–429, 1979.

82. Losowsky MS, Miloszewski KJA: Annotation, factor XIII. *Brit J Haematol* 37:1–4, 1977.

83. Skrzynia C, Reisner HM, McDonagh J: Characterization of the catalytic subunit of factor XIII by radioimmunoassay. *Blood* 60:1089–1095, 1982.

84. Nemerson Y, Bach R: Tissue factor revisited. In Spaet TH (ed): *Progress in Hemostasis and Thrombosis*. New York: Grune & Stratton, 1982, vol 6, p. 237–261.

85. Nemerson Y, Zur M, Radcliffe R: Initiation and control of coagulation by factor VII, a zymogen. (Abstract), *Blood* 58:223, 1981.

86. Zur M, Radcliffe RD, Oberdick J, et al: The dual role of factor VII in blood coagulation. Initiation and inhibition of a proteolytic system by a zymogen. *J Biol Chem* 257:5623–5631, 1982.

87. Abildgaard U: Antithrombin and related inhibitors of coagulation. In Poller L (ed): *Recent Advances in Blood Coagulation*. New York: Churchill Livingstone, 1981, vol 3, pp 151–173.

88. Marciniak E: Thrombin-induced proteolysis of human antithrombin III: An outstanding contribution of heparin. *Brit J Haematol* 48:325–336, 1981.

89. Bjork I, Jackson CM, Jornvall H, et al: The active site of antithrombin. *J Biol Chem* 257:2406–2411, 1982.

90. Matsuo T, Ohki Y, Kondo S, et al: Familial antithrombin III deficiency in a Japanese family. *Thromb Res* 16:815–823, 1979.

91. Matsuo O: Incidence of thrombosis in inherited antithrombin III deficiency. *Thromb Res* 24:509–510, 1981.

92. Manotti C, Quintavalla R, Megha A, et al: Inherited deficiency of antithrombin III in two Italian families. *Haemostasis* 12:300–308, 1982.

93. Liebman HA, Wada JK, Patch MJ, et al: Depression of functional and antigenic plasma antithrombin III (AT III) due to therapy with L-asparaginase. *Cancer* 50:451–456, 1982.

94. Lau SO, Tkachuch JY, Hasegawa DK, et al: Plasminogen and antithrombin III deficiencies in the childhood nephrotic syndrome associated with plasminogenuria and antithrombinuria. *J Pediatr* 96:390–392, 1980.

95. Buller HR, Weenink AH, Treffers PE, et al: Severe antithrombin III deficiency in a patient with pre-eclampsia. *Scand J Haematol* 25:81–86, 1980.

96. Wolf M, Boyer C, Lavergne JM, et al: A new familial variant of antithrombin III: Antithrombin III Paris. *Brit J Haematol* 51:285–295, 1982.

97. Sorensen PJ, Sas G, Peto I, et al: Distinction of two pathologic antithrombin III molecules: Antithrombin III 'Aalborg' and antithrombin III 'Budapest.' *Thromb Res* 26:211–219, 1982.

98. Sas G, Peto I, Banhegyi D, et al: Heterogeneity of the classical antithrombin III deficiency. *Thromb Haemostasis* 43:133–136, 1980.

Review Articles

Baugh RF, Hougie C: Structure and function in blood coagulation. In Poller L (ed): *Recent Advances in Blood Coagulation*. New York: Churchill Livingstone, 1981, vol 3, pp 81–107.

Davie EW, Hanahan DJ: Blood coagulation proteins. In Putnam F (ed): *The Plasma Proteins*. New York: Academic Press, 1977, pp 421–544.

Jackson CM, Nemerson Y: Blood coagulation. *Annu Rev Biochem* 49:765–811, 1980.

Mann KG, Fass DN: The molecular biology of blood coagulation. In Fairbanks VF (ed): *Current Hematology*. New York, John Wiley & Sons, 1983, pp 347–374.

Nemerson Y, Furie B: Zymogens and cofactors of blood coagulation. *CRC Crit Rev Biochem* 9:45–85, October 1980.

Ratnoff OD: Blood clotting mechanism: An overview. In Ogston D, Bennett B (eds): *Haemostasis: Biochemistry, Physiology, and Pathology*. London: John Wiley & Sons, 1977, chap 1, pp 1–24.

Ratnoff OD: The physiology of blood coagulation. *Behring Inst Mitt* 63:135–155, 1979.

Williams WJ: Biochemistry of plasma coagulation factors. In Williams WJ, Beutler E, Erslev AJ, et al (eds): *Hematology*. New York: McGraw-Hill, 1977, pp 1227–1249.

Zwaal RFA: Membrane and lipid involvement in blood coagulation. *Biochim Biophys Acta* 515:163–205, 1978.

Reference Books

Biggs, R: *Human Blood Coagulation, Haemostasis and Thrombosis* (2nd edition). Oxford, Blackwell, 1976.

Bloom AL (ed): *The Hemophilias*, vol 5 in *Methods in Hematology*. Edinburgh: Churchill Livingstone, 1982.

Bloom AL, Thomas DP: *Haemostasis and Thrombosis*. Edinburgh: Churchill Livingstone, 1981.

Colman RW, Hirsh J, Marder VJ, et al: *Hemostasis and Thrombosis*. Philadelphia: JB Lippincott, 1982.

Ingram GIC, Brozovic M, Slater NGP: *Bleeding Disorders: Investigation and Management* (2nd edition). Oxford: Blackwell Scientific Publications, 1982.

Triplett DA: *Laboratory Evaluation of Coagulation*. Chicago: American Society for Clinical Pathology, 1982.

Chapter
TWO

Fibrinolysis

The body also has a system that has the ability to lyse or dissolve a clot. It is called the fibrinolytic enzyme system. Most components of this system were identified between 1930 and 1950. In 1941, Milstone (1) showed that lysis of fibrin by the streptococcal substance described by Tillett and Garner in 1933 (2) depended on a "lytic factor" present in human serum. Subsequently, it was demonstrated that this lytic factor is an enzyme precursor that is converted to an active enzyme by the streptococcal product. The enzymatic zymogen was called plasminogen, the enzyme plasmin, and the streptococcal factor streptokinase. In 1947, Astrup and Permin (3) found that extracts of animal tissues contained a substance that activated plasminogen. This agent is now called tissue plasminogen activator (TPA). After these observations were made, inhibitors of plasmin and inhibitors of plasminogen activation were described (4). A simplified diagram of the fibrinolytic system is illustrated in Figure 1. There are a number of similarities between the fibrinolytic and the coagulation systems. For instance, intrinsic and extrinsic systems of plasminogen activation have been identified. Activation of the contact phase of the intrinsic pathway of coagulation will also lead to initiation of the intrinsic pathway of fibrinolysis.

Plasminogen and Plasmin

Human plasminogen is a single chain glycoprotein with a molecular weight of approximately 90,000 (Figure 2)(5–7). Plasminogen is present in plasma and serum at a fairly constant levels of 10 to 20 mg/dl and is presumably synthesized in the liver.

Plasminogen may be assayed immunologically or functionally (8,9). Functional assays are classically performed by use of a caseinolytic test system or on plasminogen free fibrin plates. The commercial availability of synthetic substrates, such as S-2251[R] or Chromozym PL[R] has greatly simplified the evaluation of the functional activity of plasminogen (10). In functional assay methods, plasminogen is activated to plasmin by urokinase or streptokinase. The amount of substrate hydrolyzed during a fixed period or the rate of hydrolysis is a measure of the concentration of plasminogen (Figure 3). Available laboratory procedures for evaluating components of the fibrinolytic system are summarized in Table 1 (8).

The complete structure of plasminogen has now been reported. A molecule of plasminogen has 790

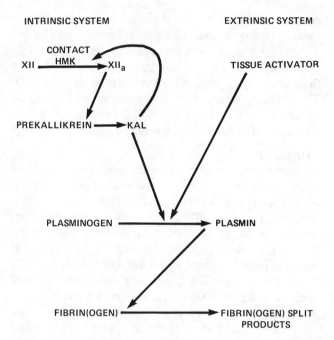

INTRINSIC SYSTEM

EXTRINSIC SYSTEM

Figure 1. Basic aspects of the fibrinolytic system are illustrated. Activation of plasminogen may be divided into two components: intrinsic and extrinsic. Intrinsic activation involves the contact system of coagulation. Activated Hageman factor (factor XIIa) generates kallikrein, which, in turn, activates plasminogen. Note that kallikrein also has a feedback function in generating additional factor XIIa. The primary physiologic inhibitor of the intrinsic system is C′-esterase inhibitor.

The extrinsic system involves tissue plasminogen activator. This activator is present in many tissues and secretions. It appears to be a serine protease and has a molecular weight of 60,000. Recently, it has been isolated from a human melanoma cell line. Efforts are under way to clone tissue activator. HMK, high-molecular-weight kininogen; KAL, kallikrein.

amino acid residues and contains 24 disulfide bridges and five triple-loop structures of "kringles" (Figure 4) (11). Comparable kringle structures have been found to be constituents of prothrombin and factor X molecules, suggesting that these related serine proteases are derived from a common ancestral molecule. Native plasminogen has an amino-terminal glutamic acid residue (Glu-plasminogen) that is easily converted by limited proteolytic degradation to modified forms with amino-terminal lysine, valine or methionine. These partially digested forms are referred to as Lys-plasminogen. Lys-plasminogen is more readily activated by urokinase and also has increased affinity for fibrin and α_2-antiplasmin (12).

The plasminogen molecule consists of two parts, one portion containing the active-site (B or light chain), and the other having lysine-binding sites (A or heavy chain) (Figure 4). The lysine-binding sites are important with respect to the interactions between plasminogen and fibrin as well as between plasmin and α_2 antiplasmin. The interaction between plasminogen and ε-aminocaproic acid (EACA) is also mediated by the lysine-binding sites. Activation of plasminogen by urokinase or other substances results from a cleavage of the peptide bond between the light and heavy chains (11). The two-chain plasmin molecule is composed of the heavy chain which originates from the amino terminal portion of plasminogen, and a light chain which constitutes the carboxy-terminal end (Figure 2). Activation of Glu-plasminogen to plasmin by urokinase occurs about 20 times slower than does activation of Lys-plasminogen. In vivo, fibrin appears to accelerate activation of plasminogen by tissue plasminogen activator and also, to a lesser extent, by urokinase.

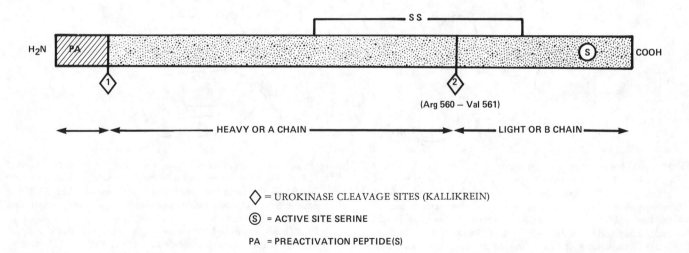

$\diamond$ = UROKINASE CLEAVAGE SITES (KALLIKREIN)

$\circledS$ = ACTIVE SITE SERINE

PA = PREACTIVATION PEPTIDE(S)

Figure 2. The prerequisite for activation of plasminogen is cleavage of a single arginine-valine bond that links the A and B chains. This cleavage is mediated by urokinase or other plasminogen activators (2 in the figure indicates this site). In addition to this cleavage, the A chain is involved in a second series of reactions; the amino-terminal end is further cleaved at the bonds between Lys-62 and Ser-63 and between Arg-67 and Met-68 and subsequently at the bond between Lys-76 and Lys-77, yielding fragments with a total molecular weight of between 4000 and 7000 (preactivation peptides). The order of bond cleavage is still a matter of controversy. Removal of the preactivation peptides may be mediated by urokinase or through plasmin auto-digestion.

PLASMINOGEN + STREPTOKINASE ──────→ PLG·SK
(PT. PLASMA)

$$\text{H}-\text{D}-\text{VAL}-\text{LEU}-\text{LYS}-\text{pNA} \xrightarrow{\text{PLG·SK}} \text{H}-\text{D}-\text{VAL}-\text{LEU}-\text{LYS}-\text{OH} + \text{pNA}$$

Figure 3. The synthetic substrate assay for plasminogen is illustrated schematically. Kabi substrate S-2251 (available in United States from Helena) is used together with streptokinase. In the first step, streptokinase is incubated with a patient's plasma. The synthetic substrate is then added, and the plasminogen-streptokinase complex (PLG·SK) converts plasminogen to plasmin, which, in turn, lyses the substrate. The *p*-nitroaniline (pNA) that is released can be quantified by measuring the color change at 405 nm with a spectrophotometer. Preferably, a recording spectrophotometer should be used. However, if one is not available, an end-point method can be used. In the end-point method, the reaction is stopped by the addition of acetic acid, and the absorbance is read against a plasma blank.

Lysine-binding sites that are found on the plasminogen molecule have been located in at least three kringles. Kinetic studies have shown that three more lysine-binding sites may exist; their exact locations are not yet known. The binding of plasminogen to fibrin is dependent upon the lysine-binding sites. Digestion of fibrin by plasmin in vitro is inhibited by ε-aminocaproic acid (EACA) or similar substances such as tranexamic acid. The ability of EACA to inhibit plasminogen (plasmin) is based on binding to the lysine-binding sites (Figure 5).

Plasminogen Activators

Intrinsic Pathway. Present knowledge of the intrinsic activation of plasminogen is still unclear. Intrinsic activation of plasminogen may occur by activation of the contact system of coagulation. Hageman factor (Factor XII), Fletcher factor (prekallikrein), and Fitzgerald factor (high molecular weight kininogen) are involved in the intrinsic pathway of plasminogen activation (13). The primary inhibitor of this pathway of fibrinolysis appears to be C'-esterase inhibitor, a naturally occuring inhibitor of the complement system (14).

Extrinsic Pathway. Plasminogen activator(s) is present in many tissues, organs, and secretions. Highly purified preparations of the activator have been obtained from porcine heart and ovaries as well as human uteri. With a histologic technique, Todd (15) demonstrated that plasminogen activator is present in the endothelial cells. Synthesis of tissue plasminogen activator by endothelial cells has been confirmed by in vitro cell culture (16,17). Tissue plasminogen activator has a molecular weight of approximately 60,000 and consists of two chains linked by disulfide bonds (18,19). The serine residue of the active site is located on the light chain. In contrast to urokinase, tissue plasminogen activator is adsorbed to fibrin and in a purified system, formation of plasmin by tissue plasminogen activator is greatly enhanced by fibrin (20).

Vascular plasminogen activator is released by the vascular endothelium under the influence of a number of specific stimuli. Epinephrine has a stimulating effect, however, its effect is blocked only partially by beta receptor blocking drugs. Intravenous injection of vasopressin raises the level of tissue plasminogen activator in

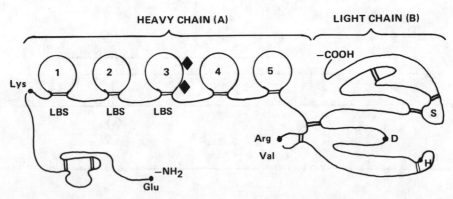

Figure 4. Plasminogen is a single-chain glycoprotein that is produced in the liver. It has a molecular weight of 90,000 and a carbohydrate content of 2%. The amino-terminal amino acid is glutamic acid; the carboxy-terminal amino acid is asparagine. Plasminogen has 790 residues and yields two chains on activation: A (Glu–Arg 560), or heavy chain, and B (Val 561–Asn 790), or light chain. The A chain has marked homologies with the nonthrombin part of prothrombin in that it possesses five triple-loop structures called "kringles" (after a Danish pastry). The kringles, each composed of approximately 80 residues, are held in a loop structure by three disulfide bridges between cysteine residues. The kringles are indicated in the figure by numbers 1 to 5. The carbohydrate groups are attached to kringle 3 and between kringles 3 and 4 (indicated by ♦).

Release of the preactivation peptides is accompanied by a conformational change in the moelcule, unmasking the lysine-binding sites (LBS). The LBS form 1:1 stoichiometric complexes with lysine, 6-aminohexanoic acid and aminomethylcylohexane. The LBS are instrumental in binding plasminogen to fibrinogen and in interacting with α_2-antiplasmin.

The B chain is homologous to thrombin and factor Xa and contains the sole active proteolytic site. The catalytic site is formed by three amino acid residues: His-602 (H), Asp-645 (D) and Ser-740 (S). The enzyme plasmin acts specifically on bonds where arginine or lysine is on the carboxyl side.

Modified from Brommer EJP, Brakman P, Haverkate F, et al: Progress in fibrinolysis. In Poller L (ed): *Recent Advances in Blood Coagulation* (vol 3). Edinburgh: Churchill Livingstone 1981, pp. 125–149.

Table 1

Laboratory Procedures for Evaluating Plasminogen/Plasmin*				
Procedure	Principle	Equipment Used	Advantages	Disadvantages
Radial immunodiffusion	Plasma sample diffuses through agar that contains antibody to plasminogen, causing formation of a precipitin ring.	None required	Technically simple; requires little technician time; specific; available in kits	No results for 48 hours; lacks sensitivity; requires high antibody concentration; does not reflect functional activity
α-Caseinolytic method	Digestion of plasmin by casein is measured by precipitating undigested casein with acid and measuring absorance of supernatant.	Spectrophotometer	Minimal laboratory instrumentation required; current reference method	Laborious and time-consuming
Fibrin plate lysis	Plasmin/plasminogen activity can be measured by zones of lysis on fibrin surface.	None required	Use of constant source of plasminogen-rich fibrin substrate yields highly reproducible degree of lysis	Tedious; 18–24 hours of incubation time; Difficult to standardize fibrin plates
Dade Protopath* synthetic fluorogenic substrate assay	Streptokinase-activated plasmin cleaves the fluorescent molecule from a synthetic substrate. (Omission of activator permits detection of free circulating plasmin.)	Dade Protopath	Available in preprogrammed kits	Requires Dade Protopath; cannot be modified
Synthetic chromogenic substrate assay†	Plasminogen converted to plasmin by streptokinase splits chromophore	Water bath, spectrophotometer	High specificity, solubility and stability	Expense; more sensitive to streptokinase activation than to urokinase activation

Table 1 *(continued)*

Laboratory Procedures for Evaluating Plasminogen/Plasmin*

Procedure	Principle	Equipment Used	Advantages	Disadvantages
	from chromogenic substrate.			
DuPont "aca" plasminogen assay	Plasminogen converted by streptokinase hydrolyzes the substrate, which releases the chromophore.	"aca"	Minimal sample size; simplicity of system; rapid turnaround time; reagent standardization; complete automation	Requires "aca" Requires "aca"
Euglobulin clot lysis time	Fibrinogen, plasminogen and plasminogen activators are precipitated by acidification and lowered ionic strength. Precipitate is redissolved and clotted; lysis time is measured.	None required	Simplicity	Low fibrinogen levels and/or presence of fibrin split products interferes with clot formation
Whole blood clot lysis	Fibrinolytic activity in serum dissolves clot after a period of time.	None required	Simplicity	Lacks specificity,* time-consuming

*Dade Division, American Hospital Supply Corp., Miami.
†Helena.
From McGann MA, Triplett DA: Laboratory evaluation of the fibrinolytic system. Lab Med 14:18–25, 1983.

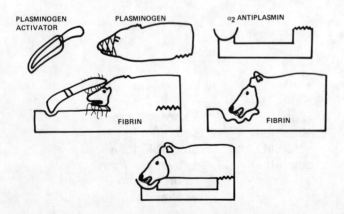

Figure 5. This schematic model illustrates various components of the fibrinolytic system. Plasminogen is converted to the serine protease plasmin by various plasminogen activators; however, this conversion occurs efficiently only on the surface of fibrin, where both activator and plasminogen are bound in proximity to each other. Plasminogen binds to fibrin by means of its lysine-binding sites (∿). Free plasmin in the blood is rapidly inactivated by α_2-antiplasmin; however, plasmin generated on the surface of fibrin is partially protected from inactivation. The interaction between plasmin and α_2-antiplasmin also involves the lysine-binding sites (∿).

Modified from: Collen D: Regulation of Fibrinolysis-Recent development. In Ménaché D, Surgenor D MacN, Anderson H, (eds): *Hemophilia and Hemostasis*. New York: Alan R. Liss, 1981, p. 224.

blood and although some analogues of vasopressin, such as DDAVP (1-desamino-8-D-arginine vasopressin) are practically devoid of vasoactive effect, they are more potent than most drugs in elevating levels of tissue plasminogen activator (21). The mode of action of DDAVP is unknown. A complex interaction between the influences on the vessel wall and those on the central nervous system has been suggested by a number of investigators. DDAVP will also elevate levels of factor VIII in the plasma.

Therapeutic Plasminogen Activators. Urokinase is a trypsin-like protease that has been isolated from human urine and cell cultures of human embryonic kidney (Table 2) (22,23). It occurs in two molecular forms, designated S-1 (molecular weight 31,600) and S-2 (molecular weight 54,000). The smaller form is thought to be a proteolytic degradation product of S-2. The antigenic characteristics and enzyme specificity of urokinase differ from those of tissue plasminogen activator. Following intravenous injection of urokinase, the half-life is approximately 10 minutes.

Streptokinase is a non-enzyme protein produced by Lancefield C stains of streptococci. This protein has a molecular weight of 47,000 and will activate the fibrinolytic system indirectly. It forms a 1:1 molar stoichiometric complex with plasminogen or plasmin. This complex is an extremely efficient activator of plasminogen (Figure 6). Presently, streptokinase is the most widely used agent in fibrinolytic therapy (Table 1). It is less expensive than urokinase, however, it is antigenic in human beings with resulting pyrogenic side effects.

Inhibitors of Plasminogen Activation. Knowledge of the inhibition of plasminogen activation is still in an embryonic stage. The presence of plasma inhibitors to

tissue plasminogen activator has been postulated since the early 1950's. There is evidence that an appreciable proportion of tissue plasminogen activator that is released into blood in vivo is cleared by mechanisms other than the actions of plasma inhibitors.

Table 2

Comparative Features of Streptokinase and Urokinase

Features	Urokinase	Streptokinase
Source	Human fetal kidney tissue culture or urine, also recombinant DNA technology.	Group C β-hemolytic streptococci
Molecular weight (daltons)	31,000–54,000	47,000
Half-life (minutes)	10 minutes	83*
Stability (°C)	4	Room temperature
Antigenicity	No	Yes
Pyrogenicity	No	Minimal
Indications	Acute pulmonary embolism	Acute pulmonary embolism, deep-vein thrombosis, occluded access shunts, arterial thrombosis
Retreatment	As needed	Wait 6–12 months
Cost	Expensive	Acceptable
Action	Direct proteolytic action on plasminogen	Indirect form, 1:1 stoichiometric complex with plasminogen or plasmin

Approximately 83 minutes in absence of antibodies; 18 minutes in presence of antibodies.
Modified from Sasahara HA, Sharma GVRK, Tow DE, et al: Clinical use of thrombolytic agents in venous thromboembolism. Arch Int Med 142:684–688, 1982.

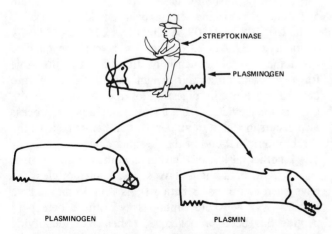

Figure 6. Streptokinase forms equimolar complexes with plasminogen (or with derivatives of plasminogen, such as plasmin and the β chain of plasmin). These stoichiometric complexes possess plasminogen activator activity and transform plasminogen within the complex to plasminogen with a functional active site but without apparent peptide bond cleavage.

Plasmin Inhibitors. α_2 Antiplasmin is a single chain polypeptide with a molecular weight of 70,000 (24). It binds plasmin very effectively, forming a 1:1 molar complex that is devoid of protease activity (Figure 5). In addition to inhibiting plasmin, α_2 antiplasmin decreases binding of Lys-plasminogen to fibrin 30 times more effectively than does ε-aminocaproic acid (25).

Complexes are formed between α_2 antiplasmin and plasmin by strong interaction between the light chain of plasmin and the inhibitor. The reaction rate between plasmin and α_2 antiplasmin is one of the fastest so far described for protein-protein interactions (11). In order for the reaction to occur, a free lysine-binding site and active serine site on the plasmin molecule are necessary.

During clotting of blood, approximately 22% of α_2 antiplasmin is covalently bound to fibrin. This binding to fibrin is mediated by factor XIII_a and requires calcium ions (26). Adsorption of α_2 antiplasmin to fibrin is an important mechanism for stabilizing the fibrin clot.

The normal plasma concentration of α_2 antiplasmin is about 60 mg/L (27). Disseminated intravascular coagulation and severe liver disease are associated with decreased plasma levels (11). During streptokinase therapy, levels of the inhibitor may be transiently exhausted (28).

In addition to acquired conditions in which there is decreased concentration of α_2 antiplasmin, a disorder that appears to be inherited in an autosomal recessive manner has been described. Patients who are homozygous for the abnormal genes have complete deficiency of α_2 antiplasmin and exhibit serious clinical bleeding similar to that of patients with hemophilia A (factor VIII deficiency) (29–33).

A natural inhibitor of fibrinolysis has recently been discovered by Lijnen and colleagues (34). This histidine rich glycoprotein interferes with binding plasminogen to fibrin by blocking one or more of the lysine-binding sites of plasminogen (35). Also, a rapidly acting plasmin inhibitor has been isolated from platelets (36).

α_2 Macroglobulin was thought to be the primary inhibitor of plasmin prior to the discovery of α_2 antiplasmin. α_2 Macroglobulin reacts very slowly with plasmin. Presently it is thought that α_2 macroglobulin inhibits plasmin formed in excess of the binding capacity of α_2 antiplasmin. Familial α_2 macroglobulin deficiency is an asymptomatic condition.

Digestion of Fibrinogen by Plasmin

Nussenzweig and colleagues first described the digestion of fibrinogen by plasmin (37). Using DEAE ion-exchange columns, they separated fibrinogen digests into five major fractions that were termed A, B, C, D, and E. Fragments D and E were described as plasmin-resistant with molecular weights of 83,000 and 33,000 respectively. Fragments D represent 50% and Fragment E 20% by weight of the original fibrinogen molecule.

Subsequent studies have further characterized the sequential digestion of fibrinogen by plasmin. The initial step involves removal of the carboxyterminal ends of the A-alpha chains (38,39). This action releases peptides of about 40,000 molecular weight, leaving the amino-terminal portion of the A-alpha chain linked by disulfide bridges to the B beta and gamma chains. The second step involves removal of peptides with molecular weight of approximately 6000 from the amino-terminal end of the B beta chains (40–42). The term Fragment X has been used to describe the remaining portion of the fibrinogen molecule following these initial steps. The molecular weight of fragment X is variable depending upon the degree of proteolysis of the amino-terminal end of the B beta chain. The third step involves an asymmetrical splitting of all three polypeptide chains at one side of the symmetrical partly digested fragment X. This lysis yields a D fragment and the remaining portion of fibrinogen referred to as the Y fragment. Subsequent lysis of Y fragment yields another D fragment together with the disulfide bonded portion of the original fibrinogen molecule referred to as fragment E (41). Thus, total digestion of fibrinogen results in two D fragments and one E fragment. The D fragments are composed of the three polypeptide chain remnants of the A alpha, B beta, and gamma chains of fibrinogen, whereas fragment E is a dimer that consists of two disulfide bonded subunits, each of which is composed of three polypeptide chains (Figure 7).

After the total primary sequence of fibrinogen had been described, investigators began to examine the structure of the molecule to locate the sites of attack by plasmin on the individual chains in the molecule (Figure 8)(43). Early plasmin degradation of the A alpha chain at its carboxy-terminal end appears to take place at A alpha Lys 208-Met-209, A alpha Lys 221-Ser-222 or A alpha Lys 232-Ala-233. These sites may be cleaved simultaneously or sequentially. In addition to the large fragments with molecular weights of 50,000 which are derived by plasmin digestion of the A alpha chain, there is some evidence that a slower degradation process also occurs in which small peptides are removed from the carboxy-terminal end of the A alpha chain.

Another early cleavage site is at the amino-terminal end of the B beta chain. Two separate sites of cleavage have been identified, B beta Arg 42-Aln 43 and B beta Lys 53-Lys 54. Radioimmunoassay of the B beta 1-42 peptide has been proposed as a means of identifying fibrinolysis in vivo (40). Conversion of fragments X and Y with release of D fragments requires cleavage of at least three peptide bonds, one each of the A alpha, β beta and gamma chain (44).

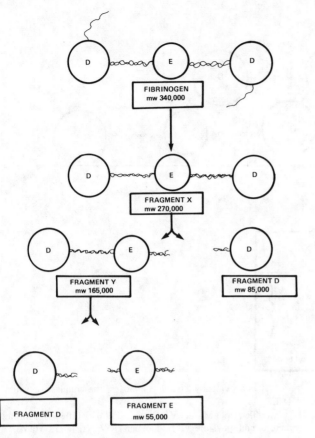

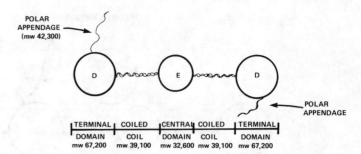

Figure 8. Fibrinogen has four major protein regions: the central domain that contains the amino-terminal disulfide knot, the thin connecting coils coiled in an alpha-helical configuration, the carboxy-terminal domains and the α-chain polar appendages. Many portions of the molecule are sensitive to plasmin, but the two most important sensitive sites are located on the polar appendage of Aα chain and on the central part of the coiled chain connecting area. Cleavage of the polar appendage gives rise to fragment X. Cleavage of the three chains of the coiled connecting area splits fragment X into fragments Y and D and fragment Y into fragments D and E.

Modified from Marder VJ, Francis CW, Doolittle RF: Fibrinogen structure and physiology. In Colman RW, Hirsh J, Marder VJ, Salzman EW (eds): *Hemostasis and Thrombosis*. Philadelphia: J.B. Lippincott, 1982, p 147.

Figure 7. The Aα polar regions are removed by plasmin to give fragment X. Cleavage of the coiled coil region involves Aα, Bβ and Y chains. This sequential cleavage gives rise to fragments D and Y and eventually to another fragment D and fragment E. Fragment E corresponds to the amino-terminal region of the fibrinogen molecule. Fragments D correspond to the carboxy-terminal portions of the symmetric fibrinogen molecule. Fragments X and Y are sometimes referred to as early fibrin split products; fragments D and E are referred to as late fibrin split products.

Modified from Marder VJ, Francis CW, Doolittle RF: Fibrinogen structure and physiology. In Colman RW, Hirsh J, Marder VJ, Salzman EW (eds): *Hemostasis and Thrombosis*. Philadelphia: J.B. Lippincott, 1982, p 149.

Digestion of Fibrin by Plasmin

When thrombin cleaves fibrinopeptide A and B from fibrinogen to give rise to fibrin monomers, there is spontaneous polymerization mediated by hydrogen bonding. Subsequently, fibrin is stabilized or cross linked in the presence of active factor XIII and calcium (Figure 9). The covalent bonds introduced by XIIIa initially occur between gamma chains to form gamma chain dimers and then more slowly between alpha chains to form alpha chain polymers. It is the formation of the high-molecular-weight alpha chain polymers that confirm a degree of plasmin resistence to the stable fibrin clot. The gamma-chain-binding sites are located near the carboxy-terminal end of the gamma chains, whereas the

alpha-chain-binding sites are located near the midportion of the alpha chains. The gamma chains are linked in an antiparallel manner.

When plasmin digests non-cross linked fibrin, the products are quite similar to those yielded by digestion of fibrinogen. The only chemical difference between the two digestion products is the absence of fibrinopeptides A and B from the fibrin fragments.

By contrast, when plasmin digests cross-linked fibrin, an electrophoretically and immunologically unique plasmin-resistant fragment is formed. This fragment has been referred to as the D-dimer. It originates from gamma chain cross-linked D fragments of a stabilized fibrin clot. The molecular weights of the D-dimer fragment have been reported to range from 63,000 to 81,000. Subsequent studies have demonstrated a D-dimer-E complex. Experimental studies suggest that the D-dimer-E complex is found in vivo more frequently than the D-dimer. However, the D-dimer expresses neoantigenicity, in contrast to the D-dimer-E complex, which does not (45,46). In addition to the D-dimer-E complex, a Y-D complex has been described.

Cell-Mediated Fibrinolysis

Recent studies suggest that polymorphonuclear neutrophils may have a role in the removal of fibrin. It appears that neutrophils contain an alternative fibrinolytic pathway in human beings. Platelets may also play a part because they have been shown to contain elastase. Also, monocytes appear to be capable of activating plasmin-

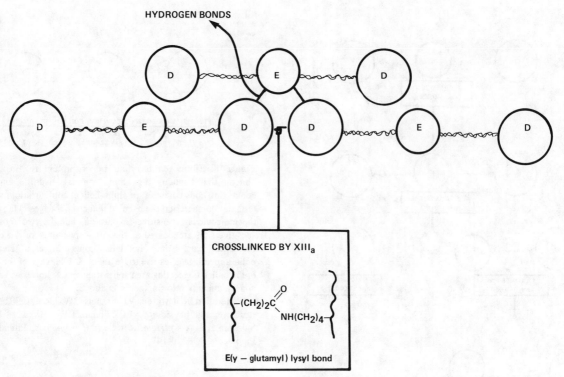

Figure 9. After thrombin cleaves fibrinopeptides A and B, fibrin monomers are formed. These monomers tend to polymerize non-covalently to give rise to fibrin dimers and then to intermediate polymers. Factor XIIIa catalyzes formation of cross-links between the γ chains of the terminal (D) domains, thus forming a stable, or cross-linked, fibrin clot. Digestion by plasmin of a fibrin clot gives rise to a series of noncovalently bound complexes, the smallest of which is DD/E.

Modified from Marder VJ, Francis CW, Doolittle RF: Fibrinogen structure and physiology. In Colman RW, Hirsh J, Marder VJ, Salzman EW (eds): *Hemostasis and Thrombosis*. Philadelphia: J.B. Lippincott, 1982, p 155.

ogen to plasmin, thereby mediating classical fibrinolysis (47,48).

Hereditary Abnormalities of Fibrinolysis

Recurrent thrombosis has been reported in a family with abnormalities of the structure and function of the plasminogen molecule (49). In this family, the proband had an abnormally low plasmin activity, but a normal level of antigenic plasminogen. Other members of the family who were heterozygous had approximately 50% of the normal functional activity of plasminogen. Five other cases of dysplasminogens have been reported (50–52). These cases were characterized by poor activation by urokinase or streptokinase. Once formed, plasmin functioned normally.

Some patients with thrombosis appear to show a lack of plasminogen activator release in response to venous occlusion or infusion of DDAVP (53–55). In addition, a number of patients with thrombotic disease appear to have substances that inhibit activation of plasminogen. However, characterization of these inhibitors has not been adequately confirmed.

Two abnormalities of the fibrinolytic system have been associated with a hemorrhagic clinical picture. The first is deficiency of α_2 antiplasmin (29–33). This condition is rare and appears to be inherited in an autosomal recessive manner. In the second disorder there is an abnormally high concentration of plasminogen activator (56).

Fibrinolytic Therapy

Although a number of therapeutic fibrinolytic agents have been described, only streptokinase and urokinase have been used with any frequency (57,58). Because of its greater availability and lower cost, streptokinase has seen wider clinical application. Recently, equimolar preparations of streptokinase-plasminogen complex have been introduced for clinical trials. (59)

Streptokinase

Tillett and Garner, in 1933, described fibrinolysis induced by filtrates of beta-hemolytic streptococcal cultures. Christensen and McLeod introduced the term streptokinase in 1945 (60). Streptokinase is a single chain protein of molecular weight 48,000. Streptokinase binds to the carboxy-terminal portion of plasminogen,

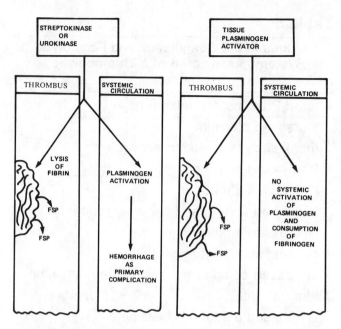

Figure 10. Conventional forms of thrombolytic therapy (streptokinase and urokinase) not only lyse a thrombus but also induce systemic fibrinolysis, resulting in consumption of fibrinogen, factor V and other components of the coagulation process. The primary complication of conventional thrombolytic therapy is hemorrhage. Tissue plasminogen activator has a high affinity for fibrin and does not induce systemic activation of plasminogen. Therefore, there are no changes in the circulating levels of fibrinogen and plasminogen, and hemorrhage is an infrequent complication.

making the active serine site more reactive. This promoting effect is achieved without cleavage of the Arg 560-Val 561 bond. This complex is then capable of converting other molecules of plasminogen to plasmin.

In addition to streptokinase, several different preparations have been described and include an equimolar complex of streptokinase and human plasminogen and an equimolar complex of human plasminogen light (B) chain-streptokinse complex (61).

After infusion of streptokinase, there is an immediate rapid clearance with a half-life of 18 minutes, which is followed by a slower disappearance phase with a half-life of approximately 83 minutes. The initial rapid clearance is attributed to immune complexing of streptokinase. Infusion of streptokinase is followed by a rapid drop in circulating levels of plasminogen and fibrinogen. With a large loading dose, the concentration of plasminogen may be decreased below 5% of the preinfusion level. Increased catabolism of fibrinogen is accompanied by the appearance of fibrinogen and fibrin degradation products. In addition, the presence of plasmin in the circulation leads to substantial reduction in the concentrations of factors V and VIII as well as digestion of the fibrin found in hemostatic plugs (Figure 10). Plasma levels of α_2 antiplasmin will also be decreased due to formation of plasmin-α_2 antiplasmin complexes.

Administration of Streptokinase
Streptokinase may be administered in a number of solutions, including saline and D_5W. The loading dose is typically 250,000 units administered intravenously over a course of 20 minutes. After the loading dose is given maintenance doses of 100,000 units per hour for 24 to 72 hours are recommended for the management of deep vein thrombosis or pulmonary embolism. A recent streptococcal infection or treatment with streptokinase is a definite indication for performance of a streptokinase resistance test so that an appropriate individualized course of therapy may be administered. Streptokinase may be given by systemic or local infusion (62–75).

In addition to the continuous regimen that has been described, various investigators have used intermittent administration of streptokinase.

Because of the antigenicity of streptokinase, corticosteroids are often administered with the loading dose of streptokinase. Some protocols use corticosteroids throughout the streptokinase treatment.

Following fibrinolytic therapy, anticoagulants are given in the majority of clinical situations. Initially heparin is administered following termination of streptokinase infusion. After heparin therapy is started, the patients are usually gradually converted to oral anticoagulants. It is important to remember that antiplatelet medication (i.e. aspirin) should not be administered during streptokinase therapy (Table 3).

Urokinase

Urokinase is a trypsin-like protease that activates plasminogen by cleaving the arg 560-Val 561 bond (76). Of the two molecular forms of urokinase, the smaller form (molecular weight 31,600) has a higher specific activity, although it is thought to be a proteolytic degradation product of S-2 (molecular weight 54,000).

The half-life of urokinase in vitro is approximately 10 minutes. The plasma inhibitors α_2 macroglobulin, α_1 antitrypsin, antithrombin III and α_2 antiplasmin all inhibit urokinase slowly.

Table 3

Precautions During Thrombolytic Therapy
Minimize physical handling
No parenteral medication
Minimize invasive procedures
Compression bandages at sites of needle punctures
Avoid concurrent anticoagulation
Avoid use of platelet-active drugs

Urokinase is usually given in a dose of 100,000–500,000 Committee on Thrombolytic Agents (CTA) units per hour. With doses in this range, there is slow and relatively mild depletion of plasminogen as well as fibrinogen (77). Continuous intravenous infusion is the most common method for the administration of urokinase.

Laboratory Monitoring of Fibrinolytic Therapy

The thrombin time has been the most frequently used test for monitoring fibrinolytic therapy; however, the prothrombin time or activated partial thromboplastin time may also be used. The thrombin time has achieved the widest acceptance because of its sensitivity to concentrations of both fibrinogen and fibrin split products. The baseline thrombin time must be obtained before therapy is instituted (Table 4). If the baseline time is between 10 to 12 seconds (normal range), the thrombin time should be maintained in a range of 20 to 70 seconds throughout the course of therapy. It has been suggested that the thrombin time be obtained at 4 hours, 12 hours, and then every 12 hours throughout therapy. When infusion has been completed, the thrombin time should again be obtained 3 to 4 hours after the last infusion. When the thrombin time has dropped to less than 20 seconds, heparin may be instituted. Occasionally, it may be necessary to perform an antistreptokinase test to titer the loading dose of streptokinase.

A rapid fibrinogen assay should also be available. Ideally, the assay should be based on clottable protein,

Table 4

Monitoring Fibrinolytic Therapy

TEST: Thrombin time (may use prothrombin or activated partial thromboplastin time)

A. Pretreatment range of thrombin time: 10–12 seconds

B. During treatment range: 20–70 seconds

C. Testing interval:

  4 hours

  12 hours

  Every 12 hours

D. When infusion is completed: Perform thrombin time after 3–4 hours; when thrombin time is <20 seconds, start heparin

Table 5

Changes in the Coagulation and Fibrinolytic Systems Associated with Thrombolytic Therapy

Altered Proteins and Inhibitors

  Increased plasmin

  Increased plasminogen activator

  Decreased plasminogen

  Decreased fibrinogen

  Increased fibrinogen-fibrin split products

  Decreased antiplasmins

  Decreased antithrombin III

  Increased complexes of plasmin-antiplasmin

Abnormal Blood Coagulation Test Results

  Decreased euglobulin lysis time

  Increased thrombin clotting time

  Increased activated partial thromboplastin time

  Increased prothrombin time

  Increased reptilase time

although the various heat precipitation techniques are probably acceptable (78–81). Changes that occur in plasma of patients receiving fibrinolytic therapy are summarized in Table 5.

Complications of Fibrinolytic Therapy

The primary complication of fibrinolytic therapy is hemorrhage. The risk for hemorrhage is related to a history of invasive procedures and also the duration of therapy.

Depending on the severity of hemorrhage, it may only be necessary to terminate therapy to achieve hemostasis. Streptokinase and urokinase are rapidly cleared and fibrinolytic activity disappears within 1 hour. To control serious clinical hemorrhage, therapy with antifibrinolytic agents such as E-aminocaproic acid or tranexamic acid may be indicated. Blood replacement or fresh frozen plasma may be needed if the concentration of fibrinogen is grossly reduced.

Other complications include pyrogenic or allergic phenomena with streptokinase therapy. Also, a transient elevation of liver enzyme levels has been reported in patients receiving streptokinase.

Table 6

Contraindications to Thrombolytic Therapy

Absolute Contraindications

    Active internal bleeding

    Recent central nervous system surgery or stroke

Relative Contraindications

    Recent major surgery

    Postpartum

    Cardiopulmonary resuscitation (rib fracture)

    Thoracentesis, paracentesis

    Recent serious trauma

    Uncontrolled coagulation defect

    Uncontrolled severe hypertension

    Pregnancy

Contraindications to Fibrinolytic Therapy

Major contraindications to fibrinolytic therapy are summarized in Table 6.

Future Perspectives in Fibrinolytic Therapy

Tissue plasminogen activator (TPA) from human melanoma cell line cultured in vitro has recently been isolated and characterized. This activator has been used to treat several patients with thrombotic disease (82). Use of this activator results in selective localized fibrinolysis without systemic fibrinogenlysis. More recently, it has been successfully cloned in Escherichia Coli (83).

Fibrinolytic Inhibitors and Antifibrinolytic Therapy

There are three distinctly different clinical situations in which antifibrinolytic therapy may be applied (84). Such therapy has been given to patients with systemic fibrinogenolysis such as occurs after administration of streptokinase or urokinase. In addition, antifibrinolytic therapy has been useful in patients with a decreased ability to form a stable hemostatic plug, such as those with hemophilia (85). Last, some patients with localized bleeding show no abnormality of hemostatic plug formation or evidence of systemic fibrinolysis (86). Neverthe-

less, in such patients, bleeding may result from an increased degree of local fibrinolysis which contributes to bleeding from injured tissue.

Mechanism of Action of Antifibrinolytic Agents

As has been discussed previously, the fibrinolytic system is fibrin oriented. Consequently, activation of plasminogen is much less efficient in the fluid phase than after binding to fibrin by means of the lysine binding sites. Plasminogen bound to fibrin is relatively protected and can be readily activated to plasmin, which then is in an excellent position for rapid digestion of the fibrin substrate. Consequently, fibrin is readily lysed in thrombi or hemostatic plugs whereas circulating fibrinogen is not attacked.

The physiologic inhibitors of plasmin include α_2 antiplasmin and α_2 macroglobulin which have been discussed previously (87). These inhibitors have not been purified for therapeutic use in human beings. Other antifibrinolytic agents include aprotinin, a polypeptide isolated from bovine parotid gland. Aprotinin is inhibitory for plasmin and other serine proteases such as trypsin and kallikrein (88). The third group of antiplasmins includes 6-aminohexanoic acid or ε-aminocaproic acid (EACA) and trans-p-aminomethylcyclohexane carboxylic acid (AMCA) which are synthetic lysine analogues (89–92) (Figure 11). The synthetic lysine analogues are structurally similar to lysine. Lysine has a five carbon chain with a carboxy group and an

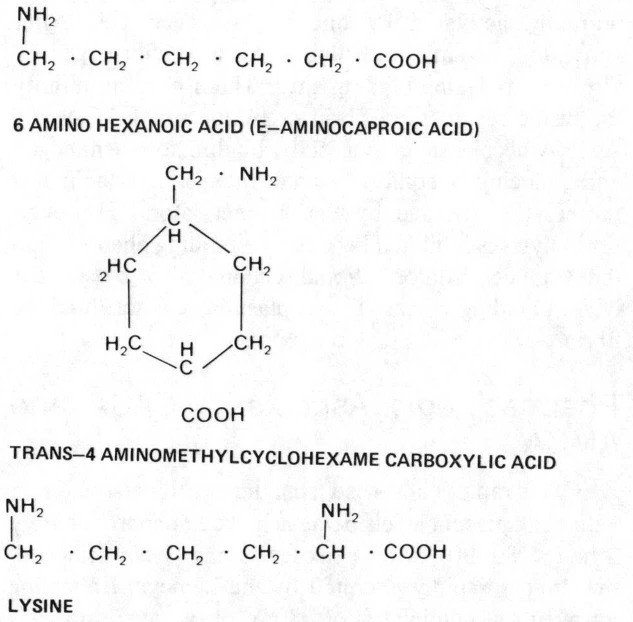

Figure 11. Lysine analogs EACA and AMCA.

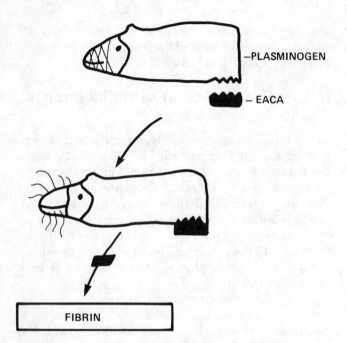

Figure 12. EACA: mechanism of action.

amino group attached to the first carbon (alpha carbon) and a second amino group attached to the fifth carbon (epsilon carbon). EACA differs from lysine only in that it lacks an alpha amino group. AMCA also lacks an alpha amino group but has two additional carbons that complete a saturated six member carbon ring.

Paradoxically, lysine analogues appear to accelerate activation of plasminogen in vitro; yet, they clearly inhibit in vivo fibrinolysis. The explanation for this apparent discrepancy is based on the interaction of EACA and AMCA with plasminogen. Plasminogen is normally activated by one or two cleavages. After activation, plasmin will bind to fibrin or fibrinogen by virtue of its lysine binding sites, which have an affinity for lysine residues on fibrin or fibrinogen. EACA and AMCA accelerate activation by binding to plasminogen and inducing a conformational change that facilitates proteolytic cleavage by various activators. However, fibrinolysis is inhibited because the binding phenomenon that induces conformational change also blocks the lysine binding sites. Thus, plasmin cannot bind to fibrin.

Pharmacologic Aspects of EACA and AMCA

EACA is rapidly absorbed from the gastrointestinal tract with peak plasma levels being achieved at approximately 2 hours (89–90). After peak levels have been achieved, the drug is rapidly excreted by the kidneys. Following intravenous administration 80% of a given dose is cleared by the kidneys within 3 hours. Usually, an intravenous loading dose of 5 grams of EACA is followed by continuous infusion of 0.5 to 1 gram per hour. EACA may also be given orally in the form of tablets or a syrup. Plasma levels of approximately 15 mg/dl are adequate for inhibition of fibrinolysis in vivo. Urinary levels are typically 75 to 100 fold higher than plasma levels; consequently, a lower dose may be effective in inhibiting urinary tract bleeding.

The plasma half-life of AMCA is similar to that of EACA and AMCA is also rapidly excreted in the urine. However, since AMCA is more potent than EACA, lower doses may achieve the same inhibitory effect on the fibrinolytic system.

Both agents have been associated with very few side effects. Patient complaints have included nasal stuffiness, nausea, vomiting, conjunctival suffusion and skin rash. Animal studies have shown teratogenicity.

A few patients who have been treated with EACA have experienced thrombotic complications. However, in all such patients, there appeared to be significant underlying prethrombotic tendencies or a low grade disseminated intravascular coagulation (93,94). Also, occasionally, EACA may produce partial renal obstruction in patients with bleeding in the upper genitourinary tract (95).

EACA and AMCA should not be used during the first trimester of pregnancy because these agents do have a teratogenic potential.

Clinical Use of Antifibrinolytic Therapy

This therapy has been used in patients with systemic fibrinolysis such as occurs with streptokinase therapy, congenital α_2 antiplasmin deficiency and after extracorporeal bypass surgery (96–98). Antifibrinolytic agents have also been used in the management of hemophilia particularly as an adjuvant therapy for controlling bleeding after dental surgery (99–100).

Last, antifibrinolytic agents have been helpful in controlling bleeding at local sites of fibrinolysis such as the prostate gland after transurethral resection.

References

1. Milstone H: A factor in normal human blood which participates in streptococcal fibrinolysis. *J Immunol* 42:109–116, 1941.
2. Tillett WS, Garner RL: The fibrinolytic activity of hemolytic streptococci. *J Exp Med* 58:485–502, 1933.
3. Astrup T, Permin PM: Fibrinolysis in the animal organism. *Nature* (London) 159:681–682, 1947.
4. Collen D: Regulation of fibrinolysis-recent development. In Menache D, Mac N Surgenor D, Anderson H: *Hemophilia and Hemostasis*. Alan R. Liss, New York, 1981, pp 221–228.

5. Sottrup-Jensen L, Claeys H, Zajdel M, et al: Primary structure of human plasminogen: isolation of two lysine-binding fragments and one "mini" plasminogen by elastase-catalyzed specific limited proteolysis. In Davidson JF, Rowan RM, Samama MM, Desnoyers PC: *Progress in Chemical Fibrinolysis and Thrombolysis.* New York, Raven Press, 1978, vol 3, pp 191–209.

6. Wallen P, Wiman B: Characterization of human plasminogen. Part II. Separation and partial characterization of different molecular forms of human plasminogen. *Biochem Biophys Acta* 272:122–134, 1972.

7. Collen D, Verstraete M: Molecular biology of human plasminogen. Part II. Metabolism in physiologic and some pathologic conditions in man. *Thromb Diath Haemorrh* 34:403–408, 1975.

8. McGann MA, Triplett DA: Laboratory evaluation of the fibrinolytic system. *Lab Med* 14:18–25, 1983.

9. Lackner H, Javid JP: Clinical significance of the plasminogen level. *Am J Clin Pathol* 60:175–181, 1973.

10. Triplett DA, Harms CS, Hermelin LI, et al: Clinical studies of the use of fluorogenic substrate assay method for determination of plasminogen, abstracted. *Thromb Haemostasis* 42:50, 1979.

11. Collen D: On regulation and control of fibrinolysis. *Thromb Haemostasis* 43:77–89, 1980.

12. Thorsen S: Differences in the binding to fibrin of native plasminogen and plasminogen modified by proteolytic degradation. *Biochim Biophys Acta* 393:55–65, 1975.

13. Gallin JI, Kaplan GP: Fletcher factor deficiency. A diminished rate of Hageman factor activation caused by absence of prekallikrein with abnormalities of coagulation, fibrinolysis, chemotactic activity and kinin generation. *J Clin Invest* 53:622–633, 1974.

14. Harpel PC: C′1 inactivator inhibition by plasmin. *J Clin Invest* 49:568–575, 1970.

15. Todd AS: The histological localization of fibrinolysin activator. *J Path Bact* 78:281–283, 1959.

16. Majno G, Joris I: Endothelium: a review. *Adv Exp Med Biol* 104:169–481, 1978.

17. Ranby M, Bergsdoff N, Nilsson T: Enzymatic properties of one and two chain form of tissue plasminogen activator. *Thromb Res* 27:175–183, 1982.

18. Rijken DC, Collen D: Purification and characterization of the plasminogen activator secreted by human melanoma cells in culture. *J Biol Chem* 256:7035–7041, 1981.

19. Atkinson T, Latter A, Electricwala A, et al: New tissue sources and types of fibrinolytic enzymes. *Lancet* 2:132–133, 1982.

20. Thorsen S, Glas-Greenwalt P, Astrup T: Differences in the binding to fibrin of urokinase and tissue plasminogen activator. *Thromb Diath Haemorrh* 28:65–74, 1972.

21. Brommer EJP, Barrett-Bergshoeff MM, Allen RA, et al: The use of desmopressin acetate (DDAVP) as a test of the fibrinolytic capacity of patients—analysis of responders and non-responders. *Thromb Haemost* 48:156–161, 1982.

22. Wun TC, Schleuning WD, Reich E: Isolation and characterization of urokinase from human plasma. *J Biol Chem* 257:3276–3283, 1982.

23. Sumi H, Toki N, Maehara S, et al: Immunochemical studies of high and low molecular forms of urokinase. *Acta Haemat* 67:263–267, 1982.

24. Mullertz S, Clemmensen I: The primary inhibitor of plasmin in human plasma. *Biochem J* 159:545–553, 1976.

25. Moroi M, Aoki A: Inhibition of plasminogen binding to fibrin by α_2-plasmin inhibitor. *Thromb Res* 10:851–856, 1977.

26. Sakata Y, Aoki N: Cross-linking of α_2 plasmin inhibitor to fibrin by fibrin-stabilizing factor. *J Clin Invest* 65:290–297, 1980.

27. Edy J, Collen D, Verstraete M: Quantitation of plasma protease inhibitor antiplasmin with chromogenic substrate S-2251. In Davidson JF, Rowan RM, Samama MM, Desnoyers PC. *Progress in Chemical Fibrinolysis and Thrombolysis.* New York, Raven Press, 1978, vol 3, pp 315–322.

28. Aoki N, Moroi M, Matsuda M, et al: The behavior of α_2 plasmin inhibitor in fibrinolytic states. *J Clin Invest* 60:365–369, 1977.

29. Vellenga E, Kluft C, Brommer EJP, et al: Deficiency of α_2 plasmin inhibitor and haemorrhage diathesis. *Eur J Clin Invest* 10:38–43, 1980.

30. Aoki N, Sakata Y, Matsuda M, et al: Fibrinolytic states in patient with congenital deficiency of α_2-plasmin inhibitor. *Blood* 55:483–488, 1981.

31. Miles LA, Plow EF, Donnelly KJ, et al: A bleeding disorder due to deficiency of α_2-antiplasmin. *Blood* 59:1246–1251, 1982.

32. Kluft C, Vellenga E, Brommer EJP, et al: A familial hemorrhagic diathesis in a Dutch family: An inherited deficiency of α_2-antiplasmin. *Blood* 59:1169–1180, 1982.

33. Yoshioka A, Kamitsuji H, Takase T, et al: Congenital deficiency of α_2-plasmin inhibitor in three sisters. *Haemostasis* 11:176–184, 1982.

34. Lijnen HR, Hoylaerts M, Collen D: Isolation and characterization of human plasma protein with affinity for lysine binding sites in plasminogen. *J Biol Chem* 225:10214–10222, 1980.

35. Heimburger N, Haupt H, Kranz T, et al: Human

serum proteine mit hoher Affinitat zu Carboxy-methylcellulose. II. Physikalischchemische und immunologische Charakterisierung eines Histidin-reichen 3.85-α_2-glykoproteins (CM-Protein I). Hoppe-Seyler's *Z Physiol Chem* 353:1133–1140, 1972.

36. Plow EF, Collen D: The presence and release of α_2-antiplasmin from human platelets. *Blood* 58:1069–1074, 1981.

37. Nussenzweig V, Seligmann M, Pelmont J, et al: Les produits de dégradation du fibrinogène humanin par la plasmine I: Separation et propriétés physicochimiques. *Ann Inst Pasteur (Par)* 100:377–389, 1961.

38. Doolittle RF: Fibrinogen and fibrin. *Sci Amer* 245: 126–135, 1981.

39. Gollwitzer R, Hafter R, Timpl R, et al: Immunological assay for a carboxyterminal peptide of the fibrinogen A α-chain in pathological human sera. *Thromb Res* 11:859–868, 1977.

40. Kudryk B, Robinson D, Netré C, et al: Measurement in human blood of fibrinogen/fibrin fragments containing the B β 15–42 sequence. *Thromb Res* 25:277–291, 1982.

41. Mosesson MW: Fibrinogen catabolic pathways. *Semin Thromb Hemostasis* 1:63–84, 1974.

42. Murano G: The molecular structure of fibrinogen. *Semin Thromb Hemostasis* 1:1–31, 1974.

43. Doolittle RF, Watt KWK, Cottrell BA, et al: The amino acid sequence of the β chain of human fibrinogen. *Nature (London)* 280:464–468, 1979.

44. Wilner GD: Molecular basis for measurement of circulating fibrinogen derivatives. In Spaet TH (ed): *Progress in Hemostasis and Thrombosis*. New York, Grune & Stratton, 1978, vol 4, pp 211–248.

45. Plow E, Edgington TS: Immunobiology of fibrinogen: Emergence of neoantigenic expressions during physiologic cleavage in vitro and in vivo. *J Clin Invest* 52:273–282, 1973.

46. Lee-Own V, Gordon YB, Chard T: The detection of neoantigenic sites on the D-dimer peptide isolated from plasmin digested cross linked fibrin. *Thromb Res* 14(1):77–84, 1979.

47. Brommer EJP, Brakman P, Haverkate F, et al: Progress in fibrinolysis. In Poller L (ed): *Recent Advances in Blood Coagulation*. Edinburgh: Churchill Livingstone, 1981, vol 3, pp 125–149.

48. Wiman B: Biochemistry of the plasminogen to plasmin conversion. In Gaffney PJ, Balkuv-Ulutin S (ed): *Fibrinolysis: Current Fundamental and Clinical Concepts*. London: Academic Press, 1978, pp 47–60.

49. Aoki N, Moroi M, Sakata Y, et al: Abnormal plasminogen. Hereditary molecular abnormality found in patient with recurrent thrombosis. *J Clin Invest* 61:1186–1195, 1978.

50. Wohl RC, Summaria L, Robbins KC: Physiological activation of the human fibrinolytic system. Isolation and characterization of human plasminogen variants, Chicago I and Chicago II. *J Biol Chem* 254:9063–9069, 1979.

51. Wohl RC, Summaria L, Chediak J, et al: Human plasminogen variant. Chicago III. *Thromb Haemostasis* 48:146–152, 1982.

52. Kazama M, Tahara C, Suzuki Z, et al: Abnormal plasminogen, a case of recurrent thrombosis. *Thromb Res* 21:517–522, 1981.

53. Pandolfi M, Isacson S, Nilsson IM: Low fibrinolytic activity in walls of veins of patients with thrombosis. *Acta Med Scand* 186:1–5, 1969.

54. Johansson L, Hedner U, Nilsson IM: Family with thromboembolic disease associated with deficient fibrinolytic activity in vessel wall. *Acta Med Scand* 203:477–480, 1978.

55. Stead NW, Bauer KA, Kinney TR, et al: Venous thrombosis in a family with defective release of vascular plasminogen activator and elevated plasma factor VIII/von Willebrand's factor. *Amer J Med* 74:33–39, 1983.

56. Booth NA, Bennett B, Wijngaards G, et al: A new life-long hemorrhagic disorder due to excess plasminogen activator. *Blood* 61:267–275, 1983.

57. Sharma GVRK, Cella G, Parisi AF, et al: Thrombolytic therapy. *N Eng J Med* 306:1268–1276, 1982.

58. Schmutzler R, Koller F: Thrombolytic therapy. In Poller L (ed): *Recent Advances in Blood Coagulation*. London: Churchill Livingstone, 1969, p 299.

59. Ling CM, Summaria L, Robbins KC: Isolation and characterization of bovine plasminogen activator from human plasminogen-streptokinase mixture. *J Biol Chem* 242:1419–1425, 1967.

60. Christensen LR, McLeod CM: A proteolytic enzyme of serum: characterization, activation and reaction with inhibitors. *J Gen Physiol* 28:559–583, 1945.

61. Summaria I, Robbins KC: Isolation of human plasmin derived functionally active, light (B) chain capable of forming with streptokinase an equimolar light (B) chain streptokinase complex with plasminogen activator activity. *J Biol Chem* 215:5810–5813, 1976.

62. Kakkar VV, Flane C, Howe CT, et al: Treatment of deep vein thrombosis: A trial of heparin streptokinase and arvin. *Br Med J* 1:806–810, 1969.

63. Robertson BR, Nilsson IM, Nylander G: Thrombolytic effect of streptokinase as evaluated by phlebography of deep venous thrombi of the leg. *Acta Chir Scand* 136:173–180, 1970.

64. Tsapogas MJ, Peabody RA, Wu KT, et al: Controlled study of thrombolytic therapy in deep vein thrombosis. *Surg* 74:973–984, 1973.

65. From the urokinase pulmonary embolism trial study group: Urokinase-streptokinase embolism trial phase 2 results. Cooperative study. *JAMA* 229:1606–1613, 1974.

66. Porter JM, Seaman AJ, Common HH, et al: Comparison of heparin and streptokinase in the treatment of venous thrombosis. *Am Surg* 41:511–519, 1975.

67. Common HH, Seaman AJ, Rosch J, et al: Deep vein thrombosis treated with streptokinase or heparin. *Follow-up of a randomized study. Angiology* 27:645–649, 1976.

68. Johansson E, Ericson K, Zetterquist S: Streptokinase treatment of deep vein thrombosis of lower extremity. *Acta Med Scand* 199:89–94, 1976.

69. Marder VJ, Soulen RL, Atichartakarn V, et al: Quantitative venographic assessment of deep vein thrombosis in the evaluation of streptokinase and heparin therapy. *J Lab Clin Med* 89:1018–1029, 1977.

70. Arenson H, Heilo A, Jakobsen E, et al: A prospective study of streptokinase and heparin in the treatment of deep vein thrombosis. *Acta Med Scand* 203:457–463, 1978.

71. Elliot MS, Immerlman EJ, Jeffery P, et al: A comparative randomized trial of heparin versus streptokinase in the treatment of acute proximal venous thrombosis: An interim report of a prospective trial. *Br J Surg* 66:838–843, 1979.

72. Gold HK, Leinbach RC: Coronary flow restoration in myocardial infarction by intracoronary streptokinase. Abstract, *Circulation* 62(Suppl III):161, 1980.

73. Stampfer MJ, Goldhaber SZ, Yusuf S, et al: Effect of intravenous streptokinase of acute myocardial infarction. *N Eng J Med* 307:1180–1182, 1982.

74. Shaw RB: Use of a fibrinolytic agent to restore function in a clotted Leveen shunt. *So Med J* 75:1285–1287, 1982.

75. Leman RB, Assey ME: Myocardial preservation by thrombolytic therapy during acute MI. *So Med J* 76:71–75, 1983.

76. Fletcher AP, Alkjaersig N, Sherry S, et al: Development of urokinase as thrombolytic agent. Maintenance of sustained thrombolytic state in man by its intravenous infusion. *J Lab Clin Med* 65:713–731, 1965.

77. Marder VJ, Donahoe JF, Bell WR, et al: Changes in plasminogen plasmin fibrinolytic system during urokinase therapy. Comparison of tissue culture urokinase with urinary source urokinase in patients with pulmonary embolism. *J Lab Clin Med* 92:721–729, 1978.

78. Babson AL, Opper CA, Crane LJ: Kinetic latex agglutinometry I. A rapid, quantitative immunologic assay for fibrinogen. *Am J Clin Path* 77:424–429, 1982.

79. Goodwin JF: An evaluation of turbidometric technics for estimation of plasma fibrinogen. *Clin Chem* 13:1057–1064, 1967.

80. Inada Y, Okamato H, Kanai S, et al: Faster determination of clottable fibrinogen in human plasma: An improved method and kinetic study. *Clin Chem* 24:351–353, 1978.

81. Jesperson J, Sidelmann J: A study of the conditions and accuracy of the thrombin time assay of plasma fibrinogen. *Acta Haemat* 67:2–7, 1982.

82. Weimer W, Stibbe J, Van Seyen AJ, et al: Specific lysis of an iliofemoral thrombus by administration of extrinsic (tissue-type) plasminogen activator. Lancet 2:1018–1020, 1981.

83. Pennica D, Holmes WE, Kohr WJ, et al: Cloning and expression of human tissue type plasminogen activator with DNA in E. coli. *Nature* 301:214–221, 1983.

84. Marder VJ, Butler FO, Barlow GH: Antifibrinolytic therapy. In Colman RW, Hirsh J, Marder VJ, Salzman EW: *Hemostasis and Thrombosis*, Philadelphia, Lippincott, 1982, pp 640–653.

85. Prentice CRM: Indications for antifibrinolysis therapy. *Thromb Diath Haemorrh* 34:634–643, 1975.

86. Nilsson IM: Local fibrinolysis as a mechanism for haemorrhage. *Thromb Diath Haemorrh* 34:623–633, 1975.

87. Aoki N: Natural inhibitors of fibrinolysis. *Prog Cardiovasc Dis* 21:267–286, 1979.

88. Kunitz M, Northrop JH: Isolation from beef pancreas of crystalline trypsinogen, trypsin, a trypsin inhibitor, and an inhibitor-trypsin compound. *J Gen Physiol* 19:991–1007, 1936.

89. Griffin JD, Ellman L: Epsilon-aminocaproic acid (EACA). *Semin Thromb Hemostasis* 5:27–40, 1978.

90. McNicol GP, Douglas AS: ε-aminocaproic acid and other inhibitors of fibrinolysis. *Brit Med Bull* 20:233–239, 1964.

91. Okamoto S, Oshiba S, Mihara H, et al: Synthetic inhibitors of fibrinolysis: In vitro and in vivo mode of action. *Ann NY Acad Sci* 146:414–429, 1968.

92. Andersson L, Nilsson IM, Nilehn JE, et al: Experimental and clinical studies on AMCA the antifibrinolytically active isomer of p aminomethyl cyclohexane carboxylic acid. *Scand J Haematol* 2:230–247, 1965.

93. Bergin JJ: The complications of therapy with epsilon amino-caproic acid. *Med Clin North Amer* 50:1669–1678, 1966.

94. Gralnick HR, Greipp P: Thrombosis with epsilon amino caproic acid therapy. *Amer J Clin Pathol* 56:151–154, 1971.
95. Prentice CRM, Lindsay RM, Barr RD, et al: Renal complications in haemophilia and Christmas disease. *Q J Med* 40:47–61, 1971.
96. Sterns LP, Lillehei CW: Effect of epsilon aminocaproic acid upon blood loss following open heart surgery. An analysis of 340 patients. *Can J Surg* 10:304–307, 1967.
97. Lambert CJ, Marengo-Rowe AJ, Leveson JE, et al: The treatment of postperfusion bleeding using ε-aminocaproic acid, cryoprecipitate, fresh-frozen plasma, and protamine sulfate. *Ann Thorac Surg* 28:440–444, 1979.
98. Kevy SV, Glickman RM, Bernhard WF, et al: The pathogenesis and control of the hemorrhagic defect in open heart surgery. *Surg Gynecol Obstet* 123:313–318, 1966.
99. Reid WO, Hodge SM, Cerutti ER: The use of EACA in preventing or reducing hemorrhages in the hemophiliac. *Thromb Diath Haemorrh* 18:179–189, 1967.
100. Forbes CD, Barr RD, Reid G, et al: Tranexamic acid in control of haemorrhage after dental extraction in haemophilia and Christmas disease. *Brit Med J* 2:311–333, 1972.

Reference Books

Gaffney PJ: The biochemistry of the degradation of fibrinogen and fibrin by plasmin. In Neri Serneri GG, Prentice CRM (eds): *Haemostasis and Thrombosis*. London: Academic Press, 1979, pp 7–26.

Gaffney PJ, Balkuv-Ulutin S: Fibrinolysis: Current Fundamental and Clinical Concepts. London: *Academic Press*, 1978.
Komttimen YP: *Fibrinolysis, Chemistry, Physiology, Pathology and Clinics*. Tampere, Finland: Oy Star AB., 1968.
Marsh N: *Fibrinolysis*. Chichester, England: John Wiley & Sons, Chichester, 1981.
Ogston D: Biochemistry of naturally occurring plasminogen activators. In Ogston D, Bennett B (eds): *Haemostasis: Biochemistry, Physiology and Pathology*. London: John Wiley & Sons, 1977, pp 221–229.
Robbins KC: Biochemistry of plasminogen and plasmin. In Ogston D, Bennett B: *Haemostasis: Biochemistry, Physiology and Pathology*. London: John Wiley & Sons, 1977, pp 208–220.

Review Articles

Aoki N: Natural inhibitors of fibrinolysis. *Prog Cardiovasc Dis* 21:267–286, 1979.
Collen D: On the regulation and control of fibrinolysis. *Thromb Haemostasis* 43:77–89, 1980.
Kwaan HC: Disorders of fibrinolysis. *Med Clin North Amer* 56:163–176, 1972.
Kwaan HC: Fibrinolysis-A perspective. *Prog Cardiovasc Dis* 21:397–403, 1979.
Robbins KC: The human fibrinolytic system: Regulation and control. *Mol Cell Biochem* 20:149–157, 1978.
Robbins KC, Summaria L: Plasminogen and plasmin. *Methods Enzymol* 45:257–273, 1976.

Chapter
THREE

Roles of Platelets and Endothelial Cells

As has been discussed in Chapter 1, hemostasis may be conveniently divided into two steps: primary and secondary hemostasis. Primary hemostasis is dependent on a blood vessel and circulating platelets whereas secondary hemostasis is dependent on coagulation proteins.

The platelets have a central role in primary hemostasis. Although platelets appear deceptively simple when viewed through a light microscope, they are found to be structurally complex when examined with transmission electron microscopy. Investigators have recently elucidated the biochemical features of the platelet response as well. The roles of the arachidonic acid pathway and of prostaglandins have been elucidated in platelets as well as endothelial cells (1–4). In addition to their central responsibility in primary hemostasis, platelets have been implicated in the pathogenesis of arterial thromboembolic disease and atherosclerosis (Figure 1) (5,6).

As early as 1820, Thackrah (7) recognized the importance of vascular integrity in hemostasis. In 1842, Donné (8) provided the first description of platelets. Subsequently, in 1883, Hayem (9) who had previously described hemocytoblasts and distinguished them from leukocytes, showed that puncture wounds in a jugular vein of a dog as well as in a mesenteric vein of a frog were occluded by "un clou hemostatique," which consisted of hemocytoblast-like "un champignon Blanchatre." (9) About the same time, Bizzozero (10) gave an extensive description of white thrombus formation. He was the first author to use the term "blood platelets." Initially, the idea that platelets played an important part in hemostasis was not accepted, but Eberth and Schimmelbusch (11) extended the work of Bizzozero and confirmed the primary role of platelets in the formation of hemostatic plugs. These investigators recognized that platelets adhered to the lips of an injured vessel, formed loose aggregates, lost their granularity and optical density and became more or less fused. Formation of fibrin at the final stage was also recognized.

After these original observations were made, researchers abandoned platelets as a fertile field of investigation and turned to the study of coagulation and the various plasma proteins involved in formation of fibrin clots. It was not until the past decade that attention was again focused on platelets and their role in normal hemostasis and thrombus formation. During the past decade, extensive information has been gained regarding the response of platelets to vascular injury as well as the

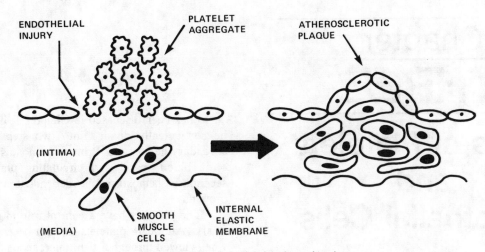

Figure 1. Role of platelets in atherosclerosis.

role of platelets in arterial thrombosis and in the development of atherosclerosis.

Before discussing the response of platelets to vascular injury, it is appropriate to review briefly the kinetics of platelet production, the anatomic structure of the circulating platelets, and the biochemical features of platelet activation.

Kinetics of Platelet Production

Circulating platelets are smooth, colorless disks that have a diameter of 2 to 4 μm and a thickness of 0.5 μm. They are anucleate and are produced by cytoplasmic partition and fragmentation of mature megakaryocytes (12). Megakaryocytes may be found in the extravascular space of the bone marrow as well as in the lungs and peripheral circulation.

During maturation, the cytoplasm of megakaryocytes develops a diffuse granularity and lines of demarcation that delineate the membranes of future platelets (13). Production of platelets appears to be related to the volume of megakaryocytes and to the quantity of their cytoplasm. The amount of cytoplasm accumulated by a megakaryocyte is roughly proportional to its ploidy value. The time required for complete differentiation of a megakaryocyte has been estimated to be approximately 3 to 5 days in human beings (14–16).

Because megakaryocytopoiesis is stimulated by thrombocytopenia or suppressed by thrombocytosis, a regulatory mechanism that involves a hormone, thrombopoietin, has been postulated (17,18). After thrombocytopenia has developed, the marrow may accelerate production of platelets as a result of three possible mechanisms: an increase in the volume of megakaryocytes, which may be related to an increase in the average number of nuclei per cell; an increase in the total number

of megakaryocytes as a result of an influx of cells from the stem cell pool; and shortening of the maturation time of megakaryocytes (17,19).

The maximal response of the bone marrow to thrombocytopenia has been suggested to be approximately eight times the basal response. Platelets released by a reactive marrow in response to thrombocytopenia are usually larger and metabolically more active than circulating platelets. There is evidence that such platelets are preferentially sequestered in the spleen for several days before they enter the bloodstream (20). In addition to being metabolically more active, younger platelets participate more effectively in the primary hemostatic response.

Isotopes that have been used to label platelets for life span determinations have included sodium chromate (^{51}Cr) and diisopropylflouorphosphate labeled with phosphorus 32 ($_{32}$P) (21). Recent studies have used indium 111 (22–25). Ideally, a radioisotope label for platelets should not alter their survival time or function in vivo and should bind irreversibly and randomly to a sample of the platelet population regardless of the volume, density or age of individual platelets. These requirements appear to be met when platelets are labeled with chromium 51 or indium 111. The disappearance patterns of labeled platelets in healthy persons are essentially linear, indicating that removal of platelets is predominantly an age-related process. In consumptive processes (e.g., autoimmune thrombocytopenia), exponential disappearance patterns reflect random removal of platelets (26). Curvilinear disappearance patterns result when senescence and consumption are combined. The importance of senescent removal of platelets is further supported by the observation that neither anticoagulants (i.e., heparin or oral anticoagulants) nor antiplatelet agents (e.g., aspirin or dipyridamole) affect the survival time of labeled platelets in healthy persons. Disappearance patterns become increasingly curvilinear with

Figure 2. Correlation between platelet function and anatomy.

Anatomic Zone	Function

Peripheral
    Exterior coat (glycocalyx)
    Unit membrane
    Submembrane area
	Adhesion and aggregation

Sol-Gel
    Microtubules
    Microfilaments
	Contraction and support

Organelles
    Dense bodies
    Alpha granules
    Lysosomes
	Storage and secretion

Membranous System
    Dense tubular system
    Surface connecting system
	Synthesis of prostaglandins and regulation of calcium

turnover rate of platelets has been estimated to be approximately 35,000 ± 4300 platelets per microliter per day.

In human beings, approximately two-thirds of the platelets are in the general circulation, and the remaining one-third are reversibly sequestered in the spleen (29). The role of the spleen in regulating the total number of circulating platelets has not been completely resolved. Changes in the platelet count after splenectomy can be attributed to removal of the splenic pool of platelets.

Morphologic Features

In the unstimulated state, platelets are small, anucleate disk-shaped cells that have an average diameter of 2 to 3

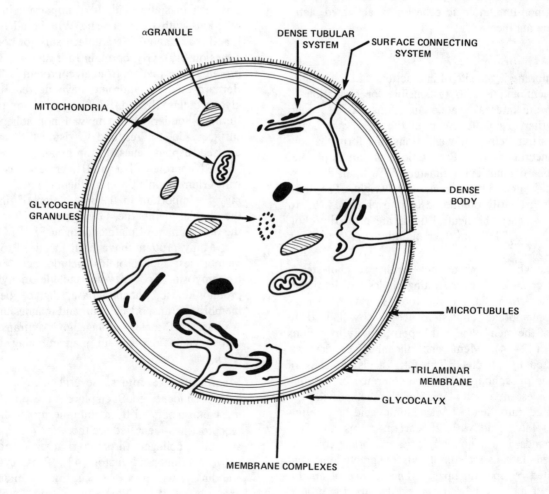

advancing age, perhaps due to the development of vascular disease (27,28).

The life span of platelets as estimated by in vitro labeling with chromium 51, ranges from 9 to 12 days in humans beings. In the steady state, production of platelets is balanced by destruction of platelets. The

μm and a volume of approximately 8 fl. In human blood, there are normally 130,000 to 400,000 platelets per microliter. When examined with transmission electron microscopy, platelets appear to be ellipsoidal or circular, depending on the plane of section (Figure 2). The platelet membrane communicates with the interior of the cell by a complex canalicular network, the surface connecting system, that provides a means of ready egress of substances secreted during the release reaction. In addition to supplying a channel of egress, the surface connecting system greatly increases the surface area of platelets (30).

For purposes of discussion, platelets may be divided into four anatomic regions: peripheral zone, sol-gel zone, organelle zone and membranous system.

Peripheral Zone

The peripheral zone consists of a membrane, a fluffy coat of mucopolysaccharide on the external surface of the membrane and a submembrane region (31). The peripheral zone mediates adhesion and aggregation of a platelet. Adhesion refers to attachment of a platelet to a damaged blood vessel or foreign surface and aggregation indicates non-immunologic cohesion of activated platelets to one another.

Platelet Membrane
The membrane is the site of interaction with the plasma environment and is also responsible for regulation of many of the internal platelet functions. As has been noted earlier, a unique aspect of the membrane is the numerous intracellular invaginations that form the surface connecting system. Preparations of human platelet membranes contain approximately 35% lipid, 8% carbohydrates, and 57% proteins by weight. The lipid bilayer is primarily composed of phospholipids (65 to 75% by weight): the neutral lipids are primarily cholesterol (20 to 25%), and the remainder is glycoproteins (2% to 5%).

Although platelets do not synthesize cholesterol, they are capable of incorporating cholesterol into their membranes from plasma lipoproteins in vivo. An increased membrane cholesterol content will lead to rigidity of the membrane and hyperreactivity to various agonists (32–34). Membrane phosphoglycerides are synthesized by platelets. The fatty acids moieties of membrane phospholipids may be saturated or unsaturated. The essential fatty acids of the diet provide the unsaturated fatty acids. Arachidonic acid, a polyunsaturated fatty acid with 20 carbon atoms and four double bonds, is a major fatty acid membrane constituent. When platelets are stimulated, free arachidonic acid is liberated by specific lipases. The release of arachidonic acid and its subsequent availability for prostaglandin synthesis is a major control point in the platelet response (35–38).

There is good evidence for an asymmetric distribution of phospholipids in the platelet membrane. Phosphatidylethanolamine, phosphatidylcholine, and phosphatidylserine are primarily oriented to the cytoplasmic aspect of the membrane. This cytoplasmic orientation

may be important in prostaglandin production following platelet stimulation. When platelets are stimulated, the lipids bilayer becomes rearranged with external orientation of phosphatidylethanolamine and phosphatidylserine. These lipids play a role in providing a surface upon which the coagulation proteins are arranged.

Membrane Glycoproteins. The membrane proteins of platelets are primarily glycoproteins which are oriented to the plasma surface of the membrane. Approximately seven major glycoproteins have been identified (39). These proteins play a major role in a number of platelet functions including cell-cell and cell-surface interactions, membrane transport, and membrane receptors and transducers. In addition, they also impart antigenicity to the platelets. Loss of membrane sialic acid is associated with platelet senescence in vivo.

Glycocalicim (GPIs), a constituent of glycoprotein I is rich in sialic acid. It is important in the platelet reactions with thrombin and Willebrand factor. Willebrand factor and GPIs are necessary for normal platelet adhesion (40). Glycoprotein Ib is an integral membrane protein that is distinct from glycoprotein Is. Patients with Bernard-Soulier syndrome have decreased membrane glycoproteins Ib and Is. Platelets from patients with Bernard-Soulier syndrome will not adhere to foreign surfaces, do not respond to ristocetin, and show decreased responsiveness to thrombin.

Glycoproteins IIb and IIIa are decreased in patients with Glanzmann's thrombasthenia. These glycoproteins may be important in the interaction of fibrinogen and the platelet membrane. Glycoprotein IIIa appears to be the determinant of platelet antigen PL^{A1} (41,42).

Many proteins have been localized to the platelet membranes; such proteins include: actin, myosin, and tropomyosin. Endoenzymes include adenylate cyclase, protein kinase, phospholipase, diglyceride lipase and membrane transport calcium and magnesium dependent ATPases. Platelet collagenglycosyltransferases are ectoenzymes involved in platelet-collagen interaction (39).

Membrane Receptors. Several membrane receptors have been identified. Such platelet receptor functions are most like mediated by membrane proteins. Among the receptor sites identified are those for ADP, epinephrine, serotonin, collagen, thrombin, Factor V and Xa as well as von Willebrand factor (43). Prostacyclin (prostaglandin I_2) which is produced by the endothelial cells exerts a potent inhibitor influence on platelet response. The receptor site for prostacyclin has not as yet been characterized, but appears to be distinct from the prostaglandin D_2 receptor (44–46).

The submembrane region constitutes the space between the unit membrane and the circumferential band of microtubules. This area contains a system of filamentous elements.

Sol-Gel Zone

Immediately beneath the platelet membrane and within the cytoplasm of the platelet is the sol gel zone which has plays a part in the support of the platelets and which also has a contractile function. In the unstimulated platelet, the microtubules main the discoid shape of the platelet by exerting an outward tension. In support of this conclusion is the assumption of a spherical shape by platelets when the microtubules are depolymerized. Microtubules are composed primarily of heterodimers of alpha and beta tubulin subunits. These subunits polymerize to form hollow tubular cylinders (47). A single tubule is approximately 25 nm in diameter. The noncovalent assembly of the microtubules is dependent upon GTP or ATP and involves phosphorylation of tubulin (48). When platelets are stimulated, there is a transient depolymerization followed by repolymerization of the microtubules.

The platelet microfilaments play an important role in the majority of platelet functions. Of these functions, the platelet release reaction and clot retraction have received the most attention. The platelet microfilaments contain actin and myosin as well as a number of other proteins. Actin is the most abundant platelet protein. In the resting platelet, actin is primarily in the nonfilamentous form. It appears that profilin will bind to actin and maintain it in the nonfilamentous form. With stimulation of platelets, actin becomes polymerized to form thin actin filaments. This gelling phenomena is promoted by actin binding protein and alpha actinin. With polymerization of actin, there is also organization into parallel arrays of microfilaments. These microfilaments are apparently linked to the platelet membrane.

The concentration of myosin in the platelet is much lower than in skeletal muscle. As a result, the actin/myosin ratio is very high. Once the light chain of myosin is phosphorylated, it interacts with actin and ATP to produce a contractile force that is related to the extent of phosphorylation. In the presence of magnesium and ATP, phosphorylation of the light chain is mediated by myosin light chain kinase which requires calcium and the regulatory protein calmodulin as cofactors (49).

Organelle Zone

The organelle zone is associated with storage and secretion of various substances contained within the three types of granules. The dense granules contain calcium, pyrophosphate, ADP, ATP, and serotonin and perhaps antiplasmin. The electron dense material which gives the granules their name is calcium. The dense granules contain the storage pool of ADP/ATP which is secreted during the platelet release reaction. This storage pool of ADP/ATP does not exchange with the metabolic pool of adenine nucleotides found in the platelet cytoplasm. The dense bodies have an important role in aggregation of platelets as evidenced by deficient aggregation in certain disease states (storage pool disease) in which the contents of the dense bodies are reduced or absent (50,51).

Alpha granules are more numerous than are dense bodies and contain a number of substances, including platelet specific proteins; namely, platelet factor 4, beta thromboglobulin, mitogenic factor (platelet derived growth factor) and thrombospondin (Table 1) (52–56). Other proteins contained within the alpha granules include: Fibronectin, factor VIII related antigen (von Willebrand factor), fibrinogen, and factor V. Platelet derived growth factor is a heat-stable basic protein that stimulates synthesis of DNA and growth of cells in tissue cultures. This protein has been implicated in the pathogenesis of atherosclerosis (53). Thrombospondin is a thrombin sensitive protein composed of three subunits linked by disulfide bonds. It is the major glycoprotein present in the alpha granules (57).

The third type of granule is similar to lysosomes in many other cells of the body. Platelet lysosomes contain proteases, hydrolases and cathepsins. Strong stimuli are required for release of the lysosomes.

In addition to the above described structures, platelets contain peroxisomes and mitochondria. The peroxisomes contain catalase and the mitochondria are necessary for ATP synthesis.

Table 1

Contents of Platelet Alpha Granules
Proteins Similar to Plasma Proteins
Albumin
Fibrinogen
Factor VIII R:Ag (von Willebrand factor)
Fibronectin
Factor V
Protease inhibitors
Platelet-Specific Proteins
Platelet factor 4
β-Thromboglobulin
Platelet-derived growth factor
Thrombospondin
Low-affinity platelet factor 4
Platelet basic protein
Bactericidal factor
Chemotactic factor

Membranous System

The membranous system is composed of the dense tubular system and the surface connecting system. The two structures frequently come in close contact to form membrane complexes. The dense tubular system is derived from smooth endoplasmic reticulum and is thought to be a major site of sequestration of calcium. The regulation of cytoplasmic ionic calcium concentration is important in mediating the major platelet functions. The dense tubular system may function in a manner similar to the system of skeletal muscle sarcotubules which controls calcium ionic flux. The dense tubular system is also the site of platelet prostaglandin synthesis.

Biochemical Properties

Platelets contain enzymes that function in the glycolytic and tricarboxylic acid cycles as well as those necessary for synthesis and catabolism of glycogen. The biochemical events that regulate aggregation of platelets and the release reaction are not completely known (58,59). Three mechanisms are presumably involved: changes in membrane adenyl cyclase activity, fluxes in platelet concentrations of calcium ions and synthesis of unstable cyclic endoperoxides and thromboxane A_2 (60–62). Perhaps the changes in cytoplasmic concentration of calcium ions represent the final common pathway in mediation of platelet activation. In addition to the above mentioned events that lead to aggregation of platelets and the release reaction, a number of investigators have recently called attention to platelet activating factor (63). This activating factor is a lysolecithin that is made available to platelets from external sources (i.e. activated basophils, neutrophils, and macrophages) as well as from platelets. This factor induces the platelet release reaction but does not activate the arachidonic acid pathway.

Prostaglandin Metabolism

Both prostaglandins and thromboxanes are involved in regulating the platelet response. Production of these compounds in platelets and endothelial cells is outlined in Figure 3.

Arachidonic acid is the usual substrate for synthesis of prostaglandin. With platelet stimulation, arachidonic acid is cleaved from the two position of membrane phosphoglycerides (phosphatidylcholine and phosphatidylinositol) (Figure 4) (64,65). There appears to be two pathways for generation of arachidonic acid from the membrane phosphoglycerides. The first pathway is dependent on a phospholipase A_2, and the second on phospholipase C. Phospholipase C cleaves phosphatidylinositol to produce a diglyceride. This diglyceride is

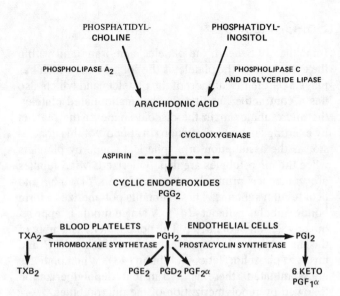

Figure 3. Synthesis of prostaglandins from arachidonic acid. Aspirin irreversibly acetylates the enzyme cyclooxygenase. Because platelets are not able to synthesize additional cyclooxygenase, they are inhibited for the remainder of their life span. Thromboxane A_2 (TXA$_2$) is a potent stimulator of platelet aggregation and a vasoconstrictor. Prostacyclin (PGI$_2$) inhibits platelet aggregation and is a vasodilator.

then acted upon by diglyceride lipase which will release arachidonic acid (66). Presumably, many inducers of platelet aggregation activate phospholipase A_2 and C directly, or promote intracellular release of the membrane bound calcium ions that are required for stimulation of phospholipases (67). After arachidonic acid is released, cyclooxygenase converts arachidonic acid to cyclic endoperoxides (prostaglandins G_2 and H_2). Alternatively, lipoxygenase enzyme may convert arachidonic acids to 12-hydroperoxy-5,8,10,14-eicosatetraenoic acid (HPETE) and 12-L-hydroxy-5,8,10-14-eicosatetraenoic acid (HETE) (68). The unstable cyclic endoperoxides are converted by thromboxane synthetase to thromboxane A_2 or may spontaneously be degraded to 12L Hydroxy-5,8,10-heptadecatrienoic acid (HHT) and malondialdehyde (MDA). Small amounts of the endoperoxides may be converted by specific synthetases to prostaglandins D_2, E_2 and $F_{2\alpha}$.

Thromboxane A_2 is an extremely potent platelet agonist and also a vasoconstrictor. It has an extremely short half-life, approximately 30 seconds, and is degraded to a nonactive product, thromboxane B_2. Thromboxane A_2 can directly cause platelets to form aggregates (in the absence of ADP release) and can also induce the release reaction. Some experimental evidence suggests that thromboxane A_2 serves as a physiologic ionophore, elevating the cytoplasmic concentration of calcium ions and thus triggering activation of platelets. Mobilized calcium in the platelet cytoplasm has at least two effects: to stimulate the release of ADP, serotonin, and other

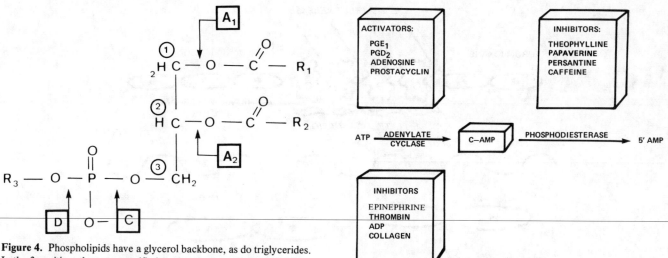

Figure 4. Phospholipids have a glycerol backbone, as do triglycerides. In the 3 position, they are esterified to phosphoric acid. Hydrocarbons are attached to the 1 and 2 positions. The hydrocarbon at the 2 position usually is a polyunsaturated fatty acid, whereas the hydrocarbon at the 1 position is a saturated fatty acid. Most phosphoric acid groups form diesters with the hydroxyl groups of choline, ethanolamine, serine or inositol.

Phospholipids can be hydrolyzed by special enzymes that are called phospholipases A_1, A_2, C and D according to their sites of action. These sites are indicated in the figure. R_1 and R_2, fatty acid residues; R_3, alcohol group.

Figure 5. Regulation of 3′, 5′-cyclic AMP.

secretory products from the platelet granules and to inhibit platelet adenyl cyclase, resulting in a fall in the intracellular concentration of 3′,5′ cyclic AMP. An increase in cytoplasmic ionic calcium concentration is also associated with activation of the interaction between actin and myosin and the enzymatic activity of phospholipases A_2 and C.

Thromboxane A_2 has been implicated in the pathogenesis of thrombotic disease. In such diseases as diabetes mellitus and certain hyperlipidemias, overproduction of thromboxane A_2 has been reported in association with "hypersensitive" platelets (69,70). Thromboxane A_2 generation has also been linked to anginal attacks.

The cyclo-oxygenase enzyme in platelets and other structures may be irreversible inactivated by aspirin. Because platelets are unable to synthesize additional protein, inactivation of the enzyme persists for their life span (71–73). Consequently, patients who have recently ingested aspirin show absence of the oxygen burst when their platelets are stimulated in vitro.

The metabolic fate of cyclic endoperoxides depends on the enzymes in the tissue in which they are generated. Endothelial cells convert prostaglandin H_2 to prostacyclin (prostaglandin I_2), the most powerful inhibitor of platelet aggregation yet described (74,75). Prostacyclin inhibits activation of platelets by elevating the level of cyclic AMP which in turn blocks mobilization of calcium ions in the platelet cytoplasm (Figure 5) (76). Prosta-

cyclin is metabolized to 6-keto prostaglandin $F_{1\alpha}$ which is essentially biologically inert (77). Thus, there appears to be a balance between production of prostacyclin by blood vessels and production of thromboxane by platelets. This balance may be a critical factor in the maintenance of blood fluidity. Also, it can be readily appreciated that aspirin inhibits cyclooxygenase activity in platelets as well as endothelial cells. Consequently, clinical trials in which doses of aspirin have been high enough to inhibit synthesis of prostacyclin cloud the interpretation of these results (78–80).

As has been noted above, a second pathway for the metabolism of arachidonic acid is the lipoxygenase pathway (81). The lipoxygenase pathway is involved in the production of HPETE and HETE. In a number of cases of myeloproliferative disorders, abnormalities of the lipoxygenase pathway have been described (82–84). Deficiencies of enzymes in this pathway could result in increased generation of thromboxane A2 through the cyclooxygenase pathway. As a result, in some instances, such platelets have been demonstrated to show "hyper-responsiveness" to arachidonic acid. It has been postulated that this defect might contribute to the thrombotic tendency that exists in some patients with myeloproliferative disorders.

Function in Primary Hemostasis

Shape Change

The processes involved in activation of platelets in vivo occur in the following sequence: shape change, adhesion to a "foreign surface," release, aggregation and platelet contraction (Figure 6).

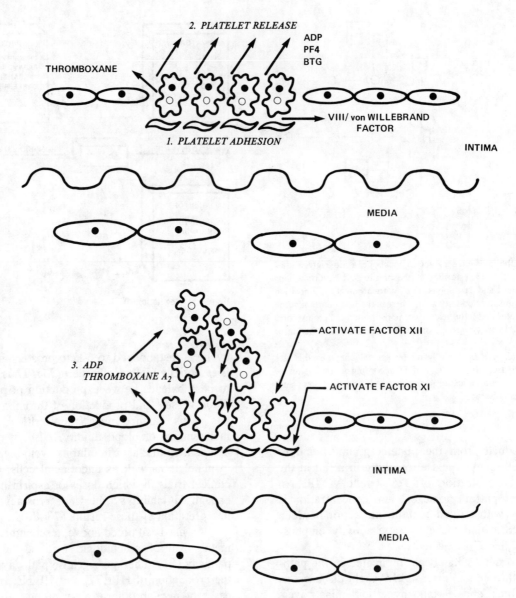

Figure 6. Sequence of platelet response.

The shape changes of platelets which involve the extrusion of pseudopods and transformation from a discoid to a spheroid configuration, seem to be the result of an actin-myosin interaction. In a recently proposed model, actin filaments anchor to the platelet membrane and, during interaction with myosin, exert a tangential force, pulling from the cell surface toward the center of the platelet (85). The increased pressure on the cytoplasm exerts tension in rigid areas of the membrane; nonrigid areas of the membrane become zones of decreased resistance that foster the development of fluid areas of the surface that flow outward to form pseudopods. Calcium ions play a central part in shape changes.

Adhesion

Under normal circumstances, platelets circulate for approximately 10 days as disk-shaped cells that are nonadherent to other elements. After endothelial damage has taken place, components of the vessel wall are exposed, and platelets adhere to various elements of the injured wall, including collagen, basement membrane and microfibrils. Adhesion of platelets to these components is regulated not only by specific properties of their membranes, but also by external variables such as the plasma concentration of von Willebrand factor and the characteristics of blood flow (86). Recently, it has been shown that thrombin stimulates adhesion of plate-

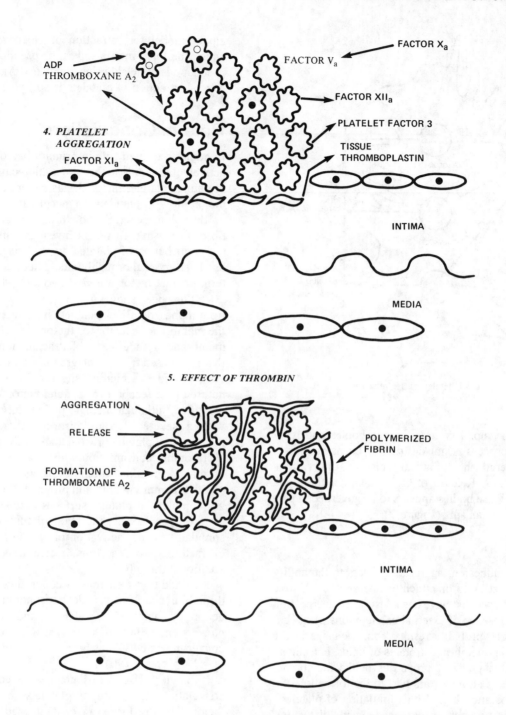

lets to tissue surfaces and increases expression of fibronectin antigen on platelet surfaces (87). Fibronectin is a protein that has been implicated in cellular adhesiveness because it has a strong affinity for collagen (88). The role of prostacyclin in the interaction of platelets with vessel walls is still debated. Of the various plasma proteins that are necessary for platelet adhesion, von Willebrand factor appears to be the most important. Specific binding sites for von Willebrand factor have been identified on platelet membranes. It appears that such binding sites may preferentially bind the higher-

molecular-weight (more active) forms of von Willebrand factor. Certain membrane glycoproteins (glycoprotein I complex) are essential for the binding of von Willebrand factor (39,41). In thrombin stimulated platelets von Willebrand factor will bind to glycoproteins IIb and III_a.

Release Reaction

After shape changes and adhesion have take place, the platelets undergo a secretory reaction, releasing the

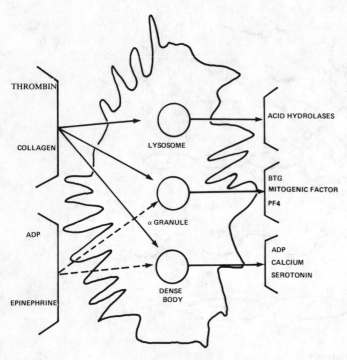

Figure 7. Platelet release reaction.

contents of the alpha granules, dense bodies and lysosomes. This process is not destructive but is similar to that encountered in individual cells of the various endocrine organs. Release of the contents of the alpha granules and dense bodies appears to be governed in part by different mechanisms (Figure 7).

Aggregation

In contrast to adhesion, aggregation refers to the ability of platelets to stick to or attach to one another. Unlike the other processes that have been described, aggregation requires the presence of external calcium ions. Aggregation of platelets, probably results from a change in the external platelet membrane proteins or lipids, causing an alteration in the physical properties of the membrane. Fibrinogen plays an important part in the formation of a primary hemostatic plug. With stimulation of platelets, fibrinogen-binding sites are exposed on platelet membranes. Platelets from patients with Glanzmann's thrombasthenia lack membrane binding sites for fibrinogen and cannot form aggregates in response to ADP, epinephrine, collagen or thrombin (41). Some ultrastructural studies have supported a bridging role for fibrin in platelet-platelet attachment (89).

Clot Retraction

In the presence of polymerizing fibrin in vitro, activation of platelets by thrombin leads to retraction of a clot. This phenomenon is a calcium-sensitive process that necessitates adherence of platelets to one another. Recently, a zipper model for retraction of clots was proposed in which the long, motile spikes, or pseudopods, reach for pseudopods of neighboring platelets (85). At present, the role of retraction of platelets is still poorly understood.

Role in Coagulation

In addition to their role in primary hemostasis, platelets actively participate in the coagulation cascade. In the old literature, platelet factor 3 was generally referred to as the ability of platelets to accelerate consumption of prothrombin, generation of thrombin, and formation of fibrin in plasma. In recent investigations, the nature of the contribution of platelets to the coagulation cascade has been more thoroughly elucidated; consequently, the term platelet factor 3 is best avoided (90,91).

It has been shown that the factor Va that is released from alpha granule of platelets has an important role as the membrane receptor for factor Xa. Thus, the platelet membrane provides a site of attachment for the factor Va that is released from alpha granules and the factor Va, in turn, provides a binding site for factor Xa (92). The nature of the receptor for platelet factor Va has not been identified, although a single patient has been described with a severe bleeding disorder characterized by a deficiency of platelet procoagulant activity and abnormal prothrombin consumption with a normal bleeding time, normal coagulation protein levels and apparently normal platelet membrane lipid and protein (93). The factor Va-Xa complex on platelet surfaces activates prothrombin to thrombin. Local generation of thrombin, of course, stimulates further activation of platelets and conversion of factor V to Va, thus accelerating production of additional thrombin.

In addition to a role in converting prothrombin to thrombin, platelets provide phospholipids in the interaction of factor IXa, calcium, and factor VIIIa for conversion of factor X to Xa. The term "factor X-converting activity" has been introduced to describe this platelet property (90).

Platelets also contribute to the contact phase of coagulation. Exposure of platelets to ADP activates factor XII and forms a "contact product" on platelet surfaces when factor XI is present. "Collagen induced coagulant activity" defines the ability of collagen-stimulated platelets to initiate intrinsic coagulation by an alternative pathway that requires factor XI but not factor XII (94). Thus, it appears that coagulation is a surface-dependent process that takes place on platelet membranes.

Role in Vascular Integrity

In addition to their role in primary hemostasis and coagulation, platelets contribute to the integrity of the vascular tree. Some electron microscope studies have indicated that platelets are taken up by endothelial cells and actually become incorporated into their cytoplasm. The nurturing or supportive role of platelets in maintaining vascular integrity originates principally from observations of patients with thrombocytopenia or platelet abnormalities. Such patients have petechiae, or purpuric hemorrhages.

In addition to the direct physical contributions of platelets to vascular integrity, a role for platelet serotonin has recently been suggested. In laboratory animals with thrombocytopenia, vascular fragility can be made less severe by injection of serotonin. Serotonin may regulate physiologic processes in endothelial cells, preventing loss of erythrocytes from capillary lumina and formation of petechiae.

Endothelial Cells

The other major component of primary hemostasis is the vascular endothelial cell. The capacity of endothelial cells to maintain blood fluidity in the face of numerous factors that predispose to the formation of thrombi has been well appreciated by investigators for many years. However, only during the past decade have major advances been made in understanding the function of endothelial cells. Improved understanding has resulted primarily from the use of techniques that have allowed researchers to culture endothelial cells in vitro (95–98).

Structure and Function

Endothelial cells form a continuous monolayer that lines all blood vessels. However, the structure and function of endothelial cells differ according to their location within the circulatory system. There may be fenestrations between endothelial cells, as is seen in hepatic sinusoids, or there may be a continuous monolayer, as is characteristic of the cerebral circulation.

In large blood vessels, endothelial cells rest on a subendothelium that is composed of elastic tissue, collagen fibers, microfibrils and basement membrane. In general, three functions have been delineated for the vascular endothelium: supplying low-molecular-weight nutrients to subendothelial structures, acting as a barrier to large macromolecular substances and particulate matter and presenting a nonthrombogenic surface for circulating blood (99).

Endothelial cells are oriented with their long axis parallel to the direction of blood flow. Typically, they are 0.5 to 1.2 μm thick and, because of their sheetlike nature, they have an extremely high surface to volume ratio (Figure 8). The luminal surface of the endothelium is covered by a mucopolysaccharide coat that is referred

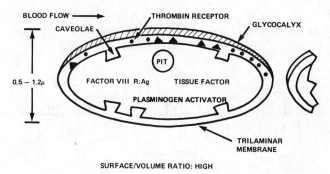

Figure 8. Endothelial cell.

to as the glycocalyx (100). An important constituent of the glycocalyx is heparan sulfate. This sulfated mucopolysaccharide is capable of weakly activating antithrombin III, thus providing one mechanism for the nonthrombogenicity of the endothelium. Beneath the glycocalyx is the plasma membrane, which is a trilaminar structure similar to other cellular membranes. This membrane contains an ADPase that degrades ADP. There are several membrane-lined structures that may be important in cellular transport. Vesicles known as caveolae intracellulares are distributed along the luminal and basal plasma membranes. These vesicles may fuse and, on occasion, form a channel from the luminal aspect of the endothelium to the subendothelium. A second type of vesicle, referred to as a "pit," measures approximately 80 to 120 nm in diameter. Apparently, pits function in the selective uptake of substances, particularly proteins, and include sites of enzymatic activity and lipoprotein receptors.

Another hypothesis has been advanced to explain the nonthrombogenicity of endothelium. Platelets and endothelium have a negative electrical charge and thus would be mutually repulsive. The negative electrical charge on endothelial cells is due primarily to the glycocalyx.

Another means by which endothelium is nonthrombogenic is the production of prostacyclin (75,76). Prostacyclin activates the adenyl cyclase of platelets, thus decreasing the concentration of calcium ions in their cytoplasm, and preventing the platelet response. Production of prostacyclin by endothelial cells is stimulated by thrombin (101).

An interesting new role for endothelium has been suggested by recent work in which thrombin has been found to bind to specific receptors on endothelial membranes (102). This binding may represent a rapid means for removing thrombin from the circulation. Thrombin also binds to a specific cofactor of endothelial membranes (thrombomodulin) (103,104). When bound to thrombomodulin, thrombin can no longer activate fibrinogen or other coagulation proteins; however, it can activate protein C to active protein C. Protein C is an effective anticoagulant that degrades factor Va and

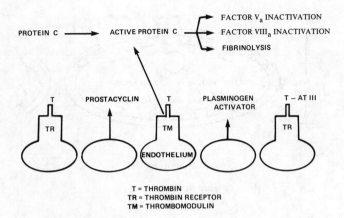

T = THROMBIN
TR = THROMBIN RECEPTOR
TM = THROMBOMODULIN

Figure 9. Endothelial cell function.

VIIIa. In addition, active protein C stimulates fibrinolysis (Figure 9).

Thrombin also stimulates endothelial cells to release plasminogen activator. This tissue plasminogen activator binds to fibrin and accelerates conversion of plasminogen to plasmin. This response could be of particular usefulness in removing hemostatic plugs after they have served their purpose.

Endothelial cells also produce a portion of the factor VIII molecule, factor VIII/R:Ag (105,106). This portion of factor VIII, may be released, allowing platelets to adhere at a site of injury. Also, factor VIII/R:Ag is present in the subendothelium, together with proteoglycans and several classes of collagen that are presumably produced by endothelial cells. The factor VIII/R:Ag (von Willebrand factor) that is found in the subendothelium is of higher molecular weight than that typically found in the plasma.

Endothelial Injury

Endothelial injury results in activation of all the major components of the hemostatic mechanism (107,108). In response to injury, there is initially rapid vasoconstriction. This phenomenon is followed by adherence of platelets to exposed subendothelial elements, with subsequent release and aggregation. Coagulation is activated concurrently by exposure of tissue factor and collagen to coagulation factors in circulating blood. Also, with injury, there is release of tissue plasminogen activator from the endothelium. Fibrinolytic removal of excess thrombus formation is necessary for re-establishing vascular patency.

References

1. Mustard JF, Kimlough-Rathbone RL: Prostaglandins and platelets. *Annu Rev Med* 31:89–96, 1980.

2. Oates JA: The 1982 Nobel prize in physiology or medicine. *Science* 218:765–768, 1982.

3. McGiff JC: Thromboxane and prostacyclin: Implications for function and disease of the vasculature. *Adv Intern Med* 25:199–216, 1980.

4. Moncada S, Vane JR: The role of prostacyclin in vascular tissue. *Fed Proc Fed Amer Soc Exp Biol* 38:66–71, 1979.

5. Ross R, Vogel A: The platelet-derived growth factor. *Cell* 14:203–210, 1978.

6. Witte LD, Kaplan KL, Nossel HL, et al: Studies of the release from human platelets of the growth factor for cultured human arterial smooth muscle cells. *Circ Res* 42:402–409, 1978.

7. Thackrah CT: An inquiry into the nature and properties of the blood as existent in health and disease. *N Engl J Med* 9:186–88, 1820.

8. Donné MA: De l'orgine des globules du sang, de leur mode de formation et de leur fin. *C R Acad Sci* 14:366–368, 1842.

9. Hayem G: Nouvelle contribution a l'étude des concrétions sanguines intra-vasculaires. *C R Acad Sci Ser D* 97:144, 1883.

10. Bizzozero J: Ueber einen neuen Formbestandtheil des Blutes und dessen Rolle bei der Thrombose und der Blutgerinnung. *Virchows Arch A* 90:261–263, 1881.

11. Eberth JD, Schimmelbusch C: Experimentelle Untersuchungen uber Thrombose. *Virchows Arch A* 103:39, 1886.

12. Wright JH: The origin and nature of the blood plates. *Boston Med Surg J* 154:643–645, 1906.

13. Paulus JM: *Platelet Kinetics*. Amsterdam: North Holland, 1971.

14. Triplett DA: The platelet in normal hemostasis and thrombosis. In Bang NU, Glover JL, Holden RW, et al (eds): *Thrombosis and Atherosclerosis*. Chicago: Year Book Medical Publishers, 1982, pp 303–321.

15. Odell TT Jr: Megakaryocytopoiesis and its response to stimulation and suppression. In Baldini MG, Effe S (eds): *Platelets: Production, Function, Transfusion and Storage*. New York: Grune & Stratton, 1974, pp 11–20.

16. Cronkhite EP: Regulation of platelet production in hemostatic mechanisms. *Brookhaven Symp Biol* 10:96, 1958.

17. Harker LA, Finch CA: Thrombokinetics in man. *J Clin Invest* 48:963–974, 1969.

18. Schulman I, Pierce M, Lukens A, et al: Studies on thrombopoiesis: I. A factor in normal human plasma required for platelet production, chronic thrombocytopenia due to its deficiency. *Blood* 16:943–957, 1960.

19. Ebbe S, Stohlman F Jr, Overcash J, et al: Megakaryocyte size in thrombocytopenia in

normal rats. *Blood* 32:383–392, 1968.

20. Shulman NR, Watkins SP Jr, Itscoitz SB, et al: Evidence that the spleen retains the youngest and hemostatically most effective platelets. *Trans Ass Amer Physicians* 81:302–313, 1968.

21. Bithell TC, Athens JW, Cartwright CE, et al: Radioactive diisopropylfluorophosphate as a platelet label: An evaluation of the in vitro and in vivo techniques. *Blood* 29:354–372, 1967.

22. Terebelo HR: III indium-labeled platelets in homocystinuria. *N Engl J Med* 308:284–285, 1983.

23. Ezekowitz MD, Wilson DA, Smith EO, et al: Comparison of indium III platelet scintigraphy and two dimensional echocardiography in the diagnosis of left ventricular thrombi. *N Engl J Med* 306:1509–1513, 1982.

24. Hill-Zobel RL, Pyeritz RE, Scheffel U, et al: Kinetics and distribution of III indium-labeled platelets in patients with homocystinuria. *N Engl J Med* 307:781–786, 1982.

25. Schmidt KG, Rasmussen JW, Lorentzen M: Function and morphology of III In-labeled platelets. *Haemostasis* 11:193–203, 1983.

26. Harker LA: Platelet survival time: Its measurement and use. In *Progress in Hemostasis and Thrombosis*. New York: Grune & Stratton, 1978, vol 4, pp 321–347.

27. Harker LA: Platelet survival and turnover in patients with thrombosis and atherosclerosis. In Bang NU, Glover JL, Holden RW, et al (eds): *Thrombosis and Atherosclerosis*. Chicago: Year Book Medical Publishers, 1982, pp 377–391.

28. Abrahamsen AF: Platelet survival studies in man; with special reference to thrombosis and atherosclerosis. *Scand J Haematol Suppl* 3:7–53, 1968.

29. Aster RH, Jandl JH: Platelet sequestration in man: I. Method. *J Clin Invest* 43:843–855, 1964.

30. White JG, Gerrard JM: The cell biology of platelets. In Weissman G (ed): *The Cell Biology of Inflammation*. Amsterdam and New York: Elsevier/North Holland, 1980, pp 83–143.

31. Triplett DA, Harms CS, Newhouse P, et al: *Platelet Function: Laboratory Evaluation and Clinical Application*. Chicago: American Society for Clinical Pathology, 1978.

32. Colman RW: Platelet function in hyperbetalipoproteinemia. *Thromb Haemostasis* 39:284–293, 1978.

33. Joist JH, Balser K, Schoenfeld G: Increased in vivo platelet function in type II and type IV hyperbetalipoproteinemia. *Thromb Res* 15:95–108, 1979.

34. Shattil SJ, Cooper RA: Role of membrane lipid composition, organization, and fluidity in human platelet function. In Spaet TH (ed): *Progress in Hemostasis and Thrombosis*. New York: Grune & Stratton, 1978, vol 4, pp 59–86.

35. Rittenhouse-Simmons S: Activation and regulation of platelet phospholipase. (Abstract) *Thromb Haemostasis* 42:432, 1979.

36. Morin RJ: The role of phospholipids in platelet function. *Ann Clin Lab Sci* 10:463–473, 1980.

37. Marcus AJ: The role of lipids in platelet function: With particular reference to the arachidonic acid pathway. *J Lipid Res* 19:793–826, 1978.

38. Smith JB, Willis AL: Formation and release of prostaglandins by platelets in response to thrombin. *Brit J Pharmacol* 40:545P–546P, 1970.

39. Nichols WL, Gerrard JM, Didisheim P: Platelet structure, biochemistry, and physiology. In Poller L (ed): *Recent Advances in Blood Coagulation*. New York: Churchill Livingstone, 1981, vol 3, pp 1–39.

40. Jenkins CS, Phillips DR, Clemetson KJ, et al: Platelet membrane glycoproteins implicated in ristocetin induced aggregation. *J Clin Invest* 57:112–124, 1976.

41. Nurden AT, Caen JP: The different glycoprotein abnormalities in thromboasthenic and Bernard Soulier platelets. *Semin Hematol* 16:234–250, 1979.

42. Jamieson GA, Okumura T, Fishback B, et al: Platelet membrane glycoproteins in thromboasthenia, Bernard Soulier and storage pool disease. *J Lab Clin Med* 93:652–660, 1979.

43. Kane WH, Lindhout MJ, Jackson CM, et al: Factor VA-dependent binding of factor XA to human platelets. *J Biol Chem* 255:1170–1174, 1980.

44. Moncada S, Vane JR: Arachidonic acid metabolites and interactions between platelets and blood vessel walls. *N Engl J Med* 300:1142–1147, 1979.

45. Cohen I: Platelet structure and function role of prostaglandins. *Ann Clin Lab Sci* 10:187–194, 1980.

46. Smith MC, Donviriyasup K, Crow JW, et al: Prostacyclin substitution for heparin in long term hemodialysis. *Amer J Med* 73:669–678, 1982.

47. White JG, Gerrard JM: Interaction of microtubules and microfilaments in platelet contractile physiology. In Gabinani G, Jasmin G, Cantini M (eds): *Methods and Achievements in Experimental Pathology*. Basel: Karger, 1979, vol 9, pp 1–39.

48. Ikeda Y, Steiner M: Phosphorylation and protein kinase activity of platelet tubulin. *J Biol Chem* 254:66–74, 1979.

49. Dabrowska R, Hartshorne DJ: A Ca^{2+} and modulator dependent myosin light chain kinase from

non-muscle cells. *Biochem Biophys Res Commun* 85:1352–1359, 1978.

50. Meyers KM, Seachord CL, Holmsen H, et al: Evaluation of the platelet storage pool deficiency in the feline counterpart of the Chediak-Higashi syndrome. *Amer J Hematol* 11:241–253, 1981.

51. Nichols WL, Didisheim P, Gerrard JM: Qualitative platelet disorders. In Poller L (ed): *Recent Advances in Blood Coagulation*. New York: Churchill Livingstone, 1981, vol 3, pp 39–80.

52. Files JC, Malpass TW, Yee EK, et al: Studies of human platelet α-granule release in vivo. *Blood* 58:607–618, 1981.

53. Weksler BB, Nachman RL: Platelets and atherosclerosis. *Amer J Med* 71:331–333, 1981.

54. Nurden AT, Kunicki TJ, Dupuis D, et al: Specific protein and glycoprotein deficiencies in platelets isolated from two patients with the gray platelet syndrome. *Blood* 59:709–718, 1982.

55. Barber AJ, Kaser-Glanzmann R, Jakabova M, et al: Characterization of chondroitin sulfate proteoglycan carrier for heparin neutralizing activity (PF4) released from human blood platelets. *Biochim Biophys Acta* 286:312–329, 1972.

56. Dawes J, Smith RC, Pepper DS: The release, distribution and clearance of human β-thromboglobulin and platelet factor 4. *Thromb Res* 12:851–861, 1978.

57. Lawler JW, Slayter HS, Coligan JE: Isolation and characterization of a high molecular weight protein from human blood platelets. *J Biol Chem* 253:8609–8616, 1978.

58. Davey MG, Luscher EF: Release reactions of human platelets induced by thrombin and other agents. *Biochim Biophys Acta* 165:490–506, 1968.

59. Fritsma G, Engelmann G, Yousuf M: Control mechanisms in platelet activation. *Amer J Med Technol* 47:813–818, 1981.

60. Hirsh PD, Campbell WB, Willerson JT, et al: Prostaglandins and ischemic heart disease. *Amer J Med* 71:1009–1026, 1981.

61. Hamburg M, Samuelsson B: Prostaglandin endoperoxides: Novel transformations of arachidonic acid in human platelets. *Proc Natl Acad Sci USA* 71:3400–3404, 1974.

62. Triplett DA, Schaeffer J: Platelets: Hyperaggregability and hypersensitivity toward secretion inducers. In Akkerman JWN (ed): *The Laboratory Diagnosis of Thrombosis*. Utrecht, The Netherlands: University of Utrecht, 1982, pp 65–93.

63. Chignard M, LeCouedic JP, Tence M, et al: The role of platelet activating factor in platelet aggregation. *Nature (London)* 279:799–800, 1979.

64. Bills TK, Smith JB, Silver MJ: Selective release of arachidonic acid from the phospholipids of human platelets in response to thrombin. *J Clin Invest* 60:1–6, 1977.

65. Vermylen J, Badenhorst PN, Deckmyn H, et al: Normal mechanisms of platelet function. *Clin Haematol* 12:107–151, 1983.

66. Bell RL, Kennerly DA, Stanford N, et al: A pathway for arachidonate release from human platelets. *Proc Natl Acad Sci USA* 76:3238–3241, 1979.

67. Flower RJ, Blackwell GJ: Anti-inflammatory steroids induce biosynthesis of a phosphilipase A_2 inhibitor which prevents prostaglandin generation. *Nature (London)* 278:456–459, 1979.

68. Michelassi F, Landa L, Hill RD, et al: Leukotriene D_4: A potent coronary artery vasoconstrictor associated with impaired ventricular contraction. *Science* 217:841–843, 1982.

69. Colwell JA, Halushka PV, Sarji K, et al: Altered platelet function in diabetes mellitus. *Diabetes* 25 (Suppl 2): 826–831, 1976.

70. Juhan I, Buonocore M, Jouve R, et al: Abnormalities of erythrocyte deformability and platelet aggregation in insulin-dependent diabetes corrected by insulin in vitro and in vivo. *Lancet* 1:535–537, 1982.

71. Masotti G, Galanti G, Poggesi L, et al: Differential inhibition of prostacyclin production and platelet aggregation by aspirin. *Lancet* 2:1213–1217, 1979.

72. Chesebro JH, Clements IP, Fuster V, et al: A platelet inhibitor drug trial in coronary artery bypass operations. *N Engl J Med* 307:73–78, 1982.

73. deGaetano G, Cerletti C, Bertele V: Pharmacology of antiplatelet drugs and clinical trials on thrombosis prevention: A difficult link. *Lancet* 2:974–977, 1982.

74. Steer ML, MacIntyre DE, Levine L, et al: Is prostacyclin a physiologically important circulating antiplatelet agent. *Nature (London)* 283:194–195, 1980.

75. Moncada SR, Gryglewski RJ, Bunting S, et al: An enzyme isolated from arteries transforms prostaglandin endoperoxides to an unstable substance that inhibits platelet aggregation. *Nature (London)* 263:663–665, 1976.

76. Rittler JM, Barrow SE, Blair IA: Release of prostacyclin in vivo and its role in man. *Lancet* 1:317–319, 1983.

77. Greaves M, Preston FE: Plasma 6-keto-prostaglandin in $F_{1\alpha}$: Factor fiction. *Thromb Res* 26:145–157, 1982.

78. Spence DJ: An approach to the use of antiplatelet agents in patients with threatened stroke. *Vas Diag Ther* 3:13–17, 1982.

79. Fox KM, Jonathan A, Selwyn AP: Effects of

platelet inhibition on myocardial ischemia. *Lancet* 2:727–730, 1982.

80. E.P.S.I.M. Research Group: A controlled comparison of aspirin and oral anticoagulants in prevention of death after myocardial infarction. *N Engl J Med* 307:701–708, 1982.

81. Bell RL, Kennerly DA, Stanford N, et al: Diglyceride lipase: A pathway for arachidonate release from human platelets. *Proc Natl Acad Sci USA* 76:3238–3241, 1979.

82. Smith IL, Martin TJ: Platelet thromboxane synthesis and release reactions in myeloproliferative disorders. *Haemostasis* 11:119–127, 1982.

83. Schafer AI: Deficiency of platelet lipoxygenase activity in myeloproliferative disorders. *N Engl J Med* 306:381–386, 1982.

84. Okuma M, Uchino H: Altered arachidonate metabolism by platelets in patients with myeloproliferative disorders. *Blood* 54:1258–1271, 1979.

85. Cohen I, Gerrard JM, Bergman RN, et al: The role of contractile filaments in platelet activation. In Peeters H (ed): *Protides of the Biological Fluids: Colloquium 26.* Oxford: Pergamon Press, 1979, pp 555–556.

86. Baumgartner HR, Tschopp TB, Weiss HJ: Platelet interaction with collagen fibrils in flowing blood: II. Impaired adhesion and aggregation and bleeding disorders. *Thromb Haemostasis* 37:17–28, 1977.

87. Ginsberg MH, Painter RG, Forsyth J, et al: Thrombin increases expression of fibronectin antigen on the platelet surface. *Proc Natl Acad Sci USA* 77:1049–1053, 1980.

88. Zucker MB, Mosesson MW, Broekman MJ, et al: Release of platelet fibronectin from alpha granules induced by thrombin or collagen: Lack of requirements for plasma fibronectin in ADP-induced platelet aggregation. *Blood* 54:8–12, 1979.

89. Shirasawa K, Barton BP, Chandler AB: Localization of ferritin-conjugated anti-fibrin/fibrinogen in platelet aggregates produced in vitro. *Amer J Pathol* 66:379–405, 1972.

90. Walsh PN: Platelet coagulant activity: Evidence for multiple different functions of platelets in intrinsic coagulation. *Ser Haematol* 6:579–592, 1973.

91. Hardisty RM, Hutton RA: Platelet aggregation and the availability of platelet factor 3. *Brit J Haematol* 12:764–776, 1966.

92. Miletich JP, Majerus DW, Majerus PW: Patients with congenital factor V deficiency have decreased factor Xa binding sites on their platelets. *J Clin Invest* 62:824–831, 1978.

93. Weiss HJ, Vicic WJ, Lages BA, et al: Isolated deficiency of platelet procoagulant activity. *Amer J Med* 67:206–213, 1979.

94. Lipscomb MS, Walsh PM: Human platelets and factor XI. *J Clin Invest* 63:1006–1014, 1979.

95. Mason RG, Sharp D, Chuang NYK, et al: The endothelium: Roles in thrombosis and haemostasis. *Arch Pathol Lab Med* 101:61–64, 1977.

96. Thorgeirsson G, Robertson AL: The vascular endothelium—Pathobiologic significance. A review. *Amer J Pathol* 93:803–847, 1978.

97. Busch C, Camcilla PA, DeBault LE: Use of endothelium cultured on microcarriers as a model for microcirculation. *Lab Invest* 47:498–504, 1982.

98. Huttner I, Gabiani G: Vascular endothelium: Recent advances and unanswered questions. *Lab Invest* 47:409–411, 1982.

99. Barnhart MI, Baechler CHA: Endothelial cell physiology: Perturbations and responses. *Semin Thromb Hemostasis* 5:50–86, 1978.

100. Wight TN: Vessel proteoglycans and thrombogenesis. *Prog Hemostasis Thromb* 5:1–39, 1980.

101. Thomas DP, Merton RE, Hiller KF, et al: Resistance of normal endothelium to damage by thrombin. *Brit J Haematol* 51:25–35, 1982.

102. Bauer PI, Machovich R, Aranyi P, et al: Mechanism of thrombin binding to endothelial cells. *Blood* 61:368–372, 1983.

103. Owen WG, Esmon CT: Functional properties of an endothelial cell cofactor for thrombin catalyzed activation of protein C. *J Biol Chem* 256:5532–5535, 1981.

104. Esmon CT, Owen WG: Identification of an endothelial cell cofactor for thrombin-catalyzed activation of protein C. *Proc Natl Acad Sci USA* 78:2249–2252, 1981.

105. Chan V, Chan TK: Characterization of factor VIII related protein synthesized by human endothelial cell: A study of structure and function. *Thromb Haemostasis* 48:177–181, 1982.

106. Rand JH, Gordon RE, Sussman IJ, et al: Electron microscopic localization of factor VIII related antigen in adult human blood vessels. *Blood* 60:627–634, 1982.

107. Reidy MA, Schwartz SM: Endothelial injury and regeneration. IV. Endotoxin: A nondenuding injury to aortic endothelium. *Lab Invest* 48:25–32, 1983.

108. Reidy MA, Schwartz SM: Endothelial regeneration. III. Time course of intimal changes after small defined injury of rat aortic endothelium. *Lab Invest* 44:301–308, 1981.

Review Articles

Harker LA, Zimmerman TS: Platelet disorders. *Clin Haematol* 12:1–355, 1983.

Marcus AJ: The role of prostaglandins in platelet function. *Prog Hematol* 11:147–171, 1979.

Nichols WL, Gerrard JM, Didisheim P: Platelet structure, biochemistry and physiology. In Poller L (ed): *Recent Advances in Blood Coagulation.* Edinburgh: Churchill Livingstone, 1981, vol 3, pp 1–39.

Vermylen J, Badenhorst PN, Deckmyn H, et al: Normal mechanisms of platelet function. *Clin Haematol* 12:107–151, 1983.

White JW: Current concepts in platelet structure. *Amer J Clin Pathol* 71:363–378, 1979.

Reference Books

Caen JP, Cronberg S, Kubisz P: *Platelets: Physiology and Pathology.* New York: Stratton Intercontinental Medical Book Corp, 1977.

Lusher JM, Barnhardt MI (eds): *Acquired Bleeding Disorders in Children. Platelet Abnormalities and Laboratory Methods.* New York: Masson Publishing, 1981.

Triplett DA, Harms CS, Newhouse P, et al: *Platelet Function: Laboratory Evaluation and Clinical Application.* Chicago: American Society for Clinical Pathology, 1978.

Chapter
FOUR

Clinical and Laboratory Approaches to Bleeding Disorders

This chapter will focus on the clinical and laboratory approaches to the diagnosis of bleeding disorders. In addition, appropriate comments will be made regarding the evaluation of patients with recurrent thromboembolic disease.

Clinical Approach

Medical History

Abnormalities of primary and secondary hemostasis typically present different patterns of bleeding (1–3). Abnormalities of primary hemostasis are characterized by bleeding of mucous membranes and many small, superficial ecchymoses. In addition, patients with deficiencies of primary hemostasis typically have abnormal intraoperative bleeding and oozing from small cuts or wounds. Thus, it appears that platelets have a primary role in capillary hemostasis. Clinical disorders associated with abnormalities of primary hemostasis include quantitative as well as qualitative abnormalities of platelets, vascular abnormalities and von Willebrand's disease (Table 1).

Patients with coagulation factor deficiencies typically have abnormal bleeding that involves large blood vessels, causing lumpy subcutaneous ecchymoses together with intramuscular hematomata and hemarthrosis. Patients with severe hemophilia A and B often have spontaneous hemorrhage into major muscle masses of the body or into articular spaces. Bleeding from superficial wounds may be delayed but difficult to control once it begins.

In obtaining a history of bleeding, it is important to question a patient carefully regarding the frequency of bleeding and to ascertain whether episodes of bleeding are associated with trauma (Table 2). Many patients attribute episodes of bleeding to other illnesses. For instance, patients with hemophilia may attribute attacks of hemarthrosis to rheumatic fever or "arthritis." Often, petechiae are described as a "rash" by unknowledgeable patients.

It is also important to attempt to quantitate the blood loss in each episode that a patient describes. Both the duration and the volume of blood loss are important in assessing the severity of a bleeding problem. A history of transfusion is particularly useful in quantitating blood loss.

When questioning a patient about previous operations, it is important to ask specifically about dental

Table 1

Clinical Manifestations in Patients with Abnormalities of Primary or Secondary Hemostasis*

Findings	Disorders of Coagulation	Disorders of Platelets or Vessels ("purpuric" disorders)
Petechiae	Rare	Characteristic
Deep dissecting hematoma	Characteristic	Rare
Superficial ecchymosis	Common; usually large, solitary and deep	Characteristic; usually small, multiple and superficial
Hemarthrosis	Characteristic	Rare
Delayed bleeding	Common (e.g., after tooth extraction, often 1–4 hours later)	Rare; usually starts immediately, responds to pressure
Bleeding from superficial cuts and scratches	Minimal, stops normally	Persistent, can be profuse
Sex of patient	Most (80% to 90%) hereditary forms occur only in males	More common in females
Mucosal bleeding	Minimal	Typical clinical picture (epistaxis, gingival bleeding, menorrhagia, etc.)
Bleeding increased by aspirin and other anti-inflammatory drugs	Yes	Yes
Positive family history	Common	Unusual
Healing of cuts	Delayed by repeated bleeding	Usually heals normally

*Modified from Bachmann F: Recognition of congenital bleeding disorders. In Green D (ed): Hemophilia. Springfield, Ill: Charles C. Thomas, 1973, pp 5–17.

Table 2

Obtaining a History

Medical History
- Spontaneous bleeding (age at onset)
  - Bruising
  - Hematoma formation (major muscles)
  - Joint bleeding
  - Mucous membrane bleeding
- Induced bleeding
  - Previous injuries
    - Duration of bleeding
    - Transfusions
    - Healing of wound (scar formation?)
  - Surgical procedures
    - Dental work
    - Circumcision
    - Tonsillectomy and adenoidectomy
    - Other surgical procedures
    - Obtain history of duration of bleeding, necessity of transfusions and wound healing
  - Menstrual history (amount and duration)
  - Medications
  - Aspirin or aspirin-containing compounds
  - Other drugs (prescribed by physician and over-the-counter)

Family History
- Prepare family tree

extractions (4). In addition, it is essential not to overlook questions regarding tonsillectomy, appendectomy, circumcision and other surgical procedures. A history of prolonged postoperative bleeding or associated transfusions with any of these procedures is suggestive of a bleeding problem.

It is also critical to document the *first* episode of abnormal bleeding. This history may be particularly helpful in differentiating a hereditary bleeding problem from an acquired abnormality.

Family History

A family history of bleeding problems is helpful in establishing a diagnosis of a hereditary abnormality of hemostasis. The pattern of inheritance may have great diagnostic relevance (Table 3). A family tree should be drawn and should include the name, age and sex of each member. Affected members should be designated by

Table 3

Clinical Diagnosis	Severity	Genetic Transmission	Frequency Per 10^6
Classical hemophilia (deficiency of antihemophilic globulin, factor VIII)	Very severe to mild	Sex-linked recessive	60–100
von Willebrand's disease	Mild to moderate, rarely severe	Autosomal dominant	Very frequent
Christmas disease (deficiency of Plasma thromboplastin component, factor IX)	Very severe to mild	Sex-linked recessive	10–20
Afibrinogenemia	Moderate	Autosomal recessive	<0.5
Dysfibrinogenemia (abnormal fibrinogen molecule)	Moderate or no disease	Autosomal dominant	1
Deficiency of prothrombin (factor II)	Mild to severe	Autosomal recessive	<0.5
Deficiency of factor V	Mild to severe	Autosomal recessive	<0.5
Deficiency of factor VII	Mild to moderate	Autosomal recessive	<0.5
Deficiency of factor X	Mild to severe	Autosomal recessive	<0.5
Plasma thromboplastin antecedent (deficiency of factor XI)	Mild to moderately severe	Autosomal recessive	1
Deficiency of fibrin-stabilizing factor (factor XIII)	Mild to moderately severe	Autosomal recessive	<0.5

Congenital Bleeding Disorders: Frequency, Mode of Inheritance and Severity*

Modified from Bachmann F: Recognition of congenital bleeding disorders. In Green D (ed): Hemophilia. Springfield, Ill: Charles C. Thomas, 1973, pp 5–17.

shading or other appropriate markers. A family tree is extremely useful in identifying the mode of inheritance (i.e., sex linked, as in hemophilia A and B, autosomal recessive, as in factor V deficiency, or autosomal dominant, as in von Willebrand's disease) (Figure 1).

Drug History

Because of the ready availability of numerous over-the-counter medications, the number of potential drug-induced bleeding disorders has been increasing. Perhaps the most common culprit is aspirin. Aspirin affects platelet function and thus may produce a clinical picture of an abnormality of primary hemostasis. It is not sufficient to ask a patient whether he or she is taking aspirin. There are approximately 600 preparations that contain aspirin; therefore, it is advisable to inquire about medications being taken for sinus trouble, headache, muscle aches, and other common problems (5,6).

Another drug that is often associated with an abnormal laboratory result is chlorpromazine hydrochloride. Patients who have taken chlorpromazine for long periods may have a prolonged activated partial thromboplastin time. This finding is due to a drug-induced "lupus anticoagulant" (7–9).

Still other drugs may affect platelet function or may be associated with specific factor inhibitors. Penicillin is an example of a drug that can have both actions (10,11). Procainamide has also been associated with an acquired lupus anticoagulant (12–14).

Physical Examination

The distribution and extent of bleeding manifestations, including bruises or purpura, should be recorded. It is important for the examiner to appreciate that many conditions can mimic petechiae (15). Venous telangiectasias are particularly important, not only because of

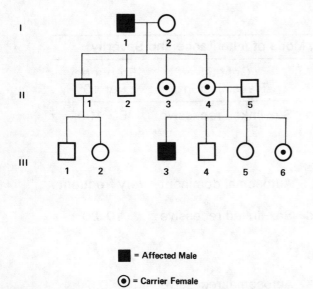

= Affected Male

= Carrier Female

Figure 1. The above pedigree is for a family with classical hemophilia A. The pattern is that of a X-linked recessive inheritance. The affected grandfather, I-1, transmits the gene to each of his daughters. The daughters are therefore carriers to hemophilia A. They, in turn, can transmit the gene to half of their sons, who will manifest the clinical picture of hemophilia A. Half of their daughters will be carriers. Male to male transmission does not occur.

their ability to simulate petechiae but also because of their association with von Willebrand's disease. Telangiectasias typically are small, flat, purple or reddish purple spots (16). They are composed of circuitous, anastomosing, thin-walled, dilated capillaries and ven-

ules. When a glass slide is pressed against a telangiectasia, the color fades markedly. Telangiectasias are found most commonly on the face, lips and inside of the mouth and nose as well as on the fingertips and toes (Table 4).

Arterial spiders may be seen in many disorders, including liver disease, and during pregnancy. Spiders typically are found over the distribution of the superior vena cava and are bright red. A spider has a central arteriole surrounded by radiating, dilated capillaries that extend outward 5 to 10 mm. Application of pressure to the central arteriole causes the redness of the entire lesion to fade.

Petechiae are associated with abnormalities of either the vascular or platelet contribution to primary hemostasis. Ecchymoses often are associated with petechiae. The finding of perifollicular petechiae in a patient with scurvy is particularly helpful in establishing this diagnosis (17). Often, the associated hair grows spirally, producing a corkscrew pattern. At an early stage, perifollicular petechiae may be bright red, but later they persist as brown spots of hemosiderin.

Laboratory Approach

As has been discussed above, the best screening tests for identifying potential hemostatic problems are thorough personal and family histories. Properly obtained histories eliminate the need for indiscriminate screening procedures and their associated costs. Unfortunately, in many

Table 4

Vascular Lesions That Mimic Petechiae*			
Lesion	Appearance	Distribution	Effect of Pressure
Osler-Weber-Rendu (telangiectasia)	Flat, round, pinpoint to 3 mm in diameter	Face, mucous membranes, palms and feet	Blanches
Cherry hemangioma (Campbell-deMorgan spot)	Flat, slightly raised, bright red, 1-3 mm in diameter	Trunk of elderly persons	Does not blanch
Spider telangiectasis	Flat or slightly raised, spider legs, bright red, 2-5 mm in diameter	Distribution of superior vena cava	Blanches, legs fill from center
Angiokeratoma (Fabry's disease)	Flat or slightly raised, dark red to blue-black, variable size	Umbilicus and buttocks	Blanches on occasion

*Modified from Wintrobe MM et al: Clinical Hematology (8th edition). Philadelphia: Lea & Febiger, 1981, p 1075.

instances, patients are screened by a "shotgun" approach to laboratory testing, and proper histories are not obtained until either a laboratory abnormality is identified or a patient has a surgical complication as the result of abnormal hemostasis.

Although patients with abnormalities of primary or secondary hemostasis often present with different clinical pictures, clinical discrimination between the two may not be precise. An excellent example of this lack of discrimination is von Willebrand's disease. In this disorder, patients may present with easy bruising and bleeding of mucous membranes, which are characteristic signs of abnormalities of primary hemostasis; if the underlying disorder is severe enough, they may present with hemarthrosis, which is a typical manifestation of abnormalities of secondary hemostasis (18). Consequently, laboratory evaluation of a potential bleeding problem is imperative once a positive clinical history has been obtained. Unfortunately, physicians are often confused by the "menu" of tests offered by the coagulation laboratory. Therefore, the initial use of a few, relatively simple screening procedures is preferred (19,20).

Screening Procedures

If six relatively simple procedures are used, the vast majority of hemorrhagic problems can be identified and an appropriate differential diagnosis established. These six procedures are examination of a peripheral smear, a platelet count and determinations of bleeding time, prothrombin time, activated partial thromboplastin time and thrombin time. These six tests should be readily available in any hospital or clinic setting. These tests and a few selected confirmatory tests are summarized in Table 5.

Examination of a Peripheral Blood Smear and Platelet Count

Examination of a peripheral blood smear may yield much information about a patient. The number of platelets should be estimated, and the estimate should be correlated with the platelet count determined by means of phase contrast microscopy or an automated instrumentation technique (21–24). The platelet estimate and the platelet count should agree. If there is disagreement, further investigation is necessary to resolve this issue. Common causes of spurious thrombocytopenia (i.e., platelet estimate normal but platelet count decreased) include the presence of giant platelets or cold agglutinins and platelet satellitosis (25). In addition to the platelet estimate, morphologic studies of red cells may be helpful in solving a clinical problem. The presence of schistocytes suggests a microangiopathic hemolytic anemia, as is seen in patients with acute disseminated intravascular coagulation (26). The presence of target cells suggests splenic hypofunction with or without concomitant liver disease.

The size and morphologic appearance of platelets may also be evaluated. Large platelets have been identified as being younger and more active metabolically as well as physiologically. A relative increase in the number of large platelets may be seen in patients with autoimmune thrombocytopenia or in situations in which there is accelerated peripheral destruction of platelets, as occurs in patients with artificial valves (27). Small platelets may be associated with iron deficiency anemia, Wiskott-Aldrich syndrome and certain forms of storage pool disease (28).

A lack of granularity of platelets is associated most often with production of dysplastic platelets in patients with underlying myeloproliferative disorders (29). Patients with myeloproliferative disorders may present with a normal, decreased or increased platelet count; consequently, the presence of atypical platelets on a peripheral smear may be an early clue to a diagnosis of an underlying myeloproliferative disorder. Interestingly, patients with myeloproliferative disorders may present with thrombosis or bleeding; rarely both problems are manifest at the time of clinical presentation.

Bleeding Time

The bleeding time is the single best procedure for evaluating primary hemostasis (30–32). In conjunction with the platelet count, determination of the bleeding time allows the examiner to make certain fundamental decisions regarding the laboratory evaluation of abnormalities of primary hemostasis. Patients with an abnormal bleeding time but a normal platelet count are arbitrarily designated as having qualitative abnormalities of platelet function. Such patients include those with von Willebrand's disease, those who have recently ingested various antiplatelet drugs (e.g., aspirin) and those with uremia (33). To further evaluate such patients, additional platelet function studies are indicated; they include platelet aggregation tests, quantification of the various components of the factor VIII complex (factor VIII R:Ag, factor VIII:C and factor VIII R:RCo), platelet retention procedures and, in a few cases, quantitation of the platelet content of ADP/ATP or electron microscopy. Qualitative abnormalities of platelets may be hereditary or acquired. Acquired abnormalities far outnumber hereditary abnormalities.

Patients with quantitative abnormalities of platelets (i.e., decreased or increased platelet count) are evaluated in a much different manner. A platelet count should be obtained before the bleeding time is determined. In many laboratories, if a platelet count is less than 50,000 cells per microliter, bleeding time is not determined (of course, depending on the clinical situation). Typically, the next procedure in such patients would be a bone marrow examination. Patients with thrombocytopenia

Table 5

	Laboratory Procedures for Diagnosing Coagulopathies*			
Procedure	Reagent Contains	Normal Range	System(s) Tested	Diseases Detected
Platelet count	None	200,000–450,000 /mm^3	Platelets	Thrombocytopenia and thrombocytosis
Template bleeding time	None	1–8 minutes	Platelets and capillaries	Thrombocytopathy, von Willebrand's disease
Activated partial thromboplastin time (APTT)	Phospholipid contact activator	<42 seconds	Intrinsic	Mild (40% to 50%) deficiencies of factors VIII, IX and XI (hemophilias), deficiency of factor XII, von Willebrand's disease, disseminated intravascular coagulation, heparin therapy
Prothrombin time (PT)	Tissue thromboplastin	10–12 seconds	Extrinsic	Factor VII deficiency (acquired or hereditary) Vitamin K deficiency
Thrombin time	Thrombin	20–24 seconds	Conversion of fibrinogen to fibrin	Hypo fibrinogenemia and dysfibrinogenemia, fibrin split products and presence of heparin
Factor assays	Specific factor-deficient substrate	50% to 150% activity (except factor XII)	Intrinsic or extrinsic	Identification and degree of specific factor deficiencies
Stypven time	Russell's viper venom	18–22 seconds	Extrinsic system (except factor VII)	Differential diagnosis of abnormalities of extrinsic system
Reptilase time	Venom of *Bothrops atrox*	18–20 seconds	Fibrinogen, fibrin	Can be used in place of thrombin time when patient is taking heparin

*From Triplett DA, Smith C: Routine testing in the coagulation laboratory in Triplett DA (ed): Laboratory Evaluation of Coagulation. Chicago: ASCP Press, 1982 pp 28–50.

may be divided into those in whom bone marrow production of platelets is decreased, those in whom peripheral sequestration of platelets is increased and those in whom peripheral destruction of platelets is increased (Table 6).

Prothrombin Time (PT)
Measurement of the prothrombin time evaluates the extrinsic system (Figure 2). This test makes use of a thromboplastin (lipoprotein) that reacts rapidly with factor VII before the final common pathway is entered. It

Table 6

Classification of Thrombocytopenia*

Decreased Production of Platelets

  Amegakaryocytic thrombocytopenia

    Aplastic anemia

    Leukemia

    Drug induced

  Megakaryocytic thrombocytopenia

    Ineffective thrombopoiesis (e.g., deficiency of vitamin B_{12} or folate)

    Preleukemia

Increased Peripheral Destruction of Platelets

  Immune system mediated

    Autoimmune

    Drug-induced antibodies

  Consumption

    Disseminated intravascular coagulation

    Thrombotic thrombocytopenic purpura

Sequestrative Thrombocytopenia

  Splenomegaly

Loss of Platelets from Body

  Extracorporeal circulation

This table is by no means inclusive. It is meant to provide guidelines concerning the primary pathophysiologic mechanisms that lead to thrombocytopenia. In evaluating thrombocytopenia, bone marrow biopsy is usually indicated. The recent introduction of mean platelet volume (MPV) on automated counters may also prove helpful in evaluating thrombocytopenia.

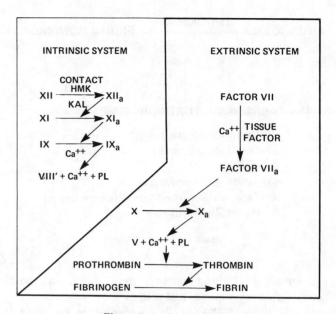

Figure 2. Prothrombin time.

deficiencies of factors VII, X, V and II and fibrinogen. The presence of a circulating anticoagulant may also prolong the prothrombin time. Spurious short results may result from cold activation of factor VII (34,40).

Activated Partial Thromboplastin Time (APTT)

The activated partial thromboplastin time is determined in two phases. The relatively slow reactions of the contact system are first initiated by incubating plasma with a particulate activator, such as kaolin, celite or micronized silica or with a "liquid" activator, such as ellagic acid. In the second phase, the remaining steps in the intrinsic system take place in the presence of a partial thromboplastin (phospholipid) (Figure 3). Ideally, the

should be emphasized that the choice of thromboplastin has some influence on the sensitivity of this test with respect to the diagnosis of various congenital coagulation abnormalities as well as acquired abnormalities secondary to either oral anticoagulant therapy or liver disease (34,35). In Europe, human brain often is used as a source of thromboplastin, whereas in the United States, rabbit brain or rabbit brain-lung combinations are commonly used (36). The choice of thromboplastin is particularly relevant in monitoring patients who are receiving long-term oral anticoagulant therapy (37,38).

The one-stage prothrombin time is probably the most common coagulation procedure currently performed. Factor VII is unique to the extrinsic system; consequently, the prothrombin time is an excellent test for monitoring oral anticoagulant therapy because factor VII is the first coagulation factor to be appreciably affected by oral anticoagulants. The prothrombin time may also be prolonged by congenital and acquired

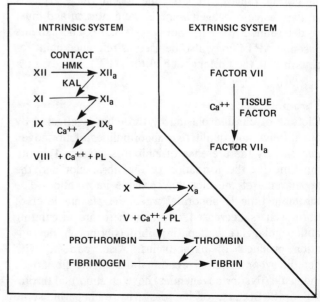

Figure 3. Activated partial thromboplastin time.

FIBRINOGEN $\xrightarrow{\text{THROMBIN}}$ FIBRIN MONOMER

ABNORMAL THROMBIN TIME

1) Hypofibrinogenemia
2) Dysfibrinogenemia
3) Heparin
4) Fibrin split products
5) Paraproteins (myeloma, Waldenströms)
6) Hyperfibrinogenemia

Figure 4. Thrombin time.

---

activated partial thromboplastin time is sensitive to factor deficiency states of less than 30% activity (normal range, 50% to 150%) (41–44). However, as has been demonstrated repeatedly, the choice of activator and the origin of the phospholipid have major influences on the sensitivity of the activated partial thromboplastin time systems (45–53). Patients with a normal prothrombin time but an abnormal activated partial thromboplastin time typically have deficiencies of factors that are unique to the intrinsic system (i.e., factors XII, XI, VIII and IX, Fletcher factor and Fitzgerald factor). In addition, it should be emphasized that patients with the lupus type of anticoagulant often present with a normal prothombin time but a prolonged activated partial thromboplastin time (54–56).

The activated partial thromboplastin time is also widely used for monitoring heparin therapy (57). Patients who are receiving full-dose heparin therapy ideally have an activated partial thromboplastin time that is two to two and one-half times longer than the upper limit of the normal range. Of course, the normal range depends on the choice of reagents and instrumentation and must be determined in each laboratory (58,59). The patients baseline APTT may also be used as reference point for determining the prolongation of the APTT.

Thrombin Time
Clotting of citrated plasma by thrombin is affected by quantitative and qualitative abnormalities of fibrinogen and also by the presence of inhibitors (Figure 4). Both the time for the formation of the fibrin clot and the appearance of the clot may provide information. The thrombin time is abnormal when the plasma level of fibrinogen is decreased or when there are circulating anticoagulants (e.g., heparin), fibrin (fibrinogen) degradation products or paraproteins. Also, patients with hereditary or acquired abnormalities of the fibrinogen molecule (dysfibrinogenemias) have an abnormal thrombin time. Because of its sensitivity to heparin, some

laboratories use a modified thrombin time for monitoring heparin therapy.

Confirmatory Tests

Fibrin (fibrinogen) Split Products
In addition to the tests that have been described, every laboratory should have available simple screening procedures for identifying fibrin split products. The most popular screening procedures make use of latex particles coated with antibodies to fibrinogen or to fibrin or fibrinogen degradation products (X, Y, D or E). These procedures are easily and rapidly performed and are relatively sensitive.

Inhibitors
In the approach to the evaluation of a patient with a prolonged activated partial thromboplastin time, it is imperative that a circulating anticoagulant be considered and appropriately ruled out. To evaluate the possibility of an inhibitor, a 1:1 mixture of normal pooled plasma and the patient's plasma is prepared, and the test is repeated on the mixture. If there is no correction after the addition of an equal aliquot of normal pooled plasma, it is appropriate to assume that an inhibitor is present. However, it should be emphasized that even in patients in whom a correction is initially demonstrated, there still may be an inhibitor that is "time dependent." Therefore, it is important that there be an incubation period with a suitable set of controls to rule out a time-dependent inhibitor in the patient's plasma (factor VIII inhibitors are typically time dependent).

Perhaps the most common inhibitor encountered in the laboratory setting is heparin. Often, this is secondary to obtaining a blood sample through an indwelling venous access line; in some instances, patients have received a bolus of heparin to maintain the patency of the venous access line. The second most frequent inhibitor encountered is the lupus anticoagulant (60). This inhibitor is seen in approximately 10% of patients with systemic lupus erythematosus; however, this nonspecific anticoagulant is often found in patients with no evidence of underlying collagen vascular disease. It is extremely important to differentiate the lupus anticoagulant from other types of inhibitors because this anticoagulant usually is not associated with clinical hemorrhage (61–63). Paradoxically, as many as 30% of patients with the lupus anticoagulant present with clinical thrombosis (64–67). The tissue thromboplastin inhibition (TTI) procedure has been suggested as a specific test for the lupus anticoagulant (60). This procedure is simply measurement of the prothrombin time performed with dilute thromboplastin. However, recent work has indicated that the tissue thromboplastin inhibition procedure is relatively insensitive (in many instances, it misses patients with the lupus anticoagulant of the IgM type) as well as nonspecific (i.e., the TTI is prolonged by inhibitors to factor VIII or V or heparin). Therefore, it is recommended that a more specific and sensitive procedure be performed. Such a procedure is the platelet neutralization procedure, which makes use of disrupted platelets prepared from platelet concentrates (68). This procedure is simple and readily differentiates the lupus anticoagulant from other causes of a prolonged activated partial thromboplastin time.

Other Procedures

Other tests that may be available in a hospital laboratory include the protamine sulfate and ethanol gel tests. These tests demonstrate fibrin monomer-fibrinogen complexes in plasma. Thus, ideally, a positive test result would provide evidence that thrombin has acted on fibrinogen. However, there are many disorders that lead to false-positive or false–negative results on these tests. The ethanol gel test is frequently negative in patients with disseminated intravascular coagulation, whereas the protamine sulfate test has a very high sensitivity but suffers from a low specificity (69). Other more recent and experimental methods (i.e., chromatographic separation) are probably too sensitive or clinically impractical.

For a discussion on other procedures, such as platelet aggregation studies and evaluation of ristocetin cofactor activity, the reader is referred to more specialized textbooks and procedural manuals (70–72).

Evaluation of Patients with Thrombotic Disease

Thrombotic disease and its complications are the most common cause of death in the Western world. Nevertheless, our understanding of the thrombotic process is still in its infancy. For the past 50 years, investigations have focused on abnormalities of hemostasis characterized by hemorrhage. Laboratory evaluation and identification of patients who are predisposed to thrombotic disease are still limited.

In the past five years, several laboratory tests have been developed to permit identification of patients who have an increased tendency to thrombosis. Such tests include antithrombin III and protein C quantitation*. Both of these proteins are physiologic inhibitors; therefore, a deficiency of either one results in an increased tendency to the development of thrombosis. Also, abnormalities of plasminogen and fibrinogen have been correlated with a thrombotic picture (i.e., dysfibrinogenimia or dysplasminogenemia).

*Recently Protein S deficiency has been found to be associated with a thrombotic predisposition.

References

1. Bachmann F: Diagnostic approach to mild bleeding disorders. *Semin Hematol* 17:292–305, 1980.
2. Ingram GIC: Investigation of a long standing bleeding tendency. *Brit Med Bull* 33:261–264, 1977.
3. Kitchens CS: The anatomic basis of purpura. *Prog Hemostasis Thromb* 5:211–244, 1980.
4. Thompson AR: Bleeding disorders. In Eisenberg MS, Copass MK (eds): *Manual of Emergency Medical Therapeutics* (2nd edition). Philadelphia: WB Saunders, 1982, p 77.
5. Leist ER, Banwell JG: Products containing aspirin. *N Engl J Med* 291:710–712, 1974.
6. Selner J: More aspirin containing medicines. *N Engl J Med* 292:372, 1975.
7. Zucker S, Zarrabi MH, Ramano GS, et al: IgM inhibitors of the contact activation phase of coagulation in chlorpromazine treated patients. *Brit J Haematol* 40:447–457, 1978.
8. Zarrabi MH, Zucker S, Miller F, et al: Immunologic and coagulation disorders in chlorpromazine-treated patients. *Ann Intern Med* 91:194–199, 1979.
9. Canoso RT, Sise HS: Chlorpromazine induced lupus anticoagulant and associated immunologic abnormalities. *Amer J Hematol* 13:121–129, 1982.
10. Andersen BR, Troup SB: Y G-antibody to human antibody to human antihemophilic globulin (factor VIII). *J Immunol* 100:175–186, 1968.
11. Green D: Spontaneous inhibitors of factor VIII. *Brit J Haematol* 15:57–75, 1968.
12. Bell WR, Boss GR, Wolfson JS: Circulating anticoagulant in procainamide-induced lupus syndrome. *Arch Intern Med* 137:1471–1473, 1977.
13. Edwards RL, Rick ME, Wakem CJ: Studies on a circulating anticoagulant in procainamide induced lupus erythematosus. *Arch Intern Med* 141:1688–1690, 1981.
14. Davis S, Furie BC, Griffin JH, et al: Circulating inhibitors of blood coagulation associated with procainamide-induced lupus erythematosus. *Amer J Hematol* 4:401–407, 1978.
15. Nydeggar UE, Miescher PA: Bleeding due to vascular disorders. *Semin Hematol* 17:178–191, 1980.
16. Osler W: On multiple hereditary telangiectases with recurring haemorrhages. *Q J Med* 1:53–58, 1907.
17. Bevelaqua A, Hasselbacher P, Schumacher HR: Scurvy and hemarthrosis. *J Amer Med Ass* 235:1874–1876, 1976.
18. Zimmerman TS, Ruggeri ZM: von Willebrand's disease. *Clin Haematol* 12:175–200, 1983.

19. Karpatkin M: Screening tests in hemostasis. *Ped Clin North Amer* 27:831–841, 1980.
20. Bowie EJW, Owen CA: The significance of abnormal preoperative hemostatic tests. *Prog Hemostasis Thromb* 5:179–209, 1980.
21. Mielke CH, Pritchard JA, Borgman B, et al: Comparative evaluation of phase, impedance and laser platelet counting. *Lab Med* 13:363–367, 1982.
22. Wertz RK, Triplett DA: A review of platelet counting performance in the United States. *Amer J Clin Pathol* 74:575–580, 1980.
23. Bessman JD: Evaluation of automated whole blood platelet counts and particle sizing. *Amer J Clin Pathol* 74:157–160, 1980.
24. Lewis SM, Skelly JV, Cousins S: Automated platelet counting—A reevaluation of the sedimentation method. *Clin Lab Haematol* 3:215–222, 1981.
25. Dale NL, Schumacher HR: Platelet satellitism—New spurious results with automated instruments. *Lab Med* 13:300–304, 1982.
26. Heene DL: Disseminated intravascular coagulation: Evaluation of therapeutic approaches. *Semin Thromb Hemostasis* 3:209–246, 1977.
27. Bessman JD, Williams LJ, Gilmer PR: Mean platelet volume: The inverse relation of platelet size and count in normal subjects and an artifact of other particles. *Amer J Clin Pathol* 76:288–293, 1981.
28. Gardner FH, Bessman JD: Thrombocytopenia due to defective platelet production. *Clin Haematol* 12:23–38, 1983.
29. Weinfield A, Branehfog I, Kubbi J: Platelets in the myeloproliferative syndrome. *Clin Haematol* 4:373–392, 1975.
30. Harker LA, Slichter SJ: The bleeding time as a screening test for evaluation of platelet function. *N Engl J Med* 287:155–159, 1972.
31. Babson SR, Babson AL: Development and evaluation of a disposable device for performing simultaneous duplicate bleeding time determinations. *Amer J Clin Pathol* 70:406–408, 1978.
32. Kumar R, Ansell JE, Canoso RT, et al: Clinical trial of a new bleeding time device. *Amer J Clin Pathol* 70:642–645, 1978.
33. Stewart JH, Castaldi PA: Uraemic bleeding: A reversible platelet defect corrected by dialysis. *Q J Med* 36:409–423, 1967.
34. Kleiner EE, Heiges L, Fukushima M: Sensitivities of thromboplastins to factor VII deficiency. *Amer J Clin Pathol* 56:162–165, 1971.
35. Denson KWE: Tissue extracts and their sensitivity to factor VII and factor X. *Thromb Diath Haemorrh* 11:146–154, 1964.
36. Loeliger EA, Van Halem-Visse LP: Biological properties of the thromboplastins and plasmas included in the ICTH/ICSH collaborative study of prothrombin time standardization. *Thromb Haemostasis* 42:1115–1127, 1979.
37. Poller L, Taberner DA: Dosage and control of oral anticoagulants: An international collaborative survey. *Brit J Haematol* 51:479–485, 1982.
38. Loeliger EA, Lewis SM: Progress in laboratory control of oral anticoagulants. *Lancet* 2:318–320, 1982.
39. Palmer RN, Gralnick HR: Cold-induced contact surface activation of the prothrombin time in whole blood. *Blood* 59:38–42, 1982.
40. Palmer RN, Kessler CM, Gralnick HR: Warfarin anticoagulation: Difficulties in interpretation of prothrombin time. *Thromb Res* 25:125–130, 1982.
41. Rapaport SI: Brief review: Preoperative hemostatic evaluation. Which tests if any? *Blood* 61:229–231, 1983.
42. Ingram GIC, O'Brien PF, North WRS: The ICTH/WFH study of the partial thromboplastin time in mild hemophilia. *Scand J Haematol* 25(Suppl 39):64–72, 1981.
43. Clarke JR, Eisenberg JM: A theoretical assessment of the value of the PTT as a preoperative screening test in adults. *Med Decision Making* 1:40–43, 1981.
44. Eisenberg JM, Clarke JR, Sussman SA: Prothrombin and partial thromboplastin time as preoperative screening tests. *Arch Surg (Chicago)* 117:48–51, 1982.
45. Stevenson KJ, Poller L: The procoagulant activity of partial thromboplastin extracts: The role of phosphatidylserine. *Thromb Res* 26:341–350, 1982.
46. Sibley C, Singer JW, Wood RJ: Comparison of activated partial thromboplastin reagents. *Amer J Clin Pathol* 59:581–586, 1973.
47. Refsum N, Collen D, Godal HC, et al: Sensitivity and precision of activated partial thromboplastin time (APTT) methods. *Scand J Haematol* 20:89–95, 1978.
48. Poller L, Thompson JM, Palmer MK: Measuring partial thromboplastin time. An international collaborative study. *Lancet* 1:842–846, 1976.
49. Itallian, CISMEL Study Group on Activated Partial Thromboplastin Time: A multicenter evaluation of commercial reagents in the diagnosis of mild hemophilia A and other coagulation defects. *Scand J Haematol* 25:308–317, 1980.
50. Hoffmann JJML, Meulendijk PN: Comparison of reagents for determining the activated partial thromboplastin time. *Thromb Hemostasis* 39:640–645, 1978.

51. Hillman CRL, Lusher JM: Determining the sensitivity of coagulation screening reagents: A simplified method. *Lab Med* 13:162–165, 1982.

52. Hathaway WE, Assmus SL, Montgomery RR: Activated partial thromboplastin time and minor coagulopathies. *Amer J Clin Pathol* 71:22–25, 1979.

53. Glynn MFX, Grady M: Comparative evaluation of reagents for the activated partial thromboplastin time in the assay of coagulation factor VIII and IX. *Can J Med Technol* 39:45–48, 1977.

54. Mannucci PM, Canciani MT, Mari D, et al: The varied sensitivity of partial thromboplastin and prothrombin time reagents in the demonstration of the lupus like anticoagulant. *Scand J Haematol* 22:422–432, 1979.

55. Hougie C: Lupus-like anticoagulants (activated partial thromboplastin time inhibitors). *Check Sample Thromb Hemostasis* 3(3), 1981.

56. Canciani MT, Maspero ML, Cattaneo M, et al: Clinical and laboratory observations in eight patients with lupus-like circulating anticoagulant. *Haematology* 64:309–321, 1979.

57. Hoffman JJML, Meulendijk PN: Plasma heparin: A simple, one sample determination of both effect and concentration based on the activated partial thromboplastin time. *Clin Chim Acta* 87:417–424, 1978.

58. Triplett DA: The College of American Pathologists (CAP) survey program. *Scand J Haematol* 25 (Suppl 37):256–257, 1981.

59. Triplett DA, Harms CS, Koepke JA: The effect of heparin on the partial thromboplastin time. *Amer J Clin Pathol* 70(Suppl):556–559, 1978.

60. Schleider MA, Nachman RL, Jaffe EA, et al: A clinical study of the lupus anticoagulant. *Blood* 48:499–509, 1976.

61. Shapiro SS, Thiagarajan P, DeMarco L: Mechanism of action of the lupus anticoagulant. *Ann NY Acad Sci* 370:359–365, 1981.

62. Coots MC, Miller MA, Glueck HI: The lupus inhibitor: A study of its heterogeneity. *Thromb Haemostasis* 46:734–739, 1981.

63. Breckenridge RT, Ratnoff OD: Studies on the site of action of a circulating anticoagulant in disseminated lupus erythematosus. *Amer J Med* 35:813–819, 1963.

64. Carreras LO, Machin SJ, Deman R, et al: Arterial thrombosis, intrauterine death and "lupus" anticoagulant. Detection of immunoglobulin interfering with prostacyclin formation. *Lancet* 1:244–246, 1981.

65. Bowie EJW, Thompson JH, Pascuzzi CA, et al: Thrombosis in systemic lupus erythematosus despite circulating anticoagulants. *J Lab Clin Med* 62:416–430, 1963.

66. Angles-Cano E, Clauvel JP, Sultan Y: Thrombophlebitis in systemic lupus erythematosus. *J Amer Med Ass* 241:2785–2786, 1979.

67. Angles-Cano E, Sultan Y, Clauvel JP: Predisposing factors to thrombosis in systemic lupus erythematosus. Possible relation to endothelial cell damage. *J Lab Clin Med* 94:312–323, 1979.

68. Triplett DA, Brandt JT, Kaczor DA, et al: Laboratory diagnosis of lupus inhibitors: A comparison of the tissue thromboplastin inhibition procedure with a new platelet neutralization procedure. *Amer J Clin Pathol* 79:678–682, 1983.

69. Gurewich V, Hutchinson E: Detection of intravascular coagulation by a serial-dilution protamine sulfate test. *Ann Intern Med* 75:895–902, 1971.

70. Triplett DA, Harms CS: *Procedures in the Coagulation Laboratory*. Chicago: American Society for Clinical Pathology, 1981, p 69.

71. Bowie EJW, Thompson JH, Didisheim D, et al: *Mayo Clinic Laboratory Manual of Hemostasis*. Philadelphia: WB Saunders, 1971.

72. Sirridge MS, Shannon R: *Laboratory Evaluation of Hemostasis and Thrombosis* (3rd edition). Philadelphia: Lea & Febiger, 1983.

Reference Books

Hathaway WE, Bonnar J: *Perinatal coagulation*. New York: Grune & Stratton, 1978.

Ingram GIC, Bruzouić M, Slater NGP: *Bleeding Disorders. Investigation and Management* (2nd edition). Oxford: Blackwell Scientific Publication, 1982.

Lewis JH, Spero JA, Hasibu U: *Bleeding Disorders: Discussions in Patient Management*. Garden City, N.Y.: Medical Examination Publishing Co., 1978.

Sirridge MS, Shannon R: *Laboratory Evaluation of Hemostasis and Thrombosis* (3rd edition). Philadelphia: Lea & Febiger, 1983.

Thompson AR, Harker LA: *Manual of Hemostasis and Thrombosis* (3rd edition). Philadelphia: FA Davis, 1983.

Thomson JM (ed): *Blood Coagulation and Haemostasis* (2nd edition). Edinburgh: Churchill Livingstone, 1980.

PART

TWO

CASE HISTORIES

PART

TWO

CASE HISTORIES

Introduction

This portion of the book deals with the application of the basic concepts of hemostasis that were presented in Part I. With a thorough understanding of the concepts presented in Chapters 1 to 4, the reader will be able to understand the terms and use of the laboratory in evaluating each case presentation. The cases have been arranged in groups; however, in many instances, closely related cases may actually be in separate categories. When there are several cases illustrating different aspects of the same bleeding disorder, they are arranged in sequence. The most comprehensive discussion and bibliography will be formed with the first case.

The format for each case presentation is consistent. Emphasis is placed on the need for an adequate history and physical examination. The importance of the history cannot be overemphasized. Often, the history provides enough information to allow the reader to arrive at an appropriate differential diagnosis.

Following the history, a few simple screening procedures are provided along with the results of such tests. The procedures that form the cornerstone of the initial evaluation include bleeding time, platelet count, prothrombin time and activated partial thromboplastin time. After these results are provided, the reader is asked several questions concerning the case.

The confirmatory test results and diagnosis are then provided, together with a discussion that answers the questions that were earlier posed to the reader. Each case also is supplemented by a bibliography and, in most instances, a number of illustrations and tables.

The normal values for this section are those used in the laboratory at Ball Memorial Hospital. They are summarized in the following table.

Normal Coagulation Values at Ball Memorial Hospital

Test	Normal Value
Tests of intrinsic system	
Activated partial thromboplastin time	<42 seconds
Tests of extrinsic system	
Prothrombin time	10–12 seconds
Tests of platelet function	
Ivy bleeding time	1–6 minutes
Mielke bleeding time (template)	1–8 minutes
Platelet retention	40% to 90%
Platelet aggregation	
Prothrombin consumption, modified procedure with inosithin	>26 seconds
Platelet count	130,000–400,000/μl
Factor assays (i.e., I, VIII and IX)	
Fibrinogen	170–410 mg/dl
Other factors	50% to 150% (Hageman as low as 30%)
Factor VIII R:Ag	50% to 150%
Factor VIII R:RCo	50% to 150%
Fibrinolysis and disseminated intravascular coagulation	
Thrombin clotting time	20–24 seconds
Euglobulin lysis	More than 2 hours for complete lysis
Protamine sulfate	No fibrin strands
Ethanol gel	No visible clot
Staphylococcal clumping (fibrin split products)	<9.0 μg/ml
Thrombo-Wellco test (fibrin split products)	<10 μg/ml
Reptilase time	18–22 seconds
Antithrombin III activity	85% to 115%
Antithrombin III antigen	23–40 mg/dl
Inhibitor studies	
Tissue thromboplastin inhibition	<1.1
Bethesda assay	0 Bethesda units
Platelet Neutralization Procedure	Normalized prolonged APTT
Platelet antibodies	<10 fg of IgG/platelet

Appendix A

Aspirin-Containing Medications

Product	Manufacturer
ACA, capsules & No. 2	Scrip
ACD	Philips Roxane
Acetabar*	Philips Roxane
Acetasem*	Philips Roxane
Acetonyl	Upjohn
Aidant	Noyes
Aidant with Dover's powder*	Noyes
Aidant with gelsemium	Noyes
Alka-Seltzer	Miles
Allylgesic*	Elder
Allylgesic with ergotamine*	Elder
Alprine*	Ulmer
Aluprin	Lemmon
Amsodyne*	Elder
Amytal with ASA*	Lilly
Anacin	Whitehall
Anexsia with codeine	Massengill
Anexsia-D*	Massengill
Anodynos	Buffington
Ansemco, Nos. 1 & 2	Massengill
APAC*	N Amer Pharm
Apamead	Spencer Mead
APC	Various manufacturers
APC with codeine*	Various manufacturers
APC with Demerol	Winthrop
APC with gelsemium*	Sutliff & Case
Aphodyne	Gold Leaf
Aphophen*	Gold Leaf
Arthra-Zene, capsules	Xttrium
ASA	Lilly
ASA, compound	Lilly
ASA, compound with codeine*	Lilly
Asalco, Nos. 1 & 2	Jenkins
Ascaphen	Schlicksup
Ascaphen, compound	Schlicksup
As-ca-phen	Ulmer
Ascodeen-30*	Burroughs Wellcome
Ascriptin	Rorer
Ascriptin with Codeine*	Rorer
Aspadine, tablets*	N Amer Pharm
Aspergum	Pharmaco
Asphac-G*	Central
Asphac-G with codeine*	Central
Asphencaf	Cole
Asphyte	Cowley
Aspirbar	Lannett
Aspir-C	Jenkins
Aspireze	Stanlabs
Aspirin (USP)	Various manufacturers
Aspirin, aluminum	Abbott

Product	Manufacturer
Aspirin, children's	Abbott
Aspirin, compound with Dover's powder	Fellows
Aspirin-Ph, tablets*	American Drug
Aspirin-secobarbital, supprettes, Nos. 1,* 2,* 3,* & 4*	Webster
Aspirin, supprettes	Webster
Aspirjen Jr, tablets	Jenkins
Aspirocal†	McNeil
Aspir-phen	Spencer-Mead & Robinson
Aspodyne	Blue Line
Aspodyne with codeine*	Blue Line
Axotal*	Warren-Teed
Babylove	Amer Pharm
Ban-O-Pain	Daniels
Bayer	Glenbrook
Bayer, children's	Glenbrook
Bayer, timed-release	Glenbrook
Brogesic*	Brothers
Bufabar*	Philips Roxane
Buff-A	Mayrand
Buffacetin	Kay & Bowman
Buff-A-Comp*	Mayrand
Buffadyne	Lemmon
Buffadyne-A-S, tablets*	Lemmon
Buffadyne with barbiturates	Lemmon
Bufferin	Bristol-Myers
Bufferin, arthritis strength	Bristol-Myers
Buffinol	Otis Clapp
Calurin	Dorsey
Cama Inlay	Dorsey
Capron	Bryant-Vitarine
Causalin*	Amfre-Grant
Cephalgesic*	Smith, Miller & Patch
Cheracol, capsules	Upjohn
Cirin	Zemmer
Clistanal*	McNeil
Codasa, tablets*	Stayner
Codempiral, Nos. 2* & 3*	Burroughs Wellcome
Codesal, Nos. 1* & 2*	Durst
Coldate	Elder
Colrex	Rowell
Colrex, compound*	Rowell
Congesprin	Bristol-Myers
Cope	Glenbrook
Coralsone, modified*	Zemmer
Cordex*	Upjohn
Cordex, forte*	Upjohn
Cordex, buffered*	Upjohn
Cordex, forte buffered*	Upjohn

Aspirin-Containing Medications

Product	Manufacturer	Product	Manufacturer
Coricidin	Schering	Hypan	Lemmon
Coricidin "D"	Schering	I-PAC*	Spencer-Mead
Coricidin Demilets	Schering	Kryl*	Ayerst
Coricidin Medilets	Schering	Liquiprin	Mitchum Thayer
Co-ryd	Daniels	Lumasprin with hyoscyamus*	Rorer
Counter Pain	Squibb	Marnal, tablets & capsules	N Amer Pharm
Covangesic	Mallinckrodt	Measurin	Breon
Darvon with ASA*	Lilly	Medadent*	Upjohn
Darvon-N with ASA*	Lilly	Medaprin*	Upjohn
Darvon, compounds 32* & 65*	Lilly	Midol	Glenbrook
DArvo-Tran*	Lilly	Multihist & APC, capsules†	Dorsey
Dasikon	Beecham-Massengill	Nembudeine, ¼*, ½* & 1*	Abbott
Dasin, capsules	Beecham-Massengill	Nembu-Gesic*	Abbott
Dasin-CS*	Beecham-Massengill	Nipirin*	Elder
Dasin, ¼ strength*	Beecham-Massengill	Norgesic*	Riker
Decagesic*	Merck Sharp & Dohme	Novahistine with APC	Dow Chemical
Delenar*	Schering	Novrad with ASA*	Lilly
Derfort*	Cole	Opacedrin	Elder
Derfule*	Cole	Opasal	Elder
Dolcin	Dolcin	Paadon*	Rorer
Dolene, compound 65*	Lederle	Pabirin	Dorsey
Dolor	Geriatric Pharm	PAC, compound, tablets	Upjohn
Doloral*	Wolly	PAC, compound with codeine*	Upjohn
Dorodol*	Durst	PAC with Cyclopal	Upjohn
Drinacet*	Philips Roxane	Palgesic*	Panamerican Pharm
Dristan, tablets	Whitehall	PC-65*	Caribe Chemical
Drocogesic, No. 3*	Century Lab	Pedidyne	Lemmon
Duopac*	Spencer-Mead	Pentagesic	Kremers-Urban
Duradyne	Durst	Pentagill	Beecham-Massengill
Duragesic	Meyer	Percobarb*	Endo
Ecotrin	Smith Kline & French	Percobarb-Demi*	Endo
Empiral*	Burroughs Wellcome	Percodan*	Endo
Empirin	Burroughs Wellcome	Percodan-Demi	Endo
Empirin, compound with codeine*	Burroughs Wellcome	Persistin	Fisons
Emprazil	Burroughs Wellcome	Phac, tablets	Cole
Emprazil-C*	Burroughs Wellcome	Phenaphen*	Robins
Epragen*	Lilly	Phenaphen with codeine	Robins
Equagesic*	Wyeth	Phencasal	Elder
Excedrin	Bristol-Myers	Phencaset, improved	Elder
Excedrin PM	Bristol-Myers	Phenergan, compound, tablets*	Wyeth
Fiorinal*	Sandoz	Phenodyne	Blue Line
Fiorinal with codeine, Nos. 1,* 2* & 3*	Sandoz	Pheno-Formasal*	First Texas
Fizrin	Glenbrook	Phensal	Dow Chemical
Formasal, capsules & tablets	First Texas	Pirseal	Fellows-Testagar
4-Way cold tablets	Bristol-Myers	Polygesic CT*	Arnar-Stone
Gelsodyne*	Blue Line	Ponodyne	Fellows-Testagar
Grillodyne*	Fellows Med	Predisal*	Mallard
Hasamal CT*	Arnar-Stone	Prolaire-B*	Stuart
Henasphen	Drug Products	Pyrasal	Philips Roxane
Histadyl & ASA compound	Lilly	Pryhist, cold	Daniels
		Pyrroxate	Upjohn

Aspirin-Containing Medications

Product	Manufacturer
Pyrroxate with codeine*	Upjohn
Rhinex	Lemmon
Robaxisal*	Robins
Robaxisal-PH*	Robins
Ryd	Daniels
Sal-Aceto	Fellows-Testagar
Sal-Fayne	Kenton
Salibar Jr*	Jenkins
Salipral*	Kenyon
Sarogesic*	Saron
Sedagesic*	Kay
Sedalgesic*	Table Rock
Sigmagen*	Schering
Sine-Off	Menley & James
Spirin, buffered	Schlicksup
Stanback	Stanback
Stero-Darvon with ASA*	Lilly
St. Joseph	Plough
St. Joseph for children	Plough
Supac	Mission
Super-Anahist	Warner-Lambert
Synalgos*	Ives
Synalgos-DC*	Ives
Synirin*	Poythress
Tetrex-APC with Bristamin*	Bristol
Thephorin-AC †	Roche
Toloxidyne	Durst
Trancogesic*	Winthrop
Trancoprin*	Winthrop
Triaminicin	Dorsey
Trigesic	Squibb
Triocin	Commerce
Vanquish	Glenbrook
Zactirin*	Wyeth
Zactirin, compound*	Wyeth

Product	Manufacturer
Unlisted Products Identified in Five Community Pharmacies	
BiAct, cold tablets	Sauter Labs
Defencin	Grove Labs
Haysma	Haysma Co.
Monacet	Rexall
Quiet World	Whitehall Labs
Saleto	Mallard
Sine-Aid	Johnson & Johnson
Soltice, cold tablets	Chatlem Drug & Chemical
Additional Aspirin-Containing Medications	
Acetidine, capsules	Merck Sharp & Dohme
Acetidine, capsules with codeine	Merck Sharp & Dohme
Acetidine, tablets with codeine	Merck Sharp & Dohme
Anahist	Warner-Lambert
Aspivite, capsules	Merck Sharp & Dohme
B-C Headache Powder	B.C. Remedy
Bristamin APC, tablets	Bristol
Cyclopal and Aspirin	Upjohn
Hydrodyne, tablets	Merck Sharp & Dohme
Monacet, compound, capsules	Rexall Drug Company
Monacet, compound, capsules with codeine	Rexall
Monacet, compound, tablets	Rexall
Monacet, compound, tablets with codeine	Rexall
Nuhist with APC	Columbia Medical
Pyrroxate, capsules	Upjohn
Pyrroxate, capsules with codeine	Upjohn
Pyrroxate, tablets	Upjohn
Riona, capsules	Merck Sharp & Dohme
Semaldyne, capsules	Massengill
Tempogen, forte, tablets	Merck Sharp & Dohme
Tempogen, tablets	Merck Sharp & Dohme
Theylene APC, capsules	Abbott

SOURCES:

Leist ER, Banwell JG: Products containing aspirin. N Engl J Med 291:710–712, 1974.

Selner J: More aspirin-containing medicines. N Engl J Med 292:372, 1975.

On prescription only.

† *Discontinued.*

Hereditary Disorders of Coagulation Proteins and Physiologic Inhibitors*

1. Deficiency of factor XII (Hageman factor)
2. Deficiency of prekallikrein (Fletcher factor)
3. Deficiency of factor XI (plasma thromboplastin antecedent)
4. Deficiency of factor IX (hemophilia B), mild
5. Deficiency of factor IX (hemophilia B), severe
6. Deficiency of factor IX (hemophilia B), moderate
7. Deficiency of factor VIII (hemophilia A), mild
8. Deficiency of factor VIII (hemophilia A), mild
9. Deficiency of factor VIII (hemophilia A), severe
10. Deficiency of factor VIII (hemophilia A), severe, with factor VIII inhibitor
11. von Willebrand's disease (type I)
12. von Willebrand's disease (type I), in association with hereditary hemorrhagic telangiectasia (Osler-Weber-Rendu disease)
13. von Willebrand's disease (type IIA)
14. von Willebrand's disease (type IIB)
15. von Willebrand's disease (type III)
16. Deficiency of factor VII
17. Deficiency of factor VII
18. Deficiency of factor X
19. Deficiency of factor V, severe
20. Afibrinogenemia
21. Hypofibrinogenemia
22. Dysfibrinogenemia
23. Hypodysfibrinogenemia
24. Deficiency of factor XIII (fibrin-stabilizing factor)
25. Deficiency of antithrombin III
26. Deficiency of α_2-antiplasmin (Miyasato disease)
27. Deficiency of protein C

Acquired Disorders of Coagulation Proteins and Physiologic Inhibitors

Vitamin K Deficiency

28. Deficiency of vitamin K; aspirin-induced qualitative abnormality of platelets
29. Hemorrhagic disease of the newborn (deficiency of vitamin K)

Liver Disease

30. Alcoholic Cirrhosis and Liver Failure (secondary to ethanol abuse)

Disseminated Intravascular Coagulation

31. Acute disseminated intravascular coagulation (due to massive burn injury)
32. Disseminated intravascular coagulation complicating preeclampsia
33. Chronic disseminated intravascular coagulation (secondary to metastatic adenocarcinoma)
34. Disseminated intravascular coagulation complicating acute promyelocytic leukemia (M-3, hypogranular variant)

Renal Disease

35. Qualitative abnormality of platelets (secondary to chronic renal insufficiency)
36. Deficiency of antithrombin III (secondary to nephrotic syndrome)
37. Deficiency of factor XII (secondary to nephrotic syndrome)

Inhibitors

38. Inhibitor of factor VIII (possibly drug [cleocin] related)
39. Lupus anticoagulant
40. Lupus anticoagulant
41. Multiple myeloma (IgG Kappa) with hyperviscosity syndrome

Miscellaneous

42. Deficiency of factor X in association with primary systemic amyloidosis
43. Polycythemia vera
44. Fibrinolysis following coronary artery bypass
45. Hematoma formation in association with streptokinase therapy

Hereditary Disorders of Platelets

46. Glanzmann's thrombasthenia
47. Bernard-Soulier syndrome
48. Storage pool disease
49. Qualitative abnormality of platelets ("aspirin-like" defect); deficiency of factor VIII (hemophilia A), mild
50. Storage pool disease in association with autosomal dominant thrombocytopenia

Acquired Disorders of Platelets

51. Acute autoimmune thrombocytopenia
52. Chronic autoimmune thrombocytopenia
53. Polycythemia vera in association with iron deficiency anemia
54. Qualitative abnormality of platelets (secondary to ticarcillin)
55. Thrombotic thrombocytopenic purpura

Complications Associated with Anticoagulant Therapy

Heparin

56. Heparin-induced thrombocytopenia
57. Disseminated intravascular coagulation complicating chronic liver disease and staphylococcal septicemia
58. Overdose of heparin
59. Decrease of antithrombin III (due to infusion of heparin)
60. Retroperitoneal hemorrhage (due to overdose of heparin)

Coumadin

61. Overdose of Coumadin (due to interaction with Seconal)
62. Adequate anticoagulation

The numbers in this and the following lists correspond to the case numbers in the text of Part Two.

CASE
1

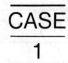

PATIENT: 42-year-old woman

CHIEF COMPLAINT: This patient was referred from a neighboring hospital for evaluation of a possible coagulopathy. She had recently experienced right upper abdominal pain, which was diagnosed by her family physician as possible cholecystitis. Subsequent cholecystography demonstrated many tiny gallstones with questionable dilatation of the cystic duct. She was then referred to a local general surgeon for further evaluation and, possibly, cholecystectomy. During the outpatient evaluation, an "abnormal" coagulation result was found. Consequently, she was referred for a coagulation workup.

MEDICAL HISTORY: The patient had undergone a number of minor surgical procedures, including tonsillectomy at 6 years of age, cesarean section at 28 years of age and hemorrhoidectomy at 38 years of age. In each instance, there was no abnormal bleeding associated with the surgical procedure. She had never required a transfusion.

FAMILY HISTORY: The patient's parents were living and well, although her father had been treated for hypertension. The patient had two children, both of whom were well.

DRUG HISTORY: The patient was taking no medication. She denied taking any drugs, except for aspirin in the remote past for headache.

PHYSICAL EXAMINATION: There was no palpable organomegaly or adenopathy.

Laboratory Results

A. Screening Procedures

Prothrombin time	11 seconds	10–12 seconds
APTT	>200 seconds	<42 seconds
Platelet count	250,000/μl	130,000–400,000/μl
Bleeding time	6 minutes and 30 seconds	1–8 minutes

Questions

1. What is the differential diagnosis?
2. What additional laboratory procedures would be helpful in further evaluating the prolonged APTT?
3. Are any precautions necessary in preparing this patient for surgical intervention?

Laboratory Results

B. Confirmatory Procedures

	Patient	Normal
APTT (50% patient plasma/50% pooled normal plasma	40 seconds	<42 seconds
APTT, 10-minute incubation	>200 seconds	
Factor XII assay	<1%	30% to 150%

DIAGNOSIS: Hereditary deficiency of factor XII

Discussion

This case is a typical example of deficiency of factor XII (Hageman factor). Despite the apparent incoagulability of blood in vitro, the patient has had no difficulty with bleeding associated with trauma or surgical procedures. The markedly prolonged APTT, together with the negative bleeding history, suggests two possibilities: acquired coagulopathy of recent origin and an abnormality of a component of the contact phase of coagulation (i.e., factor XII, prekallikrein or high-molecular-weight kininogen). To rule out the possibility of a circulating anticoagulant, a mixing study was performed; it indicated complete correction with an equal amount of pooled normal plasma. A 10-minute incubated APTT resulted in no correction, ruling out the possibility of deficiency of prekallikrein (Fletcher factor). Subsequently, a factor XII assay confirmed the diagnosis of severe deficiency of factor XII. The patient's plasma contained less than 1% activity of factor XII (normal range, 30% to 150%).*

Biochemical Aspects and Clinical Picture. Several hundred cases of deficiency of Hageman factor have been reported. The mode of inheritance is autosomal recessive. The lack of participation of Hageman factor in normal hemostasis is emphasized by the clinical observa-

*Orientals tend to have lower levels of factor XII..

HEREDITARY DEFICIENCY OF FACTOR XII

CLINICAL PICTURE

Negative bleeding history

PHYSICAL PROPERTIES OF FACTOR XII

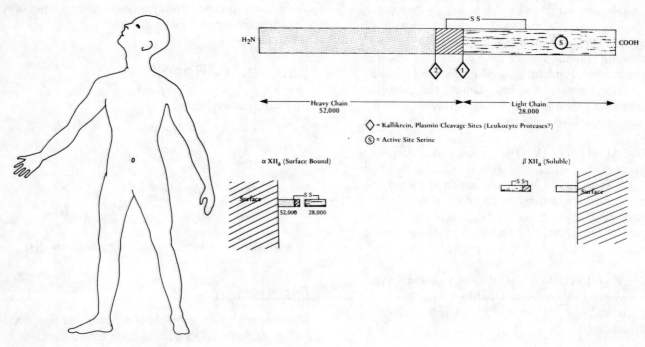

Pattern of inheritance: Autosomal recessive

LABORATORY FINDINGS

A. Screening Procedures

Test	Patient's Result	Normal Range
Prothrombin time	Normal	10–12 seconds
APTT	Abnormal	<42 seconds
Platelet count	Normal	130,000–400,000/μl
Bleeding time	Normal	1–8 minutes

B. Confirmatory Procedures

Incubated APTT (10 minutes)	No correction	<42 seconds.
Mixing APTT	Normal	<42 seconds
Factor XII assay	<1%	30% to 150%

TREATMENT

No treatment necessary

tion that patients with a complete deficiency of factor XII do not have a clinical bleeding disorder and, in several instances, have actually suffered from thrombotic disease.

Hageman factor is a single-chain beta-globulin with a molecular weight of approximately 80,000. A number of physiologic and nonphysiologic substances activate Hageman factor in the presence of other factors that participate in the contact phase of coagulation (high-molecular-weight kininogen and prekallikrein). All the substances that are involved have a negative surface charge (e.g., kaolin, ellagic acid, dextran sulfate, celite and micronized silica). The physiologic activator may be the subendothelial vascular basement membrane. Enzymatic activation of factor XII gives rise to successively smaller molecules. Activated factor XII (XIIa), in turn, cleaves prekallikrein, factor XI and factor VII proteolytically, converting them to their active forms.

Antibody neutralization studies and immunoelectrophoresis have identified a few patients with cross-reacting material. In such patients, the abnormal factor XII molecule does not function appropriately in the contact phase of coagulation. Most patients with a deficiency of factor XII do not have such cross-reacting material.

In addition to hereditary deficiency of factor XII, acquired deficiency has been reported in patients with nephrotic syndrome. There is insufficient data to determine whether deficiency of factor XII is related to the severity or the histologic type of nephrotic syndrome. Also, no correlation between acquired deficiency of factor XII and the thrombotic complications of nephrotic syndrome has been established (see Case 37).

Bibliography

Clinical Picture

Didisheim P: Hageman factor deficiency (Hageman trait): A case report and review of the literature. *Arch Intern Med* 110:170–177, 1962.

Egeberg O: New families with factor XII deficiency. *Thromb Diath Haemorrh* 23:441–448, 1970.

Kasper CK, Whissel Buechy DYE, Aggeler PM: Hageman factor (factor XII) in an affected kindred and in normal adults. *Brit. J Haematol* 14:543–551, 1976.

Biochemical Aspects

Cochrane CG, Griffin JH: Molecular assembly in the contact phase of the Hageman factor system. *Amer J Med* 67:657–663, 1979.

Goldsmith GH, Saito H, Ratnoff OD: The activation of plasminogen by Hageman factor (factor XII) and

Hageman factor fragments. *J Clin Invest* 62:54–60, 1978.

Green D, Arsever CL, Grumet KA, et al: Classic gout in Hageman factor (factor XII) deficiency. *Arch Intern Med* 142:1556–1557, 1982.

Kisiel W, Fujikawa D, Davie EW: Activation of bovine factor VII (proconvertin) by factor XIIa (activated Hageman factor). *Biochemistry* 16:4189–4194, 1977.

Cross-Reacting Material-Positive Variant of Factor XII Deficiency

Saito H, Scialla SJ: Isolation and properties of non-functional Hageman factor (HF, factor XII) from a CRM positive Hageman trait plasma. (Abstract) *Blood* (Suppl) 54:301a, 1979.

Saito H, Scott JG, Morat HZ, et al: Molecular heterogeneity of Hageman trait (factor XII deficiency): Evidence that 2 of 49 cases are cross reacting material positive (CRM+). *J Lab Clin Med* 94:256–265, 1979.

Saito H, Scott JG, Morat HZ, et al: CRM+ variants of Hageman trait. (Abstract) *Blood* (Suppl):194, 1979.

Thrombosis and Hageman Factor Deficiency

Dyerberg J, Stoffersen E: Recurrent thrombosis in a patient with factor XII deficiency. *Acta Haematol* 63:278–282, 1980.

Glueck HI, Roehill W Jr: Myocardial infarction in a patient with Hageman (factor XII) defect. *Ann Intern Med* 64:390–396, 1966.

Hoak JC, Swanson LW, Warner ED, et al: Myocardial infarction associated with severe factor XII deficiency. *Lancet* 2:884–886, 1966.

Pizzuto J, Garcia N, Regna MP, et al: Factor XII deficiency and thrombosis. (Abstract 0558) *Thromb Haemostasis* 42:236, 1979.

Ratnoff OD, Busse RJ Jr, Sheon RP: The demise of John Hageman. *N Engl J Med* 279:760–761, 1968.

Laboratory Evaluation

Gordon EM, Donaldson VH, Saito H, et al: Reduced titers of Hageman factor (factor XII) in Orientals. *Ann Intern Med* 95:697–700, 1981.

Iatridis SC, Ferguson JH: A two-stage assay method for Hageman factor activity. *Thromb Diath Haemorrh* 8:46–55, 1962.

Review Article

Ratnoff OD: A quarter century with Mr. Hageman. *Thromb Haemostasis* 43:95–98, 1980.

CASE
2

PATIENT: 62-year-old black man

CHIEF COMPLAINT: This patient was admitted with recurrent anal pruritus and pain associated with a large, thrombosed, external hemorrhoid.

MEDICAL HISTORY: The patient had no history of bleeding problems. He had undergone a number of surgical procedures, including appendectomy at 12 years of age and partial gastrectomy for recurrent duodenal ulcer disease at 55 years of age. He had not required blood components with either surgical procedure.

FAMILY HISTORY: There was no family history of hemorrhagic difficulties.

DRUG HISTORY: The patient was using Anusol suppositories and had admitted to frequent use of acetaminophen for headache.

PHYSICAL EXAMINATION: A large, thrombosed, external hemorrhoid and a questionable right inguinal hernia were noted.

Laboratory Results

A. Screening Procedures

	Patient	Normal
Prothrombin time	10 seconds	10–12 seconds
APTT	114 seconds	<42 seconds
Platelet count	180,000/μl	130,000–4000,000/μl
Bleeding time	7 minutes	1–8 minutes

Questions

1. What is the differential diagnosis?
2. What additional laboratory procedures would be helpful in further evaluating the prolonged APTT?
3. Would the choice of the activator in the APTT reagent affect the results in this patient's studies?

Laboratory Results

B. Confirmatory Procedures

	Patient	Normal
APTT (50% patient plasma/50% pooled normal plasma	42 seconds	<42 seconds
APTT, 10-minute incubation	50 seconds	<42 seconds
Factor XII assay	75%	30% to 150%
Factor XI assay	68%	50% to 150%
Prekallikrein assay	<1%	50% to 150%

DIAGNOSIS: Hereditary deficiency of prekallikrein (Fletcher factor)

Discussion

The finding of a normal prothrombin time together with a markedly prolonged APTT suggests an inherited or acquired abnormality in the intrinsic system of coagulation (factors XII and XI, Fletcher factor, Fitzgerald factor and factors VIII and IX). The possibility of an inhibitor must be considered. The mixing studies that were performed resulted in correction of the abnormal APTT, thus ruling out an inhibitor.

Because the patient had no history of bleeding problems, an abnormality of the contact phase of coagulation must be suspected. Specific assays for factors XII and XI were within normal limits; therefore, the possibility of deficiency of Fletcher factor was strongly considered. An incubated APTT resulted in correction of the abnormal APTT after 10 minutes of incubation. It should be noted that the reagent that was used contained a micronized silica as the activating substance. In the past, the possibility of different activator sensitivities has been raised in the literature. Early reagents in which ellagic acid was used as the activator were relatively insensitive to deficiency of prekallikrein. However, it appears that this problem has recently been addressed by the manufacturers of such reagents.

HEREDITARY DEFICIENCY OF PREKALLIKREIN

CLINICAL PICTURE

Negative bleeding history

Pattern of inheritance: Autosomal recessive

PHYSICAL PROPERTIES OF PREKALLIKREIN

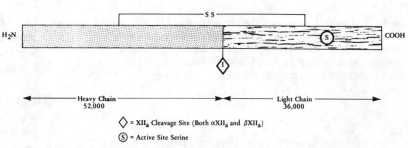

Heavy Chain
52,000

Light Chain
36,000

$\Diamond$ = XII_a Cleavage Site (Both αXII_a and βXII_a)

$\circledS$ = Active Site Serine

Circulates in plasma bound to high molecular weight kininogen (Fitzgerald factor).

LABORATORY FINDINGS

A. Screening Procedures

Test	Patient's Result	Normal Range
Prothrombin time	Normal	10–12 seconds
APTT	Abnormal	<42 seconds
Platelet count	Normal	130,000–400,000/μl
Bleeding time	Normal	1–8 minutes

B. Confirmatory Procedures

Mixing APTT	Normal	<42 seconds
Incubated APTT (10 minutes)	Marked correction	<42 seconds
Prekallikrein assay	<1%	50% to 150%

TREATMENT

No treatment necessary

Step 1:

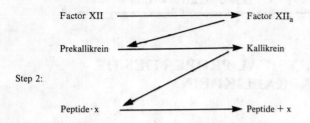

Step 2:

Figure 1. Figure 1 illustrates the chromogenic assay for plasma prekallikrein. In Step 1 the plasma sample is incubated with an activator (ellagic acid, dextran sulfate or kaolin). In Step 2 the synthetic substrate S2302 is added, and the release of paranitroaniline is monitored with a spectrophotometer. Other indicator groups include MCA and AIE.

The specific assay for Fletcher factor was performed with the synthetic substrate S-2302 (Kabi). No prekallikrein was detected in the patient's plasma (Figure 1).

Biochemical Aspects and Clinical Picture. Deficiency of prekallikrein was first described by Hathaway and colleagues in 1965. This disorder is inherited as an autosomal recessive trait. The clinical picture is similar to that of patients with a deficiency of factor XII or high-molecular-weight kininogen. Activation of prekallikrein involves cleavage of the polypeptide chain by activated Hageman factor. The active form consists of two chains linked by a disulfide bond. The light chain contains the active site, a serine residue. Activated kallikrein activates factor XII as well as plasminogen. It appears that kallikrein is the primary "intrinsic" activator of plasminogen. In addition, kallikrein activates factor IX. Kallikrein also cleaves high-molecular-weight kininogen and prorenin.

The major physiologic inhibitor of kallikrein is C'-esterase inhibitor. C'-esterase binds to the active serine residue, completely inhibiting all esterase and proteolytic activity. α_2-Macroglobulin also inhibits kallikrein, although complete inactivation does not result. In addition, antithrombin III functions as an inhibitor of plasma kallikrein in purified systems.

In addition to hereditary deficiency of prekallikrein, a number of acquired conditions characterized by a deficiency of prekallikrein have been reported. Such conditions include disseminated intravascular coagulation, liver disease, dengue fever and nephrotic syndrome. Decreased levels of prekallikrein have also been found in newborn infants.

Bibliography

Biochemical Aspects

Bouma BN, Miles LA, Beretta G, et al: Human plasma prekallikrein. Studies of its activated factor XII and of its inactivation by diisopropylphosphofluoridate. *Biochemistry* 19:1151–1160, 1980.

Brunner HR, Gavras H: Is the renin system necessary? *Amer J Med* 69:739–745, 1980.

Hathaway WE, Alsever J: The relation of "Fletcher factor" to factors XI and XII. *Brit J Haematol* 18:161–169, 1970.

Osterud B, Bouma B, Griffin JH: Human blood coagulation factor IX. Purification, properties, and mechanism of activation by activated factor XI. *J Biol Chem* 253:5946–5951, 1978.

Saito H, Ratnoff OD: Alteration of factor VII activity by activated Fletcher factor (a plasma kallikrein); A potential link between the intrinsic and extrinsic blood clotting systems. *J Lab Clin Med* 85:405–415, 1975.

Thompson RE, Mandle R Jr, Kaplan AP: Studies of the binding of prekallikrein and factor XI to high molecular weight kininogen and its light chain. *Proc Natl Acad Sci USA* 76:4862–4866, 1979.

Clinical Picture

Abildgaard CF, Harrison J: Fletcher factor deficiency: Family study and detection. *Blood* 43:641–644, 1974.

Hathaway WE, Bilhasen LP, Hathaway HS: Evidence for a new plasma thromboplastin factor I: Case report, coagulation studies and physiochemical properties. *Blood* 26:521–527, 1965.

Hathaway WE, Wuepper KD, Weston WL, et al: Clinical and physiologic studies of two siblings with prekallikrein (Fletcher factor) deficiency. *Amer J Med* 60:654–664, 1976.

Hattersley PG, Hayse D: Fletcher factor deficiency: A report of three unrelated cases. *Brit J Haematol* 18:411–416, 1970.

Wuepper KD: Prekallikrein deficiency in man. *J Exp Med* 138:1345–1355, 1973.

Contact Activation Time and Activated Partial Thromboplastin Time

Bishop RC: Ellagic acid and APTT. (Letter to editor) *Amer J Clin Pathol* 76:247, 1981.

Entes K, LaDuca FM, Tourbaf KM: Fletcher factor deficiency, source of variations of the activated partial thromboplastin time test. *Amer J Clin Pathol* 75:626–628, 1981.

Hattersley PG, Hayse D: The effect of increased contact activation time on the activated partial thromboplastin time. *Amer J Clin Pathol* 66:479–482, 1976.

Acquired Prekallikrein Deficiency

Beard MEJ, Hickton CM: Prekallikrein (Fletcher factor) deficiency in typhoid fever. *Arch Intern Med* 141:1701–1703, 1981.

Ragni MV, Lewis JH, Hasiba U, et al: Prekallikrein (Fletcher factor) deficiency in clinical disease states. *Thromb Res* 18:45–54, 1980.

Saito H, Poon MC, Vicic W, et al: Human plasma prekallikrein (Fletcher factor) clotting activity and antigen in health and disease. *J Lab Clin Med* 92:84–95, 1978.

Review Article

Colman RW: Pathophysiology of kallikrein system. *Ann Clin Lab Sci* 10:220–226, 1980.

CASE
3

PATIENT: 33-year-old man

CHIEF COMPLAINT: This patient was an enlisted man in the United States Air Force who was referred for evaluation of a possible "coagulopathy." During a routine evaluation, he was found to have a prolonged activated partial thromboplastin time (APTT).

MEDICAL HISTORY: With the exception of frequent episodes of epistaxis as a child, there was no history of spontaneous abnormal bleeding. Previous operations included hernia repair in 1953 and tonsillectomy with adenoidectomy in 1961. Also, the lower wisdom teeth had been extracted. There was no abnormal bleeding associated with any of these surgical procedures.

The patient had previously been diagnosed as having chondromalacia of the left knee and Peyronie's disease.

FAMILY HISTORY: The patient's parents and a half-sister were living and well. There was no family history of abnormal bleeding.

DRUG HISTORY: No medication

PHYSICAL EXAMINATION: Noncontributory

Laboratory Results

A. Screening Procedures

	Patient	Normal
Prothrombin time	11 seconds	10–12 seconds
APTT	80 seconds	<42 seconds
Platelet count	230,000/μl	130,000–400,000/μl
Bleeding time	2 minutes and 30 seconds	1–8 minutes

Questions

1. What is the differential diagnosis?
2. What portion of the coagulation system is abnormal?

Laboratory Results

B. Confirmatory Procedures

	Patient	Normal
APTT (50% patient plasma/ 50% pooled normal plasma)	39 seconds	<42 seconds
APTT, 10-minute incubation	71 seconds	<42 seconds
Factor XII assay	80%	30% to 150%
Factor XI assay	<2%	50% to 150%

DIAGNOSIS: Hereditary deficiency of factor XI (plasma thromboplastin antecedent)

Discussion

This case is a typical example of deficiency of factor XI. On questioning concerning ethnic background, the patient was found to be of Ashkenazic Jewish origin. His maternal and paternal grandparents had lived in European Russia.

The APTT was prolonged, but the prothrombin time was normal. Mixing studies in which pooled normal plasma and the patient's plasma were used resulted in correction of the prolonged APTT, thus ruling out the possibility of a circulating anticoagulant. Prolonged incubation of the APTT resulted in no appreciable shortening of the abnormal value, thus eliminating the possibility of deficiency of prekallikrein (Fletcher factor). The specific assay for factor XII was within normal limits, whereas the assay for factor XI was markedly abnormal, with a value of less than 2% being obtained.

Biochemical Aspects and Clinical Picture. Factor XI is a plasma protein with a molecular weight of approximately 160,000 that occurs in trace amounts, at a concentration of 4 μg/ml. Native factor XI exists as a dimer of two identical subunits linked by disulfide bonds. It circulates as a proenzyme bound to high-molecular-weight kininogen. Activation of factor XI results from cleavage of each 80,000-dalton subunit by activated factor XIIa. The major physiologic substrate of factor XIa is factor IX, which it cleaves at two sites to yield factor IXa. In addition, it has been demonstrated that factor XIa activates factor XII and plasminogen.

Deficiency of factor XI is thought to be inherited in an autosomal recessive manner. Deficiency of this factor

HEREDITARY DEFICIENCY OF FACTOR XI

CLINICAL PICTURE

PHYSICAL PROPERTIES OF FACTOR XI

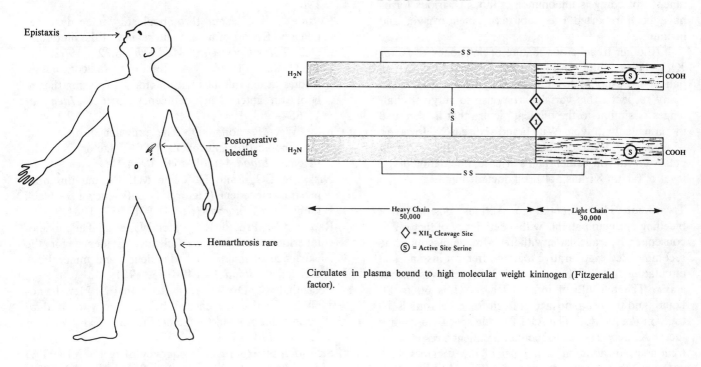

Circulates in plasma bound to high molecular weight kininogen (Fitzgerald factor).

Pattern of inheritance: Autosomal recessive

LABORATORY FINDINGS

A. Screening Procedures

Test	Patient's Result	Normal Range
Prothrombin time	Normal	10–12 seconds
APTT	Abnormal	<42 seconds
Platelet count	Normal	130,000–400,000/μl
Bleeding time	Normal	1–8 minutes

B. Confirmatory Procedures

Mixing APTT	Normal	<42 seconds
Incubated APTT (10 minutes)	No correction	<42 seconds
Factor XI assay	Abnormal	50% to 150%

TREATMENT

Indications
    Preoperative prophylaxis
    Therapeutically in bleeding patients with deficiency of plasma thromboplastin antecedent
Component
    Fresh-frozen plasma, 10–20 ml/kg per day
Adjunctive therapy
    Amicar®

is noteworthy because of the extreme variability in bleeding tendency seen in homozygous patients. In addition, there is little correlation between severity of clinical bleeding and level of factor XI activity. In many instances, patients have no history of bleeding and the deficiency comes to light in routine evaluations only because the APTT is found to be abnormal. Spontaneous bleeding is uncommon, although various forms have been reported (i.e., epistaxis, menorrhagia and hematuria).

Another treacherous feature of deficiency of factor XI is the variability in bleeding experienced by a given patient in response to different surgical procedures. In many respects, this variable response to surgical challenges is similar to the clinical picture that is observed in patients with von Willebrand's disease. However, whereas the level of factor VIII often fluctuates in patients with von Willebrand's disease, fluctuation of the level of factor XI has not been documented.

Treatment. The potential for serious postoperative bleeding exists in patients with a deficiency of factor XI; consequently, transfusion with fresh-frozen plasma is the recommended preoperative therapy. In most instances, a circulating factor XI activity of 30% achieves hemostasis. The half-life of infused factor XI is 60 to 80 hours, and the usual dosage of fresh-frozen plasma is 10 to 20 ml/kg per day. The APTT or the specific assay for factor XI may be used to monitor a patient's response to treatment. In addition, a number of investigators have suggested that ε-aminocaproic acid (EACA) be used as an adjunct to fresh-frozen plasma.

Bibliography

Biochemical Aspects

Bouma BN, Griffin JH: Human blood coagulation factor XI: Purification, properties and mechanism of activation by factor XII. *J Biol Chem* 252:6432–6437, 1977.

Jacobs A, Mannhalter C, Margalit R, et al: Contact activation of factor XI. *Brit J Haematol* 49:77–86, 1981.

Clinical Picture

Bashevkin ML, Nawabi IU: Factor XI deficiency in surgical patients. *NY State J Med* 79(9):1360–1362, August 1979.

Cavins JA, Wall RL: Clinical and laboratory studies of plasma thromboplastin antecedent deficiency (PTA). *Amer J Med* 29:444–448, 1960.

Conrad FG, Breneman WL, Grisham DB: A clinical evaluation of plasma thromboplastin antecedent

(PTA) deficiency. *Ann Intern Med* 62:885–898, 1965.

Edson JR, White JG, Krivet W: The enigma of severe factor XI deficiency without hemorrhagic symptoms. Distinction from Hageman factor and "Fletcher factor" deficiency: Family study, and problems of diagnosis. *Thromb Diath Haemorrh* 18:342–349, 1967.

Kurtides ES: Plasma thromboplastin antecedent deficiency: Report of a case and review of the literature. *Q Bull Northwest Univ Med Sch* 36:329, 1962.

Leiba H, Ramot B, Many A: Hereditary and coagulation studies in ten families with factor XI (plasma thromboplastin antecedent) deficiency. *Brit J Haematol* 11:654–663, 1965.

Muir WA, Ratnoff OD: The prevalence of plasma thromboplastin antecedent (PTA, factor XI) deficiency. *Blood* 44:569–570, 1974.

Niskanen EO, Saito H, Cline MJ: Plasma thromboplastin antecedent (factor IX) deficiency in a black family. *Arch Intern Med* 141:936–937, 1981.

Rapaport SI, Proctor RR, Patch MJ, et al: The mode of inheritance of PTA deficiency: Evidence for the existence of major PTA deficiency and minor PTA deficiency. *Blood* 18:149–165, 1961.

Rosenthal RL, Dreskin OH, Rosenthal N: New hemophilia-like disease caused by deficiency of a third plasma thromboplastin factor. *Proc Soc Exp Biol Med* 82:172–174, 1953.

Seligsohn N: High gene frequency of factor XI (PTA) deficiency in Ashkenazi Jews. *Blood* 51:1223–1228, 1978.

Slade WR, Rabiner AM: Plasma thromboplastin antecedent deficiency and subarachnoid hemorrhage. *Angiology* 24:533–537, 1973.

Todd M: Factor XI (PTA) deficiency with no hemorrhagic symptoms: Case report. *Thromb Diath Haemorrh* 11:186–194, 1964.

Laboratory Evaluation and Acquired Variation of Factor XI Activity

Andrew M, Bhogal M, Karpatkin M: Factors XI and XIII and prekallikrein in sick and healthy premature infants. *N Engl J Med* 305:1130–1133, 1981.

Iwanaga S, Kato H, Maruyama I, et al: Fluorogenic peptide substrates for proteases in blood coagulation, kallikrein-kinin and fibrinolysis systems: Substrate for plasmin and factor XIa. (Abstract #0105) *Thromb Haemostasis* 42:49, 1979.

Rapaport SI, Schiffman S, Patch MJ, et al: A simple specific one stage assay for plasma thromboplastin antecedent activity. *J Lab Clin Med* 57:771–779, 1961.

Saito H, Goldsmith GH: Plasma thromboplastin antecedent (PTA, factor XI): A specific and sensitive radioimmunoassay. *Blood* 50:377–385, 1977.

Treatment

Bick RL, Adams T, Radock K: Surgical hemostasis with a factor XI containing concentrate. *J Amer Med Ass* 229:163–165, 1974.

Robert A, Huguet H, Conrad JC, et al: Deficit congénital en facteur XI. Interêt du dépistage et du traitment en milieu chirurgical. *Anesth Analg* (Paris) 37:187–190, 1980.

Sidi A, Seligsohn U, Jones P, et al: Factor XI deficiency: Detection and management during urological survey. *J Urol* 119:528–530, 1978.

CASE
4

PATIENT: 49-year-old-man

CHIEF COMPLAINT: This patient was referred for evaluation of a possible coagulation defect. On Friday of the preceding week, he was accidently struck on the right tibia by the stock of a rifle. This accident resulted in the formation of a large hematoma over the anterior surface of the tibia.

MEDICAL HISTORY: The patient had been hospitalized on a number of occasions. The first hospitalization was in 1970, when the patient underwent hemorrhoidectomy and bled profusely after the operation. At that time, he received approximately 5 units of whole blood. The transfusion controlled the bleeding, and the patient was discharged with no further postoperative problems.

In September 1972, the patient was again admitted for gastrointestinal bleeding, which subsequently was diagnosed as being secondary to a duodenal ulcer. The patient underwent partial gastrectomy and vagotomy. Again, there was marked bleeding during and after the operation. At that time, he received 11 units of whole blood.

In January 1973, the patient was readmitted for gastrointestinal bleeding, and an exploratory laparotomy was performed. He was found to have a bleeding marginal ulcer. Again, there was marked bleeding during and after the operation, and the patient required approximately 20 units of whole blood.

In addition to the above surgical procedures, the patient had undergone several dental extractions and on each occasion had bled profusely, although a transfusion was not required. Apparently, the oral surgeon packed and meticulously stitched each extraction site. These precautions were sufficient to control the postextraction bleeding.

FAMILY HISTORY: The patient had a younger brother (47 years of age) who was diagnosed as having a deficiency of factor IX several years previously. This brother had recurrent gastrointestinal bleeding and had received numerous transfusions to control the blood loss. In addition, when 37 years of age, this brother had undergone partial gastrectomy; the operation had been complicated by operative and postoperative bleeding, which necessitated numerous transfusions.

The patient had two other siblings: a brother (41 years of age) and a sister (39 years of age). The sister had been seen on a number of occasions for recurrent sinusitis and inflammatory nasal polyps. She experienced bleeding during and after surgical intervention for the nasal polyps and subsequently was diagnosed as being a possible carrier of deficiency of factor IX. The remaining brother had no history of bleeding problems and was living and well. The patient's parents were deceased, and there was no additional family history of bleeding problems.

DRUG HISTORY: No medication

PHYSICAL EXAMINATION: There were several abdominal surgical scars. In addition, there was a large hematoma over the anterior surface of the right tibia.

Laboratory Results

A. Screening Procedures

	Patient	Normal
Prothrombin time	11 seconds	10–12 seconds
APTT	51 seconds	<42 seconds
Platelet count	210,000/μl	130,000–400,000/μl
Bleeding time	6 minutes and 30 seconds	1–8 minutes

Questions

1. What is the mode of inheritance of hereditary deficiency of factor IX?
2. What is the most likely diagnosis?
3. Would the affected brother have a similar degree of deficiency of factor IX?

Laboratory Results

B. Confirmatory Procedures

	Patient	Normal
APTT (50% patient plasma/50% pooled normal plasma)	39 seconds	<42 seconds
Factor IX activity	14%	50% to 150%
Factor IX antigen	36%	50% to 150%

DIAGNOSIS: Hereditary deficiency of factor IX (hemophilia B), mild

HEREDITARY DEFICIENCY OF FACTOR IX, MILD

CLINICAL PICTURE

Easy bruising →

Postoperative bleeding

Intramuscular hematoma formation with trauma

Traumatic hemarthrosis

Pattern of inheritance: Sex-linked recessive

PHYSICAL PROPERTIES OF FACTOR IX

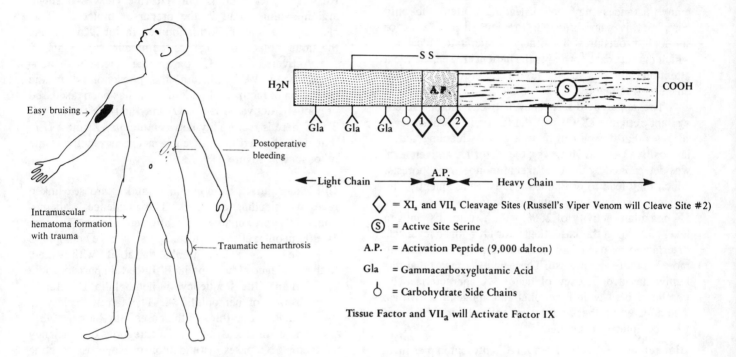

H_2N — Gla Gla Gla ◇1 ◇2 — S — COOH

←—Light Chain—→ A.P. ←—Heavy Chain—→

◇ = XI_a and VII_a Cleavage Sites (Russell's Viper Venom will Cleave Site #2)

Ⓢ = Active Site Serine

A.P. = Activation Peptide (9,000 dalton)

Gla = Gammacarboxyglutamic Acid

◯ = Carbohydrate Side Chains

Tissue Factor and VII_a will Activate Factor IX

LABORATORY FINDINGS

A. Screening Procedures

Test	Patient's Result	Normal Range
Prothrombin time	Normal	10–12 seconds
APTT	Abnormal or normal	<42 seconds
Platelet count	Normal	130,000–400,000/μl
Bleeding time	Normal	1–8 minutes

B. Confirmatory Procedures

Mixing APTT	Normal	<42 seconds
Factor IX:C activity	5% to 25%	50% to 150%
Factor IX antigen	Normal or abnormal	50% to 150%

TREATMENT

For patients with the mild form of deficiency of factor IX with non-life-threatening bleeding, the treatment of choice is fresh-frozen plasma. In patients with life-threatening (central nervous system) bleeding, prothrombin complex concentrates are the treatment of choice.

The treatment of choice for the severe form of hemophilia B is prothrombin complex concentrates.

Factor IX:C Target values for therapy.

Severe hemorrhage: 20–50% for 3–5 days.

Minor hemorrhage: 20%

Surgery: 50–70% for 1st two days.

Discussion

This case is an excellent example of mild deficiency of factor IX. Mild cases of hemophilia are often not diagnosed until late in life. Frequently, this condition comes to light when bleeding occurs in response to trauma or a surgical procedure. The medical history in many instances may be misleading. Often, the only complaint is easy bruising. Previous dental work or surgical procedures inevitably precipitate bleeding, which in most cases prompts the patients to seek medical attention. In this case, however, previous surgical bleeding was ignored.

The apparent discrepancy between factor IX co-agulant activity (IX:C) and the factor IX antigen level suggests that this patient may be a cross-reacting material-positive variant. However, the factor IX antigen level was determined by use of rocket immunoelectrophoresis, which may lead to erroneous results. Subsequently, the patient's sister was evaluated and found to have a factor IX coagulant activity of 28%, with a factor IX antigen level of 30%. In this case, the factor IX antigen level was determined by use of a radioimmunoassay that is much more accurate and precise. These values suggest that this family has a deficiency of factor IX characterized by parallel decreases in functional and antigenic activities. The affected brother and the patient's children have not been completely evaluated.

Biochemical Aspects. Factor IX is present in plasma at a relatively low concentration (approximately 4 μg/ml). The physical properties of factor IX are similar to those of prothrombin and factors VII and X. Human and bovine factor IX are single-chain glycoproteins that contain approximately 20% carbohydrate. The molecular weight of human factor IX is approximately 55,000. There are 12 γ-carboxyglutamic acid residues per molecule of factor IX. These residues are important in the binding of calcium ions and are necessary for the localization of factor IX on phospholipid surfaces.

Factor IX participates in the intrinsic pathway of coagulation. It is activated by factor XIa. In this reaction, two internal peptide bonds are hydrolyzed. This hydrolysis results in the release of an activation peptide with a molecular weight of approximately 10,000. The activation peptide contains three of the four carbohydrate chains present in the bovine zymogen. The remaining heavy and light chains of factor IX are linked by disulfide bonds. The light chain originates from the amino-terminal portion of the molecule, whereas the heavy chain originates from the carboxy-terminal region.

In addition to participating in the intrinsic pathway of coagulation, factor IX may be activated by tissue factor and factor VIIa. This pathway represents an alternate mechanism for the activation of factor IX and bypasses the contact activation system, which involves factor XIa. The rate of activation of factor IX by tissue factor and factor VIIa is about six to seven times slower than that of factor X activation. The relative physiologic importance of these pathways is unknown.

Factor IX can also be activated by a protease from Russell's viper venom. This enzyme cleaves a single arginine-valine bond in the precursor molecule. This cleavage leads to the formation of a factor IXa that has the same molecular weight as the precursor protein.

Activated factor IX participates along with activated factor VIII, calcium and phospholipid in the activation of factor X. In addition, as has been discussed previously, activated factor IX may activate factor VII. Thus, there is reciprocity between factors IX and VII in that the activated form of each factor may activate the other factor (Figure 1).

Clinical Picture. Hemophilia A and B are sex-linked recessive bleeding disorders. The incidence of hemophilia is approximately one affected person in every 10,000 people; 20% of affected persons have hemophilia B. However, there is geographic variability with respect to the incidence of hemophilia B. In certain parts of India and Indiana, the frequency of hemophilia B actually exceeds that of hemophilia A. The family history in approximately one-third of the cases may be negative.

There are at least two broad categories of deficiency of factor IX: cases with demonstrable cross-reacting material (CRM+) and those with an absence of cross-reacting material (CRM−). Approximately one-third of

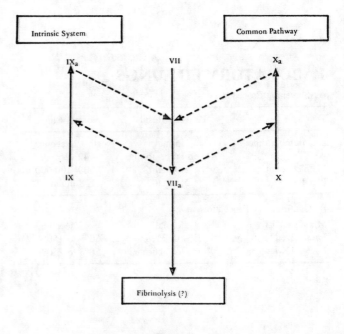

Figure 1

patients with a deficiency of factor IX have demonstrable cross-reacting material (CRM+). A number of variant forms of hemophilia B have been described and include hemophilia B_m and hemophilia B Leyden. Patients with hemophilia B_m are found to have a prolonged one-stage prothrombin time when ox brain thromboplastin is used. Early experiments suggested that such patients synthesize factor IX molecules that are devoid of procoagulant activity but that are capable of acting as an inhibitor of coagulation in the ox brain prothrombin time assay. Patients with hemophilia B Leyden characteristically show increasing levels of factor IX with advancing age. Other variants of factor IX have been described and include factor IX Alabama, Chapel Hill and Worcester.

Hemophilia B occurs in severe, moderate and mild forms, corresponding to the plasma level of factor IX activity. In the severe form, the level of factor IX activity is less than 1%; approximately one-half of patients with hemophilia B belong to this group. In the moderate form, coagulant levels of factor IX range from 1% to 5%; in the mild form, coagulant levels vary from 5% to 25%. Depending on the sensitivity of the APTT reagent, patients are occasionally encountered with mild hemophilia B in whom the APTT results are minimally prolonged, borderline or normal.

A decreased level of factor IX activity has also been found in female carriers. In fact, the frequency of bleeding among carriers of factor IX deficiency is common as compared to the frequency of bleeding among female carriers of factor VIII deficiency. Recent studies suggest that determinations of factor IX coagulant activity and factor IX antigen are helpful in identifying the carrier state of hemophilia B.

Clinical symptoms of hemophilia A and those of hemophilia B are similar. With the severe forms, patients have recurrent hemarthrosis as well as intramuscular hemorrhages. As a result of the recurrent joint hemorrhages, there may be severe damage to the cartilaginous surfaces of the affected joints, leading to chronic synovitis with destruction of the cartilage and underlying bone. In the more advanced stages, new bone formation, fibrosis and even bony ankylosis may result in complete destruction of the affected joints. In addition to the joint destruction, there often is marked atrophy of the supporting muscles around the joints, which predisposes to further joint damage. Intramuscular bleeding may lead to nerve injury, with paresis and contractures, and to the formation of pseudotumors. Also, other types of bleeding, such as hematuria and intracranial bleeding as well as retroperitoneal bleeding, may occur.

Severe or spontaneous bleeding is uncommon in patients with the mild form of hemophilia A or B. Consequently, the mild forms of hemophilia A and B may go unrecognized for many years.

Treatment. To manage the severe form of hemophilia B, prothrombin complex concentrates must be used; such concentrates (Konyne and Proplex) have been available for about 10 years. The half-life of factor IX in vivo is 18 to 40 hours; however, the in vivo recovery of factor IX after infusion is only 20% to 40% of the activity infused. This low rate of recovery is no doubt due to the wide distribution of factor IX in intravascular and extravascular sites. With joint bleeding, a plasma level of factor IX ranging from 20% to 50% of normal is recommended for the first 3 to 5 days. Subsequently, a plasma level of 10% to 20% is recommended. This level may have to be maintained for 10 days or until healing occurs. With minor hemorrhage, a plasma level of factor IX of approximately 20% is sufficient for approximately 1 week. When surgical intervention is contemplated, a plasma level of factor IX of approximately 50% to 70% is recommended during the operation and on the first postoperative day. For the following 3 days, a plasma level of 30% to 40% is adequate; during the next week, the level should be maintained at 20%.

To prevent disabling joint damage, prophylactic or home therapy has been instituted for patients with the severe form of hemophilia B.

The most serious complication in patients with hemophilia B is the development of antibodies to factor IX. Circulating inhibitors of factor IX have been reported in 10% of patients with hemophilia B. Inhibitors appear much more frequently in patients with the severe form of hemophilia B. The anticoagulants are IgG antibodies; however, extensive characterization of these antibodies has not been undertaken. In addition to the appearance of antibodies, many such patients suffer from liver disease as a result of exposure to hepatitis viruses contained in the prothrombin complex concentrates. Also recently Acquired Immune Deficiency Syndrome (AIDS) has been described in patients with both hemophilia A and hemophilia B.

Bibliography

Biochemical Aspects

Berkowitz RM, Nemerson Y: Quantitation of contact system activation using a radiometric assay for activated factor IX. *Blood* 55:528–531, 1980.

Hedner U, Davie EW: Biochemical characterization of factor IX. In Seligsohn U, Rimon A, Horoszowski H (eds): *Current Status in Haemophilia*. Turnbridge Wells, Kent, U.K.: Castle House Publications, 1981, pp 13–18.

Kingdon H, Herion J, Rausch P: Cellular activation of factor IX. *Thromb Res* 13:501–507, 1978.

Osterud B, Rapaport S: Activation of factor IX by the reaction product of tissue factor and factor VII: Additional pathway for initiating blood coagulation. *Proc Natl Acad Sci USA* 74:5260–5264, 1977.

Rapaport SI: The activation of factor IX by the tissue factor pathway. In Menache D, Surgenor DMacN, Anderson H (eds): *Hemophilia and Hemostasis*. New York: Alan R. Liss, 1981, pp 57–76.

Suomela H: Multiple forms of human factor IX in chromatography and isoelectric focusing. *Thromb Res* 7:101–112, 1975.

Tans G, Janssen-Claessen T, Dieijen G, et al: Activation of factor IX by factor XIa—A spectrophotometric assay for factor IX in human plasma. *Thromb Haemostasis* 48:127–132, 1982.

Zur M, Shastri K, Nemerson Y: Kinetics of the tissue factor pathway of coagulation: Activation of factor IX. *Blood* 52:198–202, 1978.

Clinical Picture

Aggeler PM, White SG, Glendening MB, et al: Plasma thromboplastin component (PTC) deficiency: A new disease resembling hemophilia: *Proc Soc Exp Biol Med* 79:692–694, 1952.

Biggs R, Douglas AS, Macfarlane RC, et al: Christmas disease: A condition previously mistaken for haemophilia. *Brit Med J* 2:1378–1382, 1952.

Brozovic M: Christmas disease and other functional coagulation factor deficiencies. In Ogston D, Bennett B (eds): *Haemostasis: Biochemistry, Physiology and Pathology*. London: Wiley, 1977, p 390–404.

Gendelman S, Aledort L, Hollin S: Intracranial meningioma in factor IX deficiency. *J Amer Med Ass* 239:748–749, 1978.

Muir WA, Ratnoff OD: The prevalence of plasma thromboplastin antecedent (PTA, factor IX) deficiency. *Blood* 44:569–570, 1974.

Pavlovsky A: Contribution to the pathogenesis of hemophilia. *Blood* 2:185–191, 1947.

Cross-Reacting Material-Positive Variants of Factor IX Deficiency

Bertina RM, van der Linden IK: Inhibitor neutralization assay and electroimmunoassay of human factor IX (Christmas factor). *Clin Chim Acta* 77:275–286, 1979.

Bertina RM, van der Linden IK: Factor IX Deventer-Evidence for the heterogeneity of hemophilia B$_m$. *Thromb Haemostasis* 47:136–140, 1982.

Bertina RM, Veltkamp JJ: The abnormal factor IX of hemophilia B$^+$ variants. *Thromb Haemostasis* 40:335–349, 1978.

Bertina RM, Veltkamp JJ: A genetic variant of factor IX with decreased capacity for Ca^{2+} binding. *Brit J Haematol* 42:623–635, 1979.

Bithell TC, Pizarro A, MacDiarmid WD: Variant of factor IX deficiency in female with 45-X Turner's syndrome. *Blood* 36:169–179, 1970.

Briet E, Griffith MJ, Braunstein KM, et al: Determination of the relative activities of two factor IX variants—factor IX Chapel Hill and factor IX Alabama—in a purified factor X activating system. (Abstract) *Blood* 58:212a, 1981.

Briet E, Reisner HM, Roberts HR: The study of abnormal factor IX with conformer-specific antibodies. (Abstract) *Blood* 58:212a, 1981.

Braunstein KM, Noyes CM, Griffith MJ, et al: The purification and characterization of an abnormal variant of factor IX: Factor IX Alabama. (Abstract) *Blood* 58:212a, 1981.

Chung KS, Madar DA, Goldsmith JC, et al: Purification and characterization of an abnormal factor IX (Christmas factor) molecule, factor IX Chapel Hill. *J Clin Invest* 62:1078–1085, 1978.

Denson KWE, Biggs R, Mannucci PM: An investigation of three patients with Christmas disease due to an abnormal type of factor IX. *J Clin Pathol* 21:160–165, 1968.

Hougie C, Twomey JJ: Haemophilia B$_m$ a new type of factor IX deficiency. *Lancet* 1:698–700, 1967.

Kidd P, Denson KWE, Biggs R: The Thrombotest reagent® and Christmas disease. *Lancet* 2:522–527, 1963.

Osterud B, Kasper CK, Lavine KK, et al: Purification and properties of an abnormal blood coagulation factor IX (factor IX$_{BM}$)/kinetics of its inhibition of factor X activation by factor VII and bovine tissue factor. *Thromb Haemostasis* 45:55–59, 1981.

Osterud B, Kasper CK, Prodanos C: Factor IX variants of hemophilia B. The effect of activated factor XI and the reaction product of factor VII and tissue factor on the abnormal factor IX molecules. *Thromb Res* 15:235–243, 1979.

Osterud B, Lavine K, Kasper CK, et al: Isolation and properties of the abnormal factor IX molecule of haemophilia B$_m$. (Abstract) *Thromb Haemostasis* 38:51, 1977.

Suzuki L, Thompson AR: Factor IX antigen by a rapid staphylococcal protein. A membrane binding radioimmunoassay: Results in haemophilia B patients and carriers and in fetal samples. *Brit J Haematol* 50:673–682, 1982.

Thompson AR: Factor IX antigen by radioimmunoassay. Abnormal factor IX protein in patients on warfarin therapy and with haemophilia B. *J Clin Invest* 59:900–910, 1977.

Tiarks CY, Pechet L: Immunologic survey of the factor IX molecule in hemophilia B+ patients, carriers and cord blood. *Thromb Res* 21:391–398, 1981.

Twomey JJ, Corless J, Thornton L, et al: Studies on the inheritance and nature of hemophilia B$_m$. *Amer J Med*

46:372–379, 1969.
Yang HC: Purification and immunological studies of factor IX Worcester. *Blood* 50(Suppl):289, 1977.

Carrier Detection

Didisheim P, Vandervoort RLE: Detection of carriers for factor IX (PTC) deficiency. *Blood* 20:150–154, 1962.
Orstavik KH, Veltkamp JJ: Detection of haemophilia B carriers. In Seligsohn U, Rimon A, Horoszowski H (eds): *Haemophilia*. Turnbridge Wells, Kent, U.K.: Castle House Publications, 1981, pp 29–38.

Acquired Factor IX Deficiency

Brown CH, Kvols LK, Hsu TH: Factor IX deficiency and bleeding in a patient with Sheehan's syndrome. *Blood* 39:650–657, 1972.
Handley DA, Lawrence JR: Factor IX deficiency in the nephrotic syndrome. *Lancet* 1:1079–1081, 1967.
Lechner K: Immune reactive factor IX in acquired factor IX deficiency. *Thromb Diath Haemorrh* 27:19–24, 1972.
Natelson EA, Lynch EC, Hetty RA, et al: Acquired factor IX deficiency in the nephrotic syndrome. *Ann Intern Med* 73:373–378, 1970.
Roklan BJ, Sawitsky A: Factor IX deficiency in Gaucher disease. An in vitro phenomenon. *Arch Intern Med* 136:489–492, 1976.

Treatment

Kingdon HS, Lundblad RL, Veltkamp JJ, et al: Potentially thrombogenic materials in factor IX concentrates. *Thromb Diath Haemorrh* 33:617–631, 1975.
Smith KJ, Thompson AR: Labeled factor IX kinetics in patients with hemophilia B. *Blood* 58:625–629, 1981.

Reference Book

Hilgartner MW (ed): *Hemophilia in the Child and Adult*. New York: Masson Publishing, 1982.

CASE 5

PATIENT: 22-month-old boy

CHIEF COMPLAINT: This patient was referred for an evaluation of deficiency of factor IX.

MEDICAL HISTORY: The patient's first episode of bleeding occurred at the time of circumcision. After circumcision, there was marked hemorrhage, and the boy was referred to a large hospital for evaluation of a possible coagulopathy. At that time, he was found to have a prolonged activated partial thromboplastin time (APTT) and a decreased plasma level of factor IX:C. However, the evaluating laboratory did not have an established normal range for factor IX:C in newborn infants. The patient was treated with fresh-frozen plasma, which stopped the bleeding.

Since his first hemorrhagic problem, the patient has been hospitalized on a number of occasions. When he was 4½ months of age, the boy fell and sustained a large hematoma of the right arm. He was hospitalized and received prothrombin complex concentrates. This therapy apparently corrected the bleeding problem. Subsequently, when the boy was 18 months of age, he bled into the right knee and again required factor IX concentrates. In addition to these two hospitalizations, the patient has had a number of bleeding episodes that involved the muscles of the legs.

FAMILY HISTORY: The patient had a younger brother (3 months of age). At the time of the brother's delivery, a blood sample was obtained from the umbilical cord and a factor IX:C assay performed. The factor IX activity was 25% (normal adult range, 50% to 150%).

Other family members, including four maternal uncles and one aunt, had no history of bleeding problems. Both parents were living and well with no history of bleeding abnormalities.

DRUG HISTORY: No medication

PHYSICAL EXAMINATION: Several ecchymoses were noted over the trunk and legs.

Laboratory Results

A. Screening Procedures

	Patient	Normal
Prothrombin time	11 seconds	10–12 seconds
APTT	97 seconds	<42 seconds
Platelet count	235,000/μl	130,000–400,000/μl
Bleeding time	6 minutes	1–8 minutes

Questions

1. What is the normal range for factor IX:C activity in newborn infants?
2. Is it necessary to have a separate set of normal values for newborn infants?

Laboratory Results

B. Confirmatory Procedures

	Patient	Normal
APTT* (50% patient plasma/ 50% pooled normal plasma)	41 seconds	<42 seconds
Factor IX:C activity	<1%	50% to 150%
Factor IX-Related antigen	Nondetectable	50% to 150%
Thrombotest†	>100%	80% to 100%

DIAGNOSIS: Hereditary deficiency of factor IX (hemophilia B), severe

Discussion

This case is an example of severe deficiency of factor IX. The case is unusual in that there was bleeding at the time of circumcision. Ironically, many patients with severe deficiencies of factors VIII and IX may inadvertently undergo circumcision with no bleeding problems.

Factor IX:C activity in cord blood ranges from 15% to 40% of adult values. Factor IX:C activity reaches adult levels during the second or third month of age. Therefore it is necessary to have a separate set of normal values for newborn infants. The patient's brother who had a IX:C activity of 25% was considered to be normal.

*In the past, many laboratories performed additional mixing studies utilizing barium sulfate adsorbed plasma as a source of factors I, V, VIII, XI, XII and serum as a source of factors VII, IX, X, XI and XII. Thus in factor IX deficiency, adsorbed plasma would not correct the prolonged APTT while serum would. In hemophilia A or factor VIII deficiency opposite results were obtained.

† Thrombotest (Nyegaard) is used in most circumstances to monitor the effectiveness of oral anticoagulant therapy. The reagent contains an optimal concentration of calcium, with adsorbed bovine plasma as a source of factor V and fibrinogen, and a tissue thromboplastin of bovine brain origin. It has been used to detect factor IX variants who are cross-reacting material positive. This subclass of patients (deficiency of factor IX with abnormal Thrombotest results) are designated hemophilia B_m.

HEREDITARY DEFICIENCY OF FACTOR IX, SEVERE

CLINICAL PICTURE

PHYSICAL PROPERTIES OF FACTOR IX

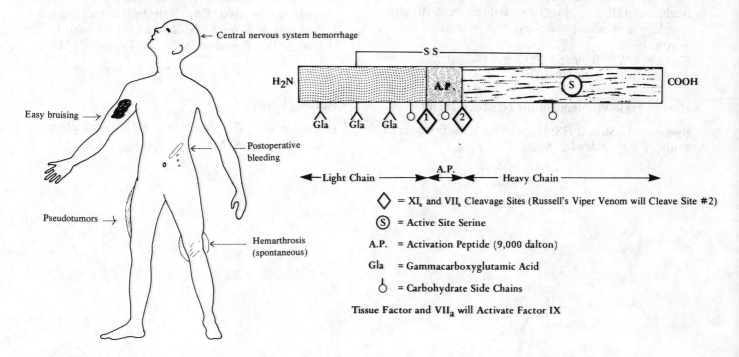

Central nervous system hemorrhage

Easy bruising

Postoperative bleeding

Pseudotumors

Hemarthrosis (spontaneous)

Pattern of inheritance: Sex-linked recessive

◇ = XI$_a$ and VII$_a$ Cleavage Sites (Russell's Viper Venom will Cleave Site #2)

Ⓢ = Active Site Serine

A.P. = Activation Peptide (9,000 dalton)

Gla = Gammacarboxyglutamic Acid

○ = Carbohydrate Side Chains

Tissue Factor and VII$_a$ will Activate Factor IX

LABORATORY FINDINGS

A. Screening Procedures

Test	Patient's Result	Normal Range
Prothrombin time	Normal	10–12 seconds
APTT	Abnormal	<42 seconds
Platelet count	Normal	130,000–400,000/μl
Bleeding time	Normal	1–8 minutes

B. Confirmatory Procedures

Mixing APTT	Normal	<42 seconds
Factor IX activity	<1%	50% to 150%
Factor IX antigen	Normal or abnormal	50% to 150%
Thrombotest	>100%	80–100%

TREATMENT

Prothrombin complex concentrates
  Proplex or Konyne
Complications of concentrates
  Hepatitis
  Thrombogenicity
  Acquired immune deficiency syndrome (AIDS)
  Antibodies to Factor IX

Bibliography

Perinatal Coagulation

Bleyer WA, Hakami N, Shepard TH: The development of hemostasis in the human fetus and in the newborn. *J Pediatr* 79:838–853, 1971.

Buchanan GR: Neonatal coagulation: Normal physiology and pathophysiology. *Clin Haematol* 7:85–109, 1978.

Hathaway WE, Bonnar J: *Perinatal Coagulation*. New York: Grune & Stratton, 1978.

Hemorrhagic Problems in the Newborn Infant

Baehner RL, Strauss HS: Hemophilia in the first year of life. *N Engl J Med* 275:524–528, 1966.

Buchanan GR: Hemorrhagic diseases. In Nathan DG, Oski FA (eds): *Hematology of Infancy and Childhood* (2nd edition). Philadelphia: WB Saunders, 1981, p 119.

Hathaway WE: Coagulation problems in the newborn infant. *Pediatr Clin North Amer* 17:929–942, 1970.

Oski FA, Naiman JL: Hematologic problems in the newborn. In Oski FA, Naiman JL (eds): *Major Problems in Clinical Pediatrics* (3rd edition). Philadelphia: WB Saunders, 1982, vol IV, pp 137–174.

Review Article

Hathaway WE: The bleeding newborn. *Semin Hematol* 12:175–188, 1975.

CASE
6

PATIENT: 11- and 6-year-old brothers

CHIEF COMPLAINT: These patients were referred for evaluation of a probable hemostatic abnormality.

MEDICAL HISTORY: When 9 years of age, the older brother was seen for a bleeding problem after a dental extraction. He was subsequently hospitalized and received 2 units of whole blood and 1 unit of fresh-frozen plasma to control the hemorrhage. Despite the transfusions, he continued to have oozing from the extraction site for approximately 5 days. He was subsequently discharged and had no difficulty in the ensuing 2 years. He was an active boy and engaged in a number of sports, including basketball. The mother volunteered that he had difficulty with "bruising of the ankles." With this exception, he had no sports-related injuries.

The younger brother had a single episode of bleeding that occurred after he sustained a cut above the right eye at 2 years of age. This injury resulted from a fall against a corner of a living room table. At the time of the injury, the mother applied a pressure bandage, which controlled the bleeding. However, 5 days later, the boy was hospitalized and given 1 unit of whole blood because the wound had not healed properly and had started to hemorrhage after apparently healing.

FAMILY HISTORY: There were three other siblings, all sisters (7, 8 and 10 years of age). The sisters had no history of bleeding problems. There was a strong family history of bleeding on the maternal side, with male members being affected (see Figure 1, family tree). An uncle was hospitalized after an industrial accident. A portion of a grinding wheel fragmented and struck him in the right temple. During hospitalization, he required an operation for subdural hematoma. The patient died after the operation. A number of units of fresh-frozen plasma and Konyne had been administered.

DRUG HISTORY: No medication. Both patients had been instructed to avoid aspirin-containing compounds.

PHYSICAL EXAMINATION: A large cicatrix was noted above the right eye of the younger brother. Joint mobility was within normal limits in both patients.

Laboratory Results

A. Screening Procedures

	11-Year-Old Brother	6-Year-Old Brother	Normal
Prothrombin time	11 seconds	11 seconds	10–12 seconds
APTT	57 seconds	60 seconds	<42 seconds
Platelet count	190,000/μl	230,000/μl	130,000–400,000/μl
Bleeding time	7 minutes	5 minutes and 30 seconds	1–8 minutes

Questions

1. On the basis of the family history, what is the differential diagnosis?
2. Is the delayed bleeding in the younger brother unusual?

Laboratory Results

B. Confirmatory Procedures

	11-Year-Old Brother	6-Year-Old Brother	Normal
APTT (50% patient plasma/50% pooled normal plasma)	<40	4%	<42
Factor IX:C activity	3%	3%	50% to 150%
Factor IX antigen	16%	13%	50% to 150%

DIAGNOSIS: Hereditary deficiency of factor IX (hemophilia B), moderate

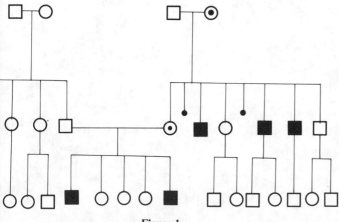

Figure 1

HEREDITARY DEFICIENCY OF FACTOR IX, MODERATE

CLINICAL PICTURE

PHYSICAL PROPERTIES OF FACTOR IX

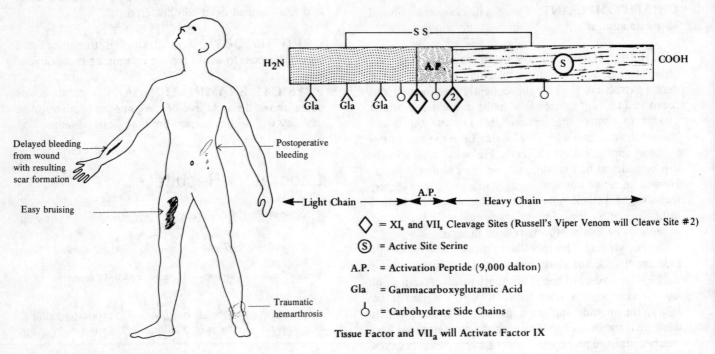

Delayed bleeding from wound with resulting scar formation

Easy bruising

Postoperative bleeding

Traumatic hemarthrosis

Pattern of inheritance: Sex-linked recessive

◆ Light Chain ◆ ——— A.P. ——— Heavy Chain ———→

◇ = XI$_a$ and VII$_a$ Cleavage Sites (Russell's Viper Venom will Cleave Site #2)

Ⓢ = Active Site Serine

A.P. = Activation Peptide (9,000 dalton)

Gla = Gammacarboxyglutamic Acid

○ = Carbohydrate Side Chains

Tissue Factor and VII$_a$ will Activate Factor IX

LABORATORY FINDINGS

A. Screening Procedures

Test	Patient's Result	Normal Range
Prothrombin time	Normal	10–12 seconds
APTT	Abnormal	<42 seconds
Platelet count	Normal	130,000–400,000/μl
Bleeding time	Normal	1–8 minutes

B. Confirmatory Procedures

Mixing APTT	Normal	<42 seconds
Factor IX:C activity	2% to 5%	50% to 150%
Factor IX antigen	Normal or abnormal	50% to 150%

TREATMENT

Non-life-threatening bleeding
   Fresh-frozen plasma
Life-threatening bleeding
   Konyne® or Proplex®

Discussion

These cases are examples of moderate deficiency of factor IX. They point out the consistency of factor assay results within a given kindred. In this instance, factor IX antigen levels were determined by radioimmunoassay. There was a slight discrepancy between factor IX antigen level and factor IX:C activity. However, it was not considered to be of sufficient degree to warrant the diagnosis of a cross-reacting material-positive variant of factor IX deficiency.

The maternal side of the family had a history of hemorrhagic problems. Of particular interest was the recent death of an uncle after an industrial accident.

One would wonder about the mother's description of "bruising of the ankles." Presumably, this complaint might signify discoloration over the ankles that was noticed by the mother. Most likely, it was the result of recurrent intraarticular hemorrhage associated with athletic activity.

The delayed bleeding noted in the younger brother is typical of hemophilia A and B. Because primary hemostasis is normal in both forms of hemophilia, platelet plugs would be expected to control immediate bleeding. However, because a primary hemostatic plug is not adequately stabilized by fibrin, hemorrhage secondary to minimal trauma to a site of injury is common. After the onset of secondary bleeding, it may be extremely difficult to stop localized bleeding. Therefore, fresh frozen plasma is often indicated in patients with a moderate deficiency of factor IX.

Bibliography

(See Bibliography for Case 4)

CASE
7

PATIENT: 18-year-old man

CHIEF COMPLAINT: This patient was referred from a small neighboring community. He had been evaluated by his family physician and was found to have weakness and loss of some sensation of the right leg. Because of the physical findings, he was referred to a neurosurgeon with a provisional diagnosis of femoral neuropathy.

MEDICAL HISTORY: The patient had not been hospitalized previously and could recall no bleeding problems. Before the onset of femoral neuropathy, the patient had fallen from a ladder while working on the family barn. He had fallen on his right buttock and right flank.

FAMILY HISTORY: An 82-year-old maternal grandfather had been told at one time that he had "hemophilia." This family member had never been hospitalized or adequately evaluated, however. Although elderly, the grandfather continued to work on his farm. The only apparent difficulty that he experienced was "swelling of the knees." To control the swelling, he wrapped each knee with Ace bandages before beginning his workday.

DRUG HISTORY: After the fall, the patient had taken aspirin on a daily basis for pain.

PHYSICAL EXAMINATION: There was some loss of sensation over the anterior and lateral aspects of the right thigh. In addition, there was weakness in flexing the right leg. A large ecchymosis was noted over the right buttock and the lateral aspect of the right hip. There was palpable firmness in this area suggestive of a deep hematoma.

Laboratory Results

Before performing a myelogram, the neurosurgeon ordered a series of screening tests.

A. Screening Procedures

	Patient	Normal
Prothrombin time	11.9 seconds	10–12 seconds
APTT	51 seconds	<42 seconds
Platelet count	330,000/µl	130,000–400,000/µl
Bleeding time	10 minutes and 15 seconds	1–8 minutes

Questions

1. What is the differential diagnosis?
2. Why is the bleeding time prolonged?
3. What caused the sudden onset of the right femoral neuropathy?

Laboratory Results

B. Confirmatory Procedures

	Patient	Normal
APTT (50% patient/50% pooled normal plasma	40 seconds	<42 seconds
Factor VIII:C activity	7.5%	50% to 150%
Factor VIII R:Ag	110%	50% to 150%
Factor VIII R:RCo	100%	50% to 150%

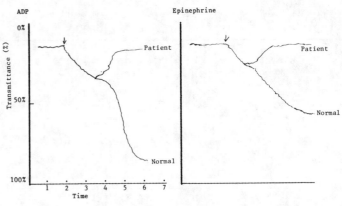

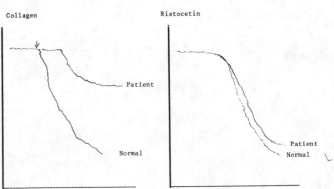

Figure 1. Platelet aggregation studies (Case 7).

HEREDITARY DEFICIENCY OF FACTOR VIII, MILD

CLINICAL PICTURE

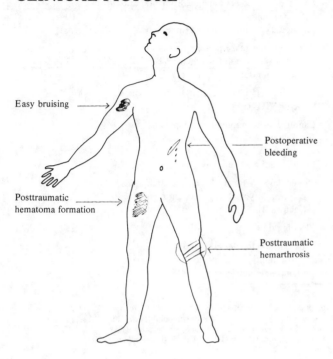

Easy bruising

Postoperative bleeding

Posttraumatic hematoma formation

Posttraumatic hemarthrosis

Pattern of inheritance: Sex-linked recessive

PHYSICAL PROPERTIES OF FACTOR VIII
See table, page 106.

LABORATORY FINDINGS

A. Screening Procedures

Test	Patient's Result	Normal Range
Prothrombin time	Normal	10–12 seconds
APTT	Abnormal	<42 seconds
Platelet count	Normal	130,000–400,000/μl
Bleeding time	Normal	1–8 minutes

B. Confirmatory Procedures

Mixing APTT	Normal	<42 seconds
Factor VIII:C activity	5% to 25%	50% to 150%
Factor VIII R:Ag	Normal	50% to 150%
FActor VIII R:RCo	Normal	50% to 150%

TREATMENT

1-Desamino-8-D-arginine vasopressin (DDAVP) may be useful in mild bleeding

Non-life-threatening bleeding:
    Cryoprecipitate

Central nervous system hemorrhage and severe bleeding:
    Factor VIII concentrates

ε-Aminocaproic acid (EACA) useful in dental surgery

Avoidance of aspirin containing compounds

Factor VIII Complex Noncovalently Bound

Property	Factor VIII:C	von Willebrand Factor
Site of production	?, Perhaps liver	Megakaryocytes and endothelial cells
Gene control	Sex chromosome	Autosome
Molecular weight	285,000 (range, 85,000–270,000)	Series of multimers ranging from 800,000 to 12,000,000 Individual multimers having three bands
Function in vivo	Secondary hemostasis (coagulation)	Primary hemostasis: platelet adhesion Carrier protein: stabilizes factor VIII:C Regulates production of factor VIII:C
Antigenic properties	Homologous or monoclonal antibodies to factor VIII:C:Ag	Heterologous or monoclonal antibodies to factor VIII R:Ag
Laboratory measurement of antigen	Radioimmunoassay or immunoradiometric assay	Laurell rocket immunoelectrophoresis Enzyme-linked immunosorbent assay Radioimmunoassay Immunoradiometric assay
Laboratory measurement of function	Factor VIII:C assay (modified APTT)	*Screening: ristocetin—platelet rich plasma confirmatory: ristocetin cofactor assay (factor VIII R:RCo)
Evaluation in vivo	—	Bleeding time
Evaluation of variants	Radioimmunoassay for factor VIII:C:Ag	Crossed immunoelectrophoresis Agarose multimer analysis Immunoradiometric assay (IRMA)

*Many people are confused about the interpretation of ristocetin induced platelet agglutination of platelet rich plasma. This procedure is a screening test and may be thought of as being analogous to the APTT in screening for a factor deficiency (e.g. VIII:C deficiency in hemophilia A). This procedure is a qualitative assay and should not be confused with the ristocetin cofactor assay which is quantitative. The ristocetin cofactor assay employs aliquots of the patient plasma which are added with ristocetin to lyophilized, washed, or formalin fixed platelets. The ristocetin cofactor activity (VIII R:RCo) is expressed as a percent of the activity found in pooled normal plasma.

Platelet aggregation studies were performed with adenosine diphosphate, epinephrine, collagen and ristocetin (see platelet aggregation tracings, Figure 1). The responses to adenosine diphosphate and epinephrine were markedly abnormal. There was a primary wave of aggregation in both instances, with an absence of a secondary wave. The response to collagen was also abnormal, with a prolonged lag phase occurring after collagen had been added to the patient's platelet-rich plasma and a 30% optical density change (control, 75% optical density change).

DIAGNOSIS: Hereditary deficiency of factor VIII (hemophilia A), mild; qualitative abnormality of platelets (secondary to ingestion of aspirin)

Discussion

This case illustrates a number of useful clinical points. The family history is equivocal, whereas that of the patient is totally negative. A thorough physical examination disclosed a hematoma over the right buttock, which raised the possibility that a hemostatic disorder might account for the clinical neuropathy. Consequently, screening tests were performed and yielded an abnormal APTT and bleeding time. These findings suggest a number of possible diagnoses, including von Willebrand's disease. Mixing studies suggested a factor deficiency. Therefore, a complete evaluation of the factor VIII molecule was undertaken, and platelet aggregation studies were performed. Factor VIII coagulant (VIII:C) activity was found to be decreased, whereas factor VIII ristocetin cofactor (VIII R:RCo) activity and the factor VIII-related antigen (VIII R:Ag) level were within normal limits. These laboratory results, together with the equivocal family history of a maternal grandfather with "hemophilia," establish the diagnosis of mild hemophilia A.

The abnormal platelet aggregation studies and the prolonged bleeding time can be explained by the recent ingestion of aspirin. Aspirin irreversibly acetylates the cyclooxygenase enzyme, resulting in inhibition of platelet function. Absence of the release reaction in the platelet aggregation studies is typical of platelets that have been exposed to aspirin. To evaluate platelet aggregation patterns adequately, it is necessary to have patients refrain from taking aspirin for at least 7 days before the studies are performed. This patient had ingested aspirin as recently as 3 days before evaluation. (For a list of aspirin-containing compounds, the reader is referred to Appendix A.)

Biochemical Aspects. Recent work indicates that factor VIII circulates in plasma as a complex of factor VIII:C activity and factor VIII:C:Ag as well as von Willebrand factor activity (factor VIII R:RCo and factor VIII R:Ag). Thus, the two entities are properties of the same macromolecule. Presumably, the complex is noncovalently bound (Table 1).

The two proteins may be physically separated by gel filtration at high ionic strength or in the presence of reducing agents or by use of chromatography with specific antibodies to the two components of the molecule. Hemophilia A in which the factor VIII coagulant protein is either absent or dysfunctional is transmitted by X chromosomal inheritance. On the other hand, quantitative and qualitative abnormalities of von Willebrand factor as seen in von Willebrand's disease are inherited in an autosomal manner.

The molecular weight of human factor VIII:C has been estimated to be 285,000. However, there are conflicting data in this area. Sodium dodecyl sulfate electrophoresis has indicated molecular weights ranging from 85,000 to 270,000. When exposed to thrombin, human factor VIII:C undergoes proteolytic degradation. Optimal exposure of factor VIII:C to thrombin increases the coagulant activity of this protein. However, prolonged exposure results in degradation of Factor VIII:C, with loss of activity. Antibodies to factor VIII:C inactivate the coagulant activity. These antibodies do not form precipitates with human von Willebrand factor, nor do they inactivate the platelet-aggregating activity of bovine factor VIII.

Table 1
Nomenclature of Factor VIII/ von Willebrand Factor

Factor VIII:C	Procoagulant activity: measured with factor VIII assay (modified APTT)
Factor VIII C:Ag	Factor VIII:C antigen; measured with homologous or monoclonal antibodies in immunoradiometric assay or radioimmunoassay
Factor VIII R:RCo	Ristocetin cofactor; activity necessary for ristocetin-induced platelet agglutination *in vitro*
Factor VIII R:Ag	Factor VIII-related antigen; reacts with heterologous antisera to factor VIII†; measured by rocket immunoelectrophoresis, radioimmunoassay or immunoradiometric assay
Factor VIII R:WF	von Willebrand factor; bleeding time factor; activity necessary for formation of in vivo platelet plug

Recently, the use of hybridoma monoclonal antibodies has permitted identification of a number of antigenic determinations on the factor VIII molecule.

The von Willebrand portion of the factor VIII molecule consists of a series of multimers that range in molecular weight from approximately 800,000 to 12,000,000. von Willebrand factor in plasma displays a marked degree of heterogeneity, as demonstrated by crossed immunoelectrophoresis. The asymmetrical pattern seen with crossed immunoelectrophoresis results from the different mobilities of multimers of different sizes (Figure 2). Small multimers migrate much more rapidly toward the anode, whereas large multimers are located in the cathodal portion of the precipitant arc. The recent introduction of sodim dodecyl sulfate agarose or agarose acrylamide has led to a more precise analysis of the multimeric composition of von Willebrand factor. After separation of the multimers in the agarose, the gels are reacted with an antibody to von Willebrand factor

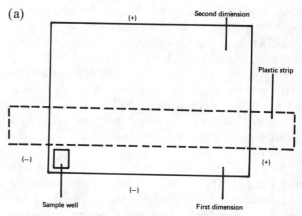

(a)

Crossed immunoelectrophoresis for factor VIII related antigen: juxtaposition of first and second dimensions on 3 X 5-in. microscopic slide.

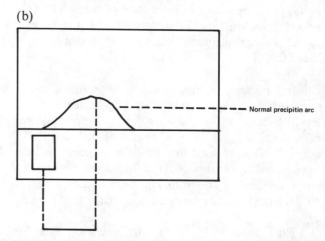

(b)

Figure 2. In the first dimension the factor VIII/von Willebrand multimers are separates according to size and electrical charge. In the second dimension the dispersed multimers are electrophorsed into an agarose that contains an antibody to factor VIII R:Ag. The broad precipitin arc indicates the heterogenicity of the multimers. If there was a homogeneous size distribution of multimers the precipitin arc would be very narrow, somewhat similar to the rockets formed in rocket immunoelectrophoresis. From Triplett DA, Harms CS: *Procedures for the Coagulation Laboratory.* Chicago: ASCP Press, 1981, pp 53, 55.

that has been labeled with ^{125}I. The gels are then developed by means of autoradiography.

Use of a discontinuous buffer system with 2% agarose has improved resolution of the multimers. This system has indicated that each multimer is composed of at least three bands. In normal plasma, the central band predominates.

The von Willebrand portion of the factor VIII complex has an important role in primary hemostasis. In a simplistic way, one may assume that this portion of the molecule is involved in "sticking" platelets to a site of injury. In the absence of this portion of the molecule, the bleeding time is prolonged. Absence of this portion also leads to the other manifestations of abnormal primary hemostasis that have been described in patients with von Willebrand's disease. The high-molecular-weight multimers are essential for this function.

von Willebrand factor is a glycoprotein. Several studies have suggested that the carbohydrate moiety plays an important part in the interaction between von Willebrand factor and platelets. In addition, carbohydrate residues apparently have an important role in the intravascular survival of von Willebrand factor. Removal of sialic acid from von Willebrand factor results in more rapid removal of this protein from plasma.

von Willebrand factor is produced in megakaryocytes and endothelial cells and is also found in alpha granules of platelets.

It is likely that von Willebrand factor serves as a "carrier protein" for factor VIII:C. In vitro, von Willebrand factor has a stabilizing effect on factor VIII:C. There is also experimental evidence that von Willebrand factor promotes production or release of factor VIII:C, although the exact site of production of factor VIII:C is as yet unknown. Studies performed with the porcine model of von Willebrand's disease suggest that the liver is the site of synthesis of factor VIII:C.

Clinical Picture. Hemophilia A is an X-linked recessive bleeding disorder that results from a decreased blood level of factor VIII:C (antihemophilic factor). As has been discussed previously, hemophilia A (deficiency of factor VIII) is at least four times more common than hemophilia B. Because of its X-linked mode of inheritance, the sons of an affected man are normal, whereas all daughters are obligatory carriers of the trait (Figure 3).

There appears to be a high mutation rate for hemophilia A; consequently, as many as one-third of affected persons have no family history of the disease. Female carriers of hemophilia A would be anticipated to have a factor VIII coagulant activity of approximately 50%; however, use of this test alone as a means of detecting the carrier state is fraught with difficulty. Factor VIII coagulant activity increases in response to a number of phenomena, including exercise, pregnancy

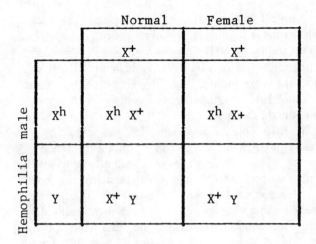

Figure 3. Inheritance pattern for hemophilia A and B.
X^+ = Normal X chromosome
Xh = Abnormal X chromosome
Y = Normal Y chromosome
$X^h\,X^+$ = Carrier female
$X^h\,Y$ = Affected male

and fever (Table 2). In addition to the biologic variables, there are important analytic variables that must be taken into consideration when the factor VIII:C assay is performed in a laboratory. Consequently, the use of factor VIII R:Ag as a means of assisting in the detection of carriers has proved extremely helpful. Because factor VIII R:Ag is controlled by an autosomal chromosome, one would expect the level of this antigen to be normal in carriers and in affected male patients with hemophilia A. Thus, the ratio of factor VIII R:Ag to factor VIII:C should be approximately 2:1 in the carrier state. Physiologic and pathologic situations that may elevate the level of factor VIII:C also proportionally elevate the

Table 2
Elevation of Factor VIII Activity

Transient	Permanent
Exercise	Age
Fever	Males > females
Surgical procedures	Blood group A
Oral contraceptive use	Diabetes mellitus
Pregnancy	Coronary artery disease
Corticosteroid administration	Postmenopausal
Hyperthyroidism	
Cushing's syndrome	
Uremia	
Coumarin (indanedione drug) administration	
Venous congestion	

level of factor VIII R:Ag, thus maintaining this ratio (Table 2).

The clinical severity of bleeding in hemophilia may be predicted from the level of factor VIII:C. Persons who have less than 1% of factor VIII:C have spontaneous hemorrhage into the major muscle masses (thighs, biceps, retroperitoneal) as well as into joint spaces. A classification of hemophilia A according to factor assay results is given in Table 3. Persons who have mild hemophilia usually have hemorrhage secondary to trauma or surgical intervention. Such cases often are not diagnosed until adult life.

In addition to recurrent hemorrhage, persons with both hemophilia A and B often have easy bruisability and a number of other clinical complications. Such complications include chronic liver disease secondary to exposure to hepatitis viruses, development of specific antibodies to factor VIII:C and, more recently, the appearance of acquired immune deficiency syndrome (AIDS). AIDS is characterized by recurrent infections, such as those caused by *Pneumocystis carinii* and atypical mycobacteria. Persons who have AIDS often exhibit generalized lymphadenopathy with hepatosplenomegaly. Recently, an immunologic thrombocytopenia has been described in such persons. Mortality of persons with AIDS has been estimated to be 70%. In addition to infection, affected persons may also suffer from lymphoproliferative disorders and Kaposi's sarcoma.

Treatment. Replacement therapy for severe hemophilia A consists of factor VIII concentrates. Patients who have mild or moderate hemophilia A usually can be treated satisfactorily with cryoprecipitate. The association of AIDS with the use of factor VIII concentrates has prompted some authors to suggest that all patients with hemophilia A should be treated with cryoprecipitate until the etiologic agent of AIDS has been identified.

Arbitrarily, the amount of factor VIII activity in 1 ml of normal plasma is accepted as one unit. The half-life of factor VIII is between 8 and 12 hours; initially, the level declines rapidly due to diffusion into extravascular spaces. The minimal hemostatic level for mild hemorrhage is 30% (0.30 units per milliliter of plasma). In patients with major hemorrhagic lesions, the level of factor VIII:C must be maintained at 50% or higher. In patients with life-threatening lesions and in those undergoing operation, the level must be maintained at 80% to 100%. A simple and reproducible dosage calculation can be made by assuming that each unit of factor VIII that is infused per kilogram of body weight will raise the level of factor VIII:C by 2%.

For monitoring therapy, the factor VIII:C assay is the procedure of choice. Clinicians should not use the APTT or another screening test in place of the factor VIII:C assay because the results may be extremely misleading.

Table 3
Clinical Classification of Hemophilia*

Severity	Factor VIII Activity	Clinical Picture	Activated Partial Thromboplastin Time
Severe	<1%	Severe hemarthrosis and spontaneous bleeding	Prolonged
Moderate	1% to 5%	Spontaneous bleeding uncommon; serious bleeding from minimal trauma	Prolonged
Mild	5% to 25%	Spontaneous bleeding rare; unsuspected bleeding after surgical intervention or trauma	Variable
Subclinical	25% to 50%	Diagnosis frequently missed; moderate bleeding after trauma or surgical intervention	Usually normal

*Modified from Wintrobe MM, et al: Clinical Hematology 8th ed. Philadelphia: Lea Febiger, 1981, p 1162.

To prevent the complications of recurrent hemarthrosis, the self-therapy, or home care, program has been introduced. Patients and their families receive instruction concerning the administration of factor VIII concentrates (or cryoprecipitate). Once this technique has been mastered, patients are allowed to administer the concentrates at home, thus eliminating visits to the emergency room for evaluation and treatment. Of course, patients are carefully instructed to refrain from taking aspirin and aspirin-containing compounds. Because aspirin inhibits platelet function, use of aspirin for its analgesic effect would only promote bleeding in patients with hemophilia A or B (Table 4). Acetaminophen is a suitable alternative.

DDAVP has been used to treat patients with mild and moderate hemophilia A and von Willebrand's disease. The mechanism of action for DDAVP is at present poorly understood. It may be administered either intravenously or intranasally.

Amicar® is also frequently used as adjunctive therapy in patients with mild and moderate hemophilia A who are undergoing dental procedures.

Table 4
Drugs to Avoid in Patients
with Hemophilia

Analgesics

  Aspirin

  Aspirin-containing compounds (see appendix A)

    Bufferin

    Anacin

    Alka Seltzer

    Darvon (propoxyphene hydrochloride)

    APC (acetylsalicylic acid, phenacetin, caffeine) in tablet form

Antihistamines

  Periactin (cyproheptadine hydrochloride)

  Chlor-Trimeton (chlorpheniramine maleate)

Cough Syrup

  Robitussin (glycerol guaiacholate ether)

Antiinflammatory Agent

  Butazolidin (phenylbutazone)

Bibliography

Clinical Picture

Aggeler PM, Hoag MS, Wallerstein RD: The mild hemophilias: Occult deficiencies of AHF, PTC and PTA frequency responsible for unexpected surgical bleeding. *Amer J Med* 30:84–94, 1961.

Birch CLaF: *Hemophilia, Clinical and Genetic Aspects*. Urbana, Illinois: University of Illinois, 1937.

Bowie EJW, Owen CA: Recognition of easily missed bleeding diseases. *Mayo Clin Proc* 57:263–264, 1982.

Buchanan GR: Hemophilia. *Pediatr Clin North Amer* 27:309–326, 1980.

Graham JB, Barrow ES, Elston RC: Carrier detection in hemophilia. (Abstract) *Amer J Hum Genet* 25:30, 1973.

Green D: Hemophilia and von Willebrand's disease: Genetic considerations. *Ann Clin Lab Sci* 10(2):123–127, 1980.

Helske T, Ikkala E, Myllyla G, et al: Joint involvement in patients with severe hemophilia A in 1957–59 and 1978–79. *Brit J Haematol* 51:643–647, 1982.

Hoyer LW, Carta CA, Mahoney MJ: Detection of hemophilia carriers during pregnancy. *Blood* 60:1407–1410, 1982.

Ikkala E, Helske T, Myllyla G, et al: Changes in the life expectancy of patients with severe hemophilia A in Finland 1930–1979. *Brit J Haematol* 52:7–12, 1982.

Kerr CV: Inheritance of factor VIII. *Thromb Diath Haemorrh Suppl* 17:173–XXX, 1965.

Kitchens CS: Occult hemophilia. *John Hopkins Med J* 146:255–259, 1980.

Nemerson Y, Zur M: Is hemophilia A disease the tissue factor pathway of coagulation? In Menache D, Surgenor DMacN, Anderson H (eds): *Hemophilia and Hemostasis*. New York: Alan R. Liss, 1981, pp 77–83.

Laboratory Measurement of Various Components of Factor VIII

Bartlett A, Dormandy KM, Hawkey CM, et al: Factor VIII-related antigen: Measurement by enzyme immunoassay. *Brit Med J* 1:994–996, 1976.

Bowie EJW, Fass DN: Factor VIII related antigen (VIII R:Ag) in hemophilia patients and in carriers. *Lancet* 2:1049–1050, 1979.

Cejka J: Enzyme immunoassay for factor VIII-related antigen. *Clin Chem* 28:1356–1358, 1982.

Crane LJ: Kinetic latex agglutinometry II: A rapid, quantitative assay for factor VIII antigen. *Clin Chem* 27:697–700, 1981.

Fishman DJ, Jones PK, Menitove JE, et al: Detection of the carrier state for classic hemophilia using an enzyme-linked immunosorbant assay (ELISA). *Blood* 59:1163–1168, 1982.

Fulcher CA, Ruggeri ZM, Zimmerman TS: Isoelectric focusing of factor VIII/von Willebrand factor in urea agarose gels. (Abstract) *Circulation* 62:170, 1980.

Furlong RA, Peake IR: Studies on the stability of factor VIII coagulant antigen (VIII:CAg) in the presence of VIII:C antibodies. *Brit J Haematol* 53:55–63, 1983.

Furlong RA, Peake IR, Blood AL: Factor VIII clotting antigen (VIII:CAg) in haemophilia measured by two immunoradiometric assays (IRMA) using different antibodies, and the measurement of inhibitors to procoagulant factor VIII (VIII:C) by IRMA. *Brit J Haematol* 48:643–650, 1981.

Gralnick HR, Coller BS, Sultan Y: Studies of the human factor VIII/von Willebrand factor protein. *J Clin Invest* 56:814–827, 1975.

Hoyer LW, Breckenridge RT: Immunologic studies of anti-hemophilic factor (AHF factor VIII): Cross reacting material in a genetic variant of hemophilia A. *Blood* 32:962–971, 1968.

Langdell RD, Wagner RH, Brinkhous KM: Effect of antihemophilic factor on one-stage clotting tests: A presumptive test for hemophilia and a simple one-stage antihemophilic factor assay procedure. *J Lab Clin Med* 41:637–639, 1953.

Lazardrick J, Hoyer LW: Immunoradiometric measurement of factor VIII procoagulant antigen. *J Clin Invest* 62:1048–1052, 1978.

Muller HP, van Tilburg NH, Bertina RM, et al: Immunoradiometric assay of procoagulant factor VIII antigen (VIII:CAg). *Clin Chim Acta* 107:11–19, 1980.

Reisner HM, Barrow ES, Graham JB: Radioimmunoassay for coagulant factor VIII related antigen (VIII:CAg). *Thromb Res* 14(1):235–239, 1979.

Rick ME: Activation of factor VIII by factor IXa. *Blood* 60:744–751, 1982.

Peake IR, Newcombe RG, Davies BL, et al: Carrier detection of haemophilia A by immunological measurement of factor VIII related antigen (VIII R:Ag) and factor VIII clotting antigen (VIII:CAg). *Brit J Haematol* 48:651–660, 1981.

Yorde LD, Hussey VC, Yorde DE, et al: Competitive enzyme linked immunoassay for factor VIII antigen. *Clin Chem* 25:1924–1927, 1979.

Variation in Factor VIII Level

Bennett B, Oxford SC, Douglas AS, et al: Studies on antihemophilic factor (AHF, factor VIII) during labor in normal women, in patients with premature separation of the placenta, and in a patient with von Willebrand's disease. *J Lab Clin Med* 84:851–860, 1974.

Bennett B, Ratnoff OD: Changes in antihemophilic factor (AHF, factor VIII) procoagulant activity and AHF antigen in normal pregnancy and following exercise and pneumoencephalography. *J Lab Clin Med* 80:256–263, 1972.

Crowell EB, Clatanoff DU, Kiekhofer W: The effect of oral contraceptives on factor VIII levels. *J Lab Clin Med* 77:551–557, 1971.

Gader AMA: The potentiating effect of cortisone (prednisolone) on the fibrinolytic and clotting factor VIII responses to intravenous infusion of adrenaline in man. *Haemostasis* 12:353–356, 1982.

Ingram GIC: Increase in antihaemophilic globulin activity following infusion of adrenaline. *J Physiol (London)* 156:217–219, 1961.

Kasper CK, Hoag MS, Aggeler PM, et al: Blood clotting factors in pregnancy: Factor VIII concentration in normal and AHF deficient woman. *Obstet Gynecol* 24:242–247, 1964.

Ludlam CA, Peake IR, Allen N, et al: Factor VIII and fibrinolytic response to deamino-8-D arginine vasopressin in normal subjects and dissociate response in some patients with haemophilia and von Willebrand's disease. *Brit J Haematol* 45:499–511, 1980.

Maisonneuve P, Sultan Y: Modification of factor VIII complex properties in patients with liver disease. *J Clin Pathol* 30:221–227, 1977.

Mannucci PM, Ruggeri AM, Gagnatelli G: Nervous regulation of factor VIII levels in man. *Brit J Haematol* 20:195–207, 1971.

Schiffman S, Rapaport SI: Increased factor VIII levels in suspected carriers of hemophilia A taking contraceptives by mouth. *N Engl J Med* 275:599–603, 1966.

Strauss HS, Diamond LK: Elevation of factor VIII (antihemophilic factor) during pregnancy in normal persons and in a patient with von Willebrand's disease. *N Engl J Med* 269:1251–1254, 1963.

Treatment

Aledort LM: The availability of plasma products and the care of hemophilia patients. *J Amer Med Ass* 246:157, 1981.

Biggs R: Thirty years of haemophilia treatment at Oxford. *Brit J Haematol* 13:452–463, 1967.

Hilgartner MW: Factor replacement therapy. In Hilgartner MW (ed): *Hemophilia in the Child and Adult*. New York: Masson Publishing, 1982, pp 63–84.

Review Articles

Aledort LM: Current concepts in diagnosis and management of hemophilia. *Hosp Pract* 17(10):77–92, 1982.

Bloom AL: Factor VIII: New clinical and genetic aspects. *Schweiz Med Wochenschr* 109:1357–1361, 1979.

Boxer GJ: Hemophilia. *J Indiana State Med Ass* 70:573–580, 1977.

Rick ME, Hoyer LW: The molecular structure of factor VIII and IX. In Hilgartner MW (ed): *Hemophilia in the Child and Adult*. New York: Masson Publishing, 1982, pp 1–28.

Acquired Immune Deficiency Syndrome

Bussel J, Welte C, Fitzgerald P, et al: Defective cellular immunity in homosexual hemophiliacs: Correction in vitro with interleukin 2. (Abstract) *Blood* 60(Suppl):209a, 1982.

Davis KC, Horsburgh CR, Hasiba U, et al: Acquired immunodeficiency syndrome in a patient with hemophilia. *Ann Intern Med* 98:284–286, 1983.

DesForges JF: AIDS and preventive treatment. (Editorial) *Hemophilia* 308:94–95, 1983.

Ehrenkranz NJ, Rubini J, Gunn R, et al: CDC. Pneumocystis carinii pneumonia among persons with hemophilia A. *Morbid Mortal Weekly Rep* 31:365–367, 1982.

Elliott JL, Hoppes WL, Platt MS, et al: The acquired immunodeficiency syndrome and Mycobacterium avium intracellular bacteremia in a patient with hemophilia. *Ann Intern Med* 98:290–293, 1983.

Goldsmith JC, Moseley PL, Monick M, et al: T-lymphocyte subpopulation abnormalities in apparently healthy patients with hemophilia. *Ann Intern Med* 98:294–296, 1983.

Lederman MM, Ratnoff OD, Scillian JJ, et al: Impaired cell mediated immunity in patients with classic hemophilia. *N Engl J Med* 308:79–83, 1983.

Luban NLC, Kelleher JF, Reaman GH: Altered distribution of T-lymphocyte subpopulations in children and adolescents with haemophilia. *Lancet* 1:503–505, 1983.

Menitove JE, Aster RH, Casper TJ, et al: T-lymphocyte subpopulations in patients with classic hemophilia treated with cryoprecipitate and lyophilized concentrates. *N Engl J Med* 308:83–86, 1983.

Ragni M, Lewis J, Spero JA, et al: Acquired immunodeficiency like syndrome in two haemophiliacs. *Lancet* 1:213–214, 1983.

Ratnoff OD, Menitove JE, Aster RH, et al: Coincident classic hemophilia and "idiopathic" thrombocytopenic purpura in patients under treatment with concentrates of antihemophilic factor (factor VIII). *N Engl J Med* 308:439–442, 1983.

Small CB, Klein RS, Friedland GH, et al: Community-acquired opportunistic infections and defective cellular immunity in heterosexual drug abusers and homosexual men. *Amer J Med* 74:433–441, 1983.

White GC, Lesesne HR: Hemophilia, hepatitis, and the acquired immunodeficiency syndrome. (Editorial) *Ann Intern Med* 98:403–404, 1983.

CASE 8

PATIENT: 32-year-old man

CHIEF COMPLAINT: This patient was a construction worker who had fallen while working on the basement of a new home. He presented to the emergency room with a swollen, tender left knee. An emergency room intern saw the patient and aspirated the left knee. The aspirate was "bloody."

MEDICAL HISTORY: The patient had a lifelong history of easy bruising that occasionally occurred spontaneously. In addition, he had a history of bleeding after dental extractions on several occasions. However, the patient was unable to provide detailed information regarding the quantity of blood loss after the dental procedures. The patient had not previously received transfusions or been hospitalized.

FAMILY HISTORY: There was no family history of bleeding problems.

DRUG HISTORY: The patient was taking no medication at the time of the accident.

PHYSICAL EXAMINATION: There was a swollen, tender left knee.

Laboratory Results

A. Screening Procedures

	Patient	Normal
Prothrombin time	12 seconds	10–12 seconds
APTT	60 seconds	<42 seconds
Platelet count	560,000/μl	200–450,000/μl
Bleeding time	7 minutes and 45 seconds	1–8 minutes

Questions

1. What is the differential diagnosis?
2. What additional laboratory procedures are indicated?
3. Why is the platelet count elevated?

Laboratory Results

B. Confirmatory Procedures

	Patient	Normal
APTT (50% patient plasma/50% pooled normal plasma)	40 seconds	<42 seconds
Factor VIII:C	20%	50% to 150%
Factor VIII R:Ag	118%	50% to 150%
Factor VIII R:RCo	110%	50% to 150%

DIAGNOSIS: Hereditary deficiency of factor VIII (hemophilia A), mild

Discussion

This case is an example of mild hemophilia A at a late stage in life. Many authors have emphasized that hemophilia is not necessarily a disease limited to the pediatric age group. Mild or moderate hemophilia A or B often is diagnosed during early adulthood but occasionally is encountered in later life. Such cases represent diagnostic problems for primary care physicians as well as specialists. In many instances, the diagnosis is entertained only after serious hemorrhage has occurred in response to trauma or surgical intervention. In this patient, the bloody aspirate from the knee raised the possibility of a hemostatic abnormality. Results of screening procedures included a slightly prolonged APTT and normal bleeding and prothrombin times.

Mixing studies ruled out the possibility of a circulating anticoagulant. The specific assay for factor VIII:C revealed an activity compatible with a diagnosis of mild hemophilia A. This diagnosis was confirmed by normal results in assays for factor VIII R:Ag and factor VIII R:RCo. The elevated platelet count, which was noted when the patient was seen in the emergency room, illustrates the rapid response of the platelet count to acute hemorrhage. In addition, elevated platelet counts are seen in some patients who have iron deficiency anemia, an underlying myeloproliferative disorder or an underlying disseminated malignant disease.

This case also emphasizes another important clinical point. Approximately one-third of persons with hemophilia A or B have no family history of the disease.

HEREDITARY DEFICIENCY OF FACTOR VIII, MILD

CLINICAL PICTURE

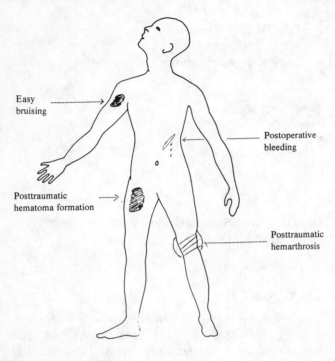

Easy bruising

Postoperative bleeding

Posttraumatic hematoma formation

Posttraumatic hemarthrosis

Pattern of inheritance: Sex-linked recessive

PHYSICAL PROPERTIES OF FACTOR VIII
See table, page 115.

LABORATORY FINDINGS

A. Screening Procedures

Test	Patient's Result	Normal Range
Prothrombin time	Normal	10–12 seconds
APTT	Abnormal	<42 seconds
Platelet count	Normal	130,000–400,000/μl
Bleeding time	Normal	1–8 minutes

B. Confirmatory Procedures

Mixing APTT	Normal	<42 seconds
Factor VIII:C	5% to 25%	50% to 150%
Factor VIII R:Ag	Normal	50% to 150%
Factor VIII R:RCo	Normal	50% to 150%

TREATMENT

Non-life-threatening bleeding
1-Desamino-8-D-arginine vasopressin (DDAVP)
   Cryoprecipitate
Central nervous system hemorrhage and severe bleeding
   Factor VIII concentrates
ε-Aminocaproic acid (EACA) useful in dental surgery
Avoidance of aspirin containing compounds

Factor VIII Complex

Property	Factor VIII:C	von Willebrand Factor
Site of production	?, Perhaps liver	Megakaryocytes and endothelial cells
Gene control	Sex chromosome	Autosome
Molecular weight	285,000 (range, 85,000–270,000)	Series of multimers ranging from 800,000 to 12,000,000 Individual multimers having three bands
Function in vivo	Secondary hemostasis (coagulation)	Primary hemostasis: platelet adhesion Carrier protein: stabilizes factor VIII:C Regulates production of factor VIII:C
Antigenic properties	Homologous or factor monoclonal antibodies to factor VIII:C:Ag	Heterologous or monoclonal antibodies to factor VIII R:Ag
Laboratory measurement of antigen	Radioimmunoassay or immunoradiometric assay	Laurell rocket immunoelectrophoresis Enzyme-linked immunosorbent assay Radioimmunoassay Immunoradiometric assay
Laboratory measurement of function	Factor VIII:C assay (modified APTT)	Screening: ristocetin + platelet rich plasma Confirmatory: ristocetin cofactor assay (factor VIII R:RCo)
Evaluation in vivo	—	Bleeding time
Evaluation of variants	Radioimmunoassay for factor VIII:C:Ag	Crossed immunoelectrophoresis Agarose multimer analysis Immunoradiometric assay

Bibliography

(See Bibliography for Case 7)

CASE
9

PATIENT: 7-day-old boy

CHIEF COMPLAINT: This patient was referred for evaluation of a possible hereditary hemostatic abnormality. On the second day after delivery, the patient was circumcised; he bled for 4 days. The bleeding eventually subsided without specific treatment. At that time, he was also noted to have several bruises over the trunk and arms.

MEDICAL HISTORY: This newborn infant was a product of an uneventful 9-month gestation. The mother was 18 years old and primagravida.

FAMILY HISTORY: A maternal uncle was diagnosed as having hemophilia A in 1968. At that time, the uncle was 18 months of age and was admitted with a hematoma of the left cheek and eyelid. The hematoma had resulted from a fall. On admission, his laboratory values included an activated partial thromboplastin time (APTT) of 88 seconds (normal, <42 seconds). Factor VIII:C activity was less than 1% (normal, 50% to 150%). He was treated with cryoprecipitate and subsequently discharged. However, he continued to have frequent episodes of bleeding and required factor VIII concentrates approximately twice each month.

Another maternal uncle apparently had no bleeding problems.

DRUG HISTORY: No medication

PHYSICAL EXAMINATION: Bruises were noted over the trunk and arms.

Laboratory Results

A. Screening Procedures

	Patient	Normal
Prothrombin time	12 seconds	10–12 seconds
APTT	111 seconds	<42 seconds
Platelet count	210,000/μl	200,000–450,000/μl
Bleeding time	Not performed	1–8 minutes

Questions

1. Is it common for patients with classical hemophilia A to bleed at the time of circumcision?

2. What is the most likely diagnosis?
3. If this patient bleeds, what would be the treatment of choice?
4. Should this patient be considered for home therapy at a later date?

Laboratory Results

B. Confirmatory Procedures

	Patient	Normal
APTT (50% patient plasma/50% pooled normal plasma	41 seconds	<42 seconds
Factor VIII:C	<1%	50% to 150%
Factor VIII R:Ag	80%	50% to 150%
Factor VIII R:RCo	76%	50% to 150%

DIAGNOSIS: Hereditary deficiency of factor VIII (hemophilia A), severe

Discussion

This case is an example of severe hemophilia A. The family history revealed that severe hemophilia A had been diagnosed in a maternal uncle in 1968. This case illustrates the consistency of factor VIII:C activity in a given family. The mother was subsequently evaluated and was found to be a carrier of hemophilia A (factor VIII:C, 19%; factor VIII R:Ag, 80%; factor VIII R:RCo 75%).

If this patient required treatment, cryoprecipitate would be the treatment of choice. Administration of cryoprecipitate is accompanied by a low risk for the development of hepatitis as a complication, and this treatment should be given until the patient can be vaccinated for hepatitis B. After vaccination, the patient could be treated with factor VIII concentrates. It is anticipated that a new heat treatment processing step will make hepatitis-free factor VIII concentrates available in the near future. However, recent cases of acquired immune deficiency syndrome (AIDS) in patients with hemophilia cloud the use of factor VIII concentrates. Until the etiologic agent (agents?) responsible for AIDS is identified, factor VIII concentrates should be used with caution.

HEREDITARY DEFICIENCY OF FACTOR VIII, SEVERE

CLINICAL PICTURE

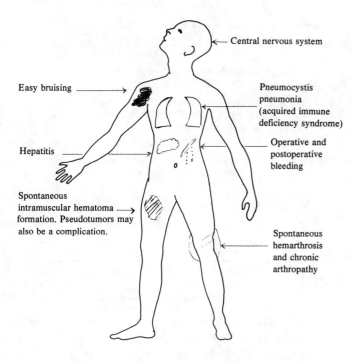

- Central nervous system
- Easy bruising
- Pneumocystis pneumonia (acquired immune deficiency syndrome)
- Hepatitis
- Operative and postoperative bleeding
- Spontaneous intramuscular hematoma formation. Pseudotumors may also be a complication.
- Spontaneous hemarthrosis and chronic arthropathy

Pattern of inheritance: Sex-linked recessive

PHYSICAL PROPERTIES OF FACTOR VIII
See table, page 118.

LABORATORY FINDINGS

A. Screening Procedures

Test	Patient's Result	Normal Range
Prothrombin time	Normal	10–12 seconds
APTT	Abnormal	<42 seconds
Platelet count	Normal	130,000–400,000/μl
Bleeding time	Normal	1–8 minutes

B. Confirmatory Procedures

Mixing APTT	Normal	<42 seconds
Factor VIII:C	<1%	50% to 150%
Factor VIII R:Ag	100%	50% to 150%
Factor VIII R:RCo	Normal	50% to 150%

TREATMENT

Factor VIII concentrates and cryoprecipitate
Avoidance of aspirin-containing drugs
Appropriate multidisciplinary support care (e.g., dentistry, orthopedics)

Factor VIII Complex

Property	Factor VIII:C	von Willebrand Factor
Site of production	?, Perhaps liver	Megakaryocytes and endothelial cells
Gene control	Sex chromosome	Autosome
Molecular weight	285,000 (range, 85,000–270,000)	Series of multimers varying from 800,000 to 12,000,000 Individual multimers having three bands
Function in vivo	Secondary hemostasis (coagulation)	Primary hemostasis: platelet adhesion Carrier protein: stabilizes factor VIII:C Regulates production of factor VIII:C
Antigenic properties	Homologous or monoclonal antibodies to factor VIII:C:Ag	Heterologous or monoclonal antibodies to factor VIII R:Ag
Laboratory measurement of antigen	Radioimmunoassay or immunoradiometric assay	Laurell rocket immunoelectrophoresis Enzyme-linked immunosorbent assay Radioimmunoassay Immunoradiometric assay
Laboratory measurement of function	Factor VIII:C assay (modified APTT)	Screening: ristocetin + platelet rich plasma Confirmatory: ristocetin cofactor assay (factor VIII R:RCo)
Evaluation in vivo	—	Bleeding time
Evaluation of variants	Radioimmunoassay for factor VIII:C:Ag	Crossed immunoelectrophoresis Agarose multimer analysis Immunoradiometric assay

Although this patient bled at the time of circumcision, it is not uncommon for children with a severe deficiency of factor VIII or IX to undergo circumcision without bleeding. Typically, children with severe hemophilia manifest easy bruising during the first 6 months of life and some bleeding associated with teething. The deficiency often is first diagnosed at the time an affected child begins to walk. As a consequence of falls, the child may be brought to a hospital with a large hematoma of the tongue or, occasionally, of the head. At that time, simple screening studies readily establish the diagnosis.

Bibliography

Perinatal Factor VIII

Fukui H, Takase T, Ikari H, et al: Factor VIII procoagulant activity, factor VIII related antigen and von Willebrand factor in newborn cord blood. *Brit J Haematol* 42:637–641, 1979.

Henriksson P, Holmberg L: Factor VIII activity and antigen in sick newborns with pathological proteolysis in blood. *Acta Paediatr Scand* 67:83–87, 1978.

Reference Books

Green D: *Hemophilia*. Springfield, Illinois: Charles C Thomas, 1973.

Hathaway WE, Bonnar J: *Perinatal Coagulation*. New York: Grune & Stratton, 1978.

Hilgartner MW (ed): *Hemophilia in the Child and the Adult*. New York: Masson Publishing, 1982.

CASE
10

PATIENT: 50-year-old man

CHIEF COMPLAINT: This patient was admitted with symmetric swelling of the upper aspect of the right thigh, with tenderness, induration and acute discoloration of the overlying skin. The swelling had appeared spontaneously.

MEDICAL HISTORY: During his childhood in Cincinnati, Ohio, the patient was diagnosed as having severe hemophilia A. He had a history of numerous episodes of bleeding into the knees, ankles and elbows. He had been hospitalized on a number of occasions in Cincinnati and several other communities. Because of recurrent hemarthrosis with destruction of the knee joints, the patient had been confined to a wheelchair.

FAMILY HISTORY: A number of male relatives (uncles and cousins) on the maternal side of the family had been diagnosed as having hemophilia A.

DRUG HISTORY: The patient had taken Talwin (pentazocine) for pain before admission.

PHYSICAL EXAMINATION: In addition to the swelling noted in the upper portion of the right thigh, both knees were noted to be deformed as a result of multiple hemarthroses and destruction of cartilage. There was also limitation of motion of the ankles and elbows. The liver was slightly palpable approximately two fingerbreadths below the right costal margin. The patient was noted to be pale and somewhat dyspneic.

Laboratory Results

A. Screening Procedures

	Patient	Normal
Prothrombin time	12 seconds	10–12 seconds
APTT	131 seconds	<42 seconds
Platelet count	480,000/µl	200,000–450,000/µl
Bleeding time	6 minutes and 30 seconds	1–8 minutes
Hemoglobin level	5.8 g/dl	14–18 g/dl

HOSPITAL COURSE: After admission, the patient received 4 units of packed red cells, which elevated the hemoglobin level to 11 g/dl. In addition, he received 24 units of cryoprecipitate over a course of 4 days (6 units per day). The activated partial thromboplastin time (APTT) did not respond to this replacement therapy; the lowest value for the APTT (88 seconds) was obtained on the second hospital day. Therefore, the patient received factor VIII concentrates, which were again unsuccessful in shortening the APTT. Factor VIII:C activity measured 2 hours after infusion of the factor VIII concentrates was less than 1%.

Questions

1. Why did the patient not respond to factor VIII replacement therapy?
2. What additional laboratory procedures are indicated?
3. What therapeutic modalities should be considered?

Laboratory Results

B. Confirmatory Procedures

	Patient	Normal
APTT (50% patient/ 50% pooled normal plasma)	100 seconds	<42 seconds

A screening procedure for circulating anticoagulants was performed:

APTT (patient plasma/ pooled normal plasma)	15-Minute Incubation	30-Minute Incubation	60-Minute Incubation
9:1	89 seconds	91 seconds	93 seconds
5:5	85 seconds	88 seconds	93 seconds
1:9	52 seconds	59 seconds	74 seconds

An appropriate series of controls was also performed. It included mixtures of 9 parts of pooled normal plasma to 1 part of buffer, 5 parts of pooled normal plasma to 5 parts of buffer and 1 part of pooled normal plasma to 9 parts of buffer.

	Patient	Normal
Factor VIII:C*	<1%	50% to 150%
Bethesda assay	250 units	<1 unit

DIAGNOSIS: Hereditary deficiency of factor VIII (hemophilia A), severe with factor VIII inhibitor

One hour after infusion of factor VIII concentrates.

HEREDITARY DEFICIENCY OF FACTOR VIII, SEVERE, WITH FACTOR VIII INHIBITOR

CLINICAL PICTURE

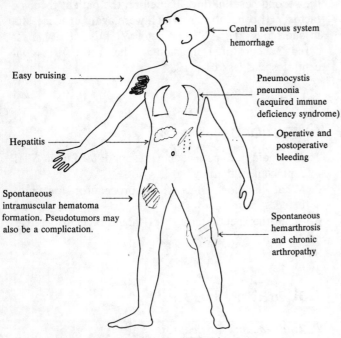

Central nervous system hemorrhage

Easy bruising

Pneumocystis pneumonia (acquired immune deficiency syndrome)

Hepatitis

Operative and postoperative bleeding

Spontaneous intramuscular hematoma formation. Pseudotumors may also be a complication.

Spontaneous hemarthrosis and chronic arthropathy

Bleeding episodes not responsive to factor VIII replacement

Pattern of inheritance: Sex-linked recessive

PHYSICAL PROPERTIES OF FACTOR VIII
See table, page 121.

LABORATORY FINDINGS

A. Screening Procedures

Test	Patient's Result	Normal Range
Prothrombin time	Normal	10–12 seconds
APTT	Abnormal	<42 seconds
Platelet count	Normal	130,000–400,000/μl
Bleeding time	Normal	1–8 minutes

B. Confirmatory Procedures

Mixing APTT	Abnormal	<42 seconds
Factor VIII:C	<1%	50% to 150%
Bethesda assay	Inhibitor present	Inhibitor absent

TREATMENT

Depends on nature of inhibitor (i.e., high or low responder)
Low responder: factor VIII concentrates
High responder:
    Prothrombin complex concentrates (activated Autoplex, FEIBA)
    Plasmapheresis may be helpful in acute bleeding
    Porcine factor VIII:C concentrates
    Immunosuppressive agents (rarely useful)
    Massive doses of factor VIII concentrates

Factor VIII Complex

Property	Factor VIII:C	von Willebrand Factor
Site of production	?, Perhaps liver	Megakaryocytes and endothelial cells
Gene control	Sex chromosome	Autosome
Molecular weight	285,000 (range, 85,000–270,000)	Series of multimers varying from 800,000 to 12,000,000 Individual multimers having three bands
Function in vivo	Secondary hemostasis (coagulation)	Primary hemostasis: platelet adhesion Carrier protein: stabilizes factor VIII:C Regulates production of factor VIII:C
Antigenic properties	Homologous or monoclonal antibodies to factor VIII:C:Ag	Heterologous or monoclonal antibodies to factor VIII R:Ag
Laboratory measurement of antigen	Radioimmunoassay or immunoradiometric assay	Laurell rocket immunoelectrophoresis Enzyme-linked immunosorbent assay Radioimmunoassay Immunoradiometric assay
Laboratory measurement of function	Factor VIII:C assay (modified APTT)	Screening: ristocetin + platelet rich plasma Confirmatory: ristocetin cofactor assay (factor VIII R:RCo)
Evaluation in vivo	—	Bleeding time
Evaluation of variants	Radioimmunoassay for factor VIII:C:Ag	Crossed immunoelectrophoresis Agarose multimer analysis Immunoradiometric assay

Discussion

This case is an example of antibodies to factor VIII:C arising in a patient with severe hemophilia A. The age of presentation of this patient is unusual because most persons with severe hemophilia A who have antibodies to factor VIII:C manifest this problem before 20 years of age (Table 1). Antibodies to factor VIII:C may also be encountered in clinical situations other than hemophilia A. Such antibodies are characteristically referred to as spontaneous inhibitors of factor VIII:C.

According to a variety of sources, the incidence of antibodies to factor VIII:C has been reported to vary between 5% and 15% of persons with severe hemophilia A. In more than 97% of cases, antibodies to factor VIII:C develop in persons whose factor VIII:C activity is less than 3% before the development of the inhibitor. In a recent cooperative study, it was found that in approximately 70% of cases, inhibitors in persons with hemophilia A develop by the time an affected person is 20 years of age.

Biochemical Aspects. Antibodies to factor VIII:C in persons with hemophilia are almost exclusively of the IgG class. There appears to be a predilection for the IgG$_4$ subclass. In instances in which light-chain typing has been accomplished, the antibodies have usually been of the kappa light-chain type. The antibodies form a

Table 1
Inhibitors of Factor VIII:C

	Hemophilia A	Spontaneous Inhibitors
Clinical picture	Severe hemophilia A	Collagen vascular diseases, pregnancy, etc.
Age	Pediatric (<20 years of age)	Adult
Immunoglobulin	IgG$_4$ kappa chains	IgG (kappa or lambda chains), IgA, IgM
Kinetics	Time dependent	Rapid initial inhibition, then equilibrium
Anamnestic response	Yes—strong	No
Spontaneous remission	Rare	Yes (postpartum, drug allergy)
Quantification	Bethesda unit	?Bethesda unit
Treatment	Various modalities	May respond to factor VIII concentrates

complex with factor VIII:C in a time- and temperature-dependent neutralization reaction that may take 1 to 2 hours to reach completion. The antibodies inactivate factor VIII:C activity but have no effect on factor VIII R:RCo or factor VIII R:Ag. The etiologic basis of antibodies to factor VIII:C is obscure. Development of the antibodies is related to exposure to infused factor VIII:C. Seventy-five percent of persons with inhibitors have more than 100 days of exposure to factor VIII. There appears to be an increased incidence of inhibitors in brother pairs. In addition, there is a higher than expected representation of inhibitors in persons whose blood group is AB.

In the past, antibodies to factor VIII:C were measured by a variety of mixing assays that made use of a patient's plasma and a source of factor VIII:C. To introduce uniformity into the measurement of factor VIII inhibitors, a standard inhibitor assay has been developed. The level of the inhibitor is expressed in Bethesda units. By definition, an inhibitor plasma that contains 1 Bethesda unit of antibody per milliliter will neutralize 50% of factor VIII:C activity in an equal volume of pooled normal plasma after incubation of the mixture at 37°C for 2 hours.

Clinical Picture. When antibodies to factor VIII develop in persons with severe hemophilia A, there is no apparent effect on the frequency of hemorrhagic episodes. By contrast, persons with mild hemophilia A in whom antibodies to factor VIII develop will have a severe bleeding diathesis that resembles severe hemophilia; the inhibitor often is of low titer and occasionally disappears spontaneously or may not recur when an affected person is again exposed to blood products that contain factor VIII. By contrast, inhibitors of factor VIII:C tend to persist in persons with severe hemophilia A.

The patterns of response of antibodies on exposure to factor VIII:C may be classified into two main types: "high" responder and "low" responder. Approximately 50% to 60% of patients with inhibitors may be classified as high responders. Typically, high responders show a rise in the titer of antibodies to factor VIII:C on the third or fourth day after infusion of blood products that contain factor VIII. The titer reaches a maximum within 2 to 3 weeks and then gradually falls to the preinfusion level over several months in the absence of a rechallenge with factor VIII:C. Low responding patients tend not to show increases in inhibitor titers in excess of 2 to 5 Bethesda units. It is exceedingly important to make the distinction between high and low responders. Patients who are low responders may be effectively treated with factor VIII replacement therapy. In some cases, such patients may even be maintained on a home therapy program with factor VIII concentrates.

Treatment. A number of regimens have been proposed for treating patients with inhibitors of factor VIII:C. Such regimens have included continuous infusion of high doses of factor VIII:C in an effort to neutralize the antibodies. Also, patients have been treated with factor VIII

concentrates prepared from a bovine or porcine source. More recently, a new porcine preparation of factor VIII has been tested in Europe. This preparation consists of only the coagulant portion of the factor VIII molecule and does not have the unpleasant side effect of thrombocytopenia that was seen with early porcine factor VIII concentrates, which contained the entire factor VIII complex. Exchange plasmapheresis has also been used to reduce the titer of circulating inhibitors, as has immunosuppressive therapy combined with infusion of high doses of factor VIII concentrates.

Prothrombin complex concentrates and activated prothrombin complex concentrates have been used in an effort to bypass the contribution of factor VIII:C to intrinsic coagulation. These concentrates have proved effective in treating patients with inhibitors of factor VIII:C.

Because large quantities of commercially prepared factor VIII are used to treat some patients with inhibitors, clinicians should be aware of the possibility of serious hemolysis in patients whose blood group is A, B or AB as a result of the measurable titers of anti-A and anti-B in such products. The titer of factor VIII:C inhibitor may also rise as a result of infusion of prothrombin complex concentrates, presumably because of the small amount of factor VIII procoagulant antigen (Factor VIII:C:Ag) contained in such preparations.

Bibliography

Clinical Picture

Gawryl MS, Hoyer LW: Inactivation of factor VIII coagulant activity by two different types of human antibodies. *Blood* 60:1103–1109, 1982.

Lavergne JM, Meyer D, Girma JP, et al: Precipitating anti-VIII:C antibodies in two patients with haemophilia A. *Brit J Haematol* 50:135–146, 1982.

Laboratory Evaluation of Factor VIII Inhibitors

Austen DEG, Lechner K, Rizza CR, et al: A comparison of the Bethesda and New Oxford methods of factor VIII antibody assay. *Thromb Haemostasis* 47:72–75, 1982.

Ewing NP, Kasper CK: In vitro detection of mild inhibitors to factor VIII in hemophilia. *Amer J Clin Pathol* 77:749–752, 1982.

Kasper CK, Aledort LM, Counts RB, et al: A more uniform measurement of factor VIII inhibitors. *Thromb Diath Haemorrh* 34:869–872, 1975.

Lossing TS, Kasper CK, Feinstein DI: Detection of factor VIII inhibitors with the partial thromboplastin time. *Blood* 49:793–797, 1977.

Treatment

Aronstam A, McLellan DS, Mbatha PS, et al: The use of an activated factor IX complex (Autoplex®) in the management of hemarthroses in haemophiliacs with antibodies to factor VIII. *Clin Lab Haematol* 4:231–238, 1982.

Brackmann HH, Gormsen J: Massive factor VIII infusion in haemophiliac with factor VIII inhibitor, high responder. *Lancet* 2:933–937, 1977.

Edson JR, McArthur JR, Branda RF, et al: Successful management of a subdural hematoma in a hemophiliac with an anti-factor VIII antibody. *Blood* 41:113–122, 1973.

Erskine JG: Plasma exchange in patients with inhibitors to factor VIII:C. *Plasma Ther Trans Tech* 3:1123–1130, 1982.

Francesconi M, Korninger C, Thaler E, et al: Plasmaphoresis: Its value in the management of patients with antibodies to factor VIII. *Haemostasis* 11:79–86, 1982.

Hewitt P, Mackie IJ, Machin SJ: Highly purified porcine factor VIII in haemophilia A. *Lancet* 1:741–742, 1982.

Hilgartner MW, Knatterud GL: FEIBA study group. The use of factor eight inhibitor by-passing activity (FEIBAImmuno) product for treatment of bleeding episodes in hemophiliacs with inhibitors. *Blood* 61:36–40, 1983.

MacFarlane RG, Biggs R, Bidwell E: Bovine antihaemophilic globulin in the treatment of haemophilia. *Lancet* 1:1316–1320, 1954.

Rizza CR, Biggs R: The treatment of patients who have factor VIII antibodies. *Brit J Haematol* 24:65–82, 1973.

Rizza CR, Matthews JM: Effect of frequent factor VIII replacement on the level of factor VIII antibodies in haemophiliacs. *Brit J Haematol* 52:13–24, 1982.

Salmassi S, Ilangovan S, Kasprisin DO: Treatment of hemophilia A with factor VIII inhibitor by plasma exchange transfusion. *Plasma Ther Trans Tech* 3:131–136, 1982.

Schimf K, Zeltsch C, Zeltsch P: Myocardial infarction complicating activated prothrombin complex concentrate substitution in patients with haemophilia A. (Letter to the editor) *Lancet* 2:1043, 1983.

Sjamsoedin LJM, Heijnen L, Mauser-Bunschoten EP, et al: The effect of activated prothrombin complex concentrate (FEIBA) on joint and muscle bleeding in patients with hemophilia A and antibodies of factor VIII. *N Engl J Med* 305:717–721, 1981.

Spero JA, Lewis JH, Hasiba U: Corticosteroid therapy for acquired F VIII:C inhibitors. *Brit J Haematol* 48:635–642, 1981.

Review Articles

Kasper CK: Management of inhibitors to factor VIII. In Brown EB (ed): *Progress in Hematology*. New York: Grune & Stratton, 1981, vol XII, pp 143–163.

White GC, McMillen CW, Blatt PM, et al: Factor VIII inhibitors: A clinical overview. *Amer J Hematol* 13:335–342, 1982.

CASE
11

PATIENT: 5-year-old boy

CHIEF COMPLAINT: This patient was referred by his pediatrician because of a marked bruising tendency of the arms and legs. The mother related that the bruising typically appeared without serious trauma.

MEDICAL HISTORY: There was no bleeding at the time of circumcision or in association with separation of the umbilical cord. When 20 months of age, the boy underwent corrective eye surgery for strabismus. At that time, the opthalmologist noted no unusual bleeding. No preoperative evaluation was obtained, and the patient did well postoperatively. When 3 years of age, the boy had an episode of marked epistaxis that necessitated admission to a hospital and transfusion of 1 unit of whole blood. After packing and transfusion, the epitaxis was satisfactorily controlled.

FAMILY HISTORY: There was a history of bleeding on the maternal side of the family. The patient's mother, maternal grandmother and maternal greatgrandmother had experienced episodes of abnormal bleeding. The bleeding was characterized by recurrent epistaxis and "easy bruising" together with menorrhagia. Little information was available regarding the nature of the hemorrhagic episodes, except that the mother had required 9 units of whole blood at the time of delivery of the patient. The patient was an only child.

DRUG HISTORY: No medication

PHYSICAL EXAMINATION: A number of bruises were noted over the arms and legs.

Laboratory Results

A. Screening Procedures

	Patient	Normal
Prothrombin time	12 seconds	10–12 seconds
APTT	41.5 seconds	<42 seconds
Platelet count	360,000/μl	200,000–450,000/μl
Bleeding time (Ivy)	>10 minutes	1–6 minutes

Questions

1. The family history suggests what pattern of inheritance?

2. Does the pattern of clinical bleeding suggest an abnormality of primary hemostasis or an abnormality of secondary hemostasis?
3. What additional laboratory procedures are indicated?
4. If this patient requires surgical intervention, what would be the treatment of choice for a bleeding complication?

Laboratory Results

B. Confirmatory Procedures

	Patient	Normal
Factor VIII:C	28%	50% to 150%
Factor VIII R:Ag	34%	50% to 150%
Factor VIII R:RCo	30%	50% to 150%
Platelet retention (glass-bead column)	46%	40% to 90%

Platelet aggregation studies were also performed (Figure 1). There was a normal aggregation response to adenosine diphosphate (ADP) and epinephrine. In both

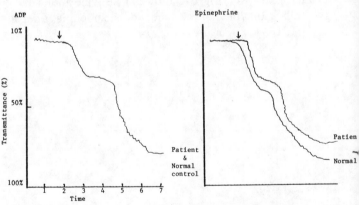

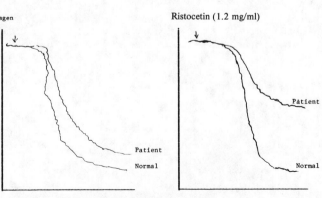

Figure 1

VON WILLEBRAND'S DISEASE (TYPE I)

CLINICAL PICTURE

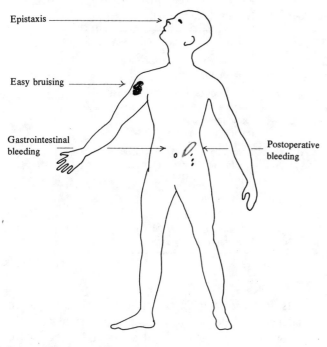

Epistaxis

Easy bruising

Gastrointestinal
bleeding

Postoperative
bleeding

Pattern of inheritance: Autosomal dominant

PHYSICAL PROPERTIES OF FACTOR VIII
See table, page 126.

LABORATORY FINDINGS

A. Screening Procedures

Test	Patient's Result	Normal Range
Prothrombin time	Normal	10–12 seconds
APTT	Abnormal or normal	<42 seconds
Platelet count	Normal	130,000–400,000/μl
Bleeding time	Abnormal or normal	1–8 minutes

B. Confirmatory Procedures

Factor VIII:C*	Abnormal	Normal
Factor VIII R:Ag	Abnormal	Normal
Factor VIII R:RCo	Abnormal	Normal
Crossed immunoelectrophoresis	Normal	Normal
Platelet aggregation	Normal ADP, epinephrine, collagen, normal or abnormal ristocetin	

*Evaluation of the various properties of factor VIII may vary from time to time in a given patient. Typical findings are indicated. The crossed immunoelectrophoresis may be normal in multimeric distribution; however, the amount of VIII R:Ag is of course decreased in a Type I von Willebrand's disease.

TREATMENT

DDAVP

Cryoprecipitate, 1 bag per 10 kg of body weight twice a day

ε-Aminocaproic acid (EACA) in dental surgery

Avoidance of aspirin containing compounds

Factor VIII Complex

Property	Factor VIII:C	von Willebrand Factor
Site of production	?, Perhaps liver	Megakaryocytes and endothelial cells
Gene control	Sex chromosome	Autosome
Molecular weight	285,000 (range, 85,000–270,000)	Series of multimers varying from 800,000 to 12,000,000 Individual multimers having three bands
Function in vivo	Secondary hemostasis (coagulation)	Primary hemostasis: platelet adhesion Carrier protein: stabilizes factor VIII:C Regulates production of factor VIII:C
Antigenic properties	Homologous or monoclonal antibodies to factor VIII:C:Ag	Heterologous or monoclonal antibodies to factor VIII R:Ag
Laboratory measurement of antigen	Radioimmunoassay or immunoradiometric assay	Laurell rocket immunoelectrophoresis Enzyme-linked immunosorbent assay Radioimmunoassay Immunoradiometric assay
Laboratory measurement of function	Factor VIII:C assay (modified APTT)	Screening: ristocetin + platelet rich plasma Confirmatory: risocetin cofactor assay (factor VIII R:RCo)
Evaluation in vivo	—	Bleeding time
Evaluation of variants	Radioimmunoassay for factor VIII:C:Ag	Crossed immunoelectrophoresis Agarose multimer analysis Immunoradiometric assay

instances, a biphasic curve was seen. Ristocetin-induced agglutination was slightly decreased, and collagen aggregation was within normal limits.

The factor VIII molecule was further evaluated by means of crossed immunoelectrophoresis. Although there was a decreased amount of factor VIII R:Ag, the rate of migration and the cathodal portion of the arc were within normal limits, thus ruling out the possibility of a qualitative abnormality of von Willebrand factor (factor VIII R:Ag, factor VIII R:RCo).

DIAGNOSIS: von Willebrand's disease (type I)

Discussion

This case is an example of a classical autosomal dominant form of von Willebrand's disease. The levels of all three components of the factor VIII molecule are concordantly decreased. In addition, crossed immunoelectrophoresis demonstrated a normal rate of migration, with the high-molecular-weight multimers in the cathodal portion of the arc. These findings establish the diagnosis of a concordant, type I form of von Willebrand's disease.

Several aspects of this case should be pointed out. The activated partial thromboplastin time (APTT) was at the upper limit of the normal range. Many investigators have mentioned the variability of laboratory test results in patients with von Willebrand's disease. In some instances, due to this variability, a normal value for any component of factor VIII (factor VIII R:Ag, factor VIII:C) as well as a normal APTT or bleeding time may be seen. In this patient, the APTT was borderline, whereas the bleeding time was markedly prolonged.

In addition to variability of laboratory test results, there may be variability of the clinical picture in von Willebrand's disease. This clinical variability is illustrated by the medical history of this patient. At 20 months of age, the patient underwent elective surgery for strabismus. This surgical procedure was associated with no bleeding problem, in marked contrast to the episode of epistaxis, which was controlled only with packing and transfusion in a hospital setting. Tonsillectomy, performed at a later age, was associated with profound bleeding, both intraoperatively and postoperatively. This bleeding episode was controlled with difficulty despite transfusion of cryoprecipitate.

Biochemical Aspects. Some of the biochemical aspects of the factor VIII complex have been discussed previously (case 7). von Willebrand factor consists of a series of multimers that range in molecular weight from approximately 800,000 to more than 12,000,000. Recent studies have provided convincing evidence that factor VIII:C and von Willebrand factor are distinct molecular entities that circulate as a complex in plasma. The delineation of the molecular basis of von Willebrand's disease has been complicated by the existence of several variants of the disease.

Several laboratory tests have been proposed to measure the activity of von Willebrand factor. The only direct test is determination of bleeding time in vivo. In vitro tests include retention of platelets in a column of glass beads and ristocetin-induced platelet agglutination as well as a quantitative assay of ristocetin cofactor activity. It should be emphasized that ristocetin-induced platelet agglutination is a screening procedure and may be *normal* in patients with the mild (type I) form of von Willebrand's disease. In addition, there are a number of other false-negative as well as false-positive test results (Table 1). More recently, an increased response of platelet-rich plasma to ristocetin has been described in two disease states: the type IIB form of von Willebrand's disease and pseudo-von Willebrand's disease (Table 2). In the latter case, a platelet abnormality results in increased binding of normal factor VIII/von Willebrand factor to platelets in the presence of ristocetin.

Perhaps the most physiologic in vitro test is measurement of the ability of platelets to adhere to the exposed subendothelium of an everted rabbit aorta or human renal artery. Adhesion of platelets is reduced in patients with von Willebrand's disease. This defective adhesion is most evident at high shear rates, which prevail in small-caliber blood vessels.

Quantitative estimation of ristocetin cofactor activity involves the use of washed normal platelets that are reacted with different dilutions of a patient's plasma. In addition to washed normal platelets, formalin-fixed platelets and lyophilized platelets have been used. Quantitative measurement of ristocetin cofactor activity does, however, suffer from lack of reliability and reproducibility. Also, quantification of ristocetin cofactor activity in vitro does not necessarily correlate with determination of bleeding time in vivo. Therefore, some investigators have suggested that another property of the factor VIII molecule might be designated factor VIII:BT (BT = bleeding time).

Factor VIII R:Ag is quantitated by use of specific heterologous antibodies. A number of techniques have been used. Such techniques include rocket immunoelectrophoresis, radioimmunoassay and immunoradiometric assay. A single quantification of the antigen by means of one of these assay systems may misrepresent the activity of von Willebrand factor in vivo. For instance, in patients with the type II form of von Willebrand's disease, high-molecular-weight multimers of factor VIII may be decreased or lacking in plasma even though there may be a normal total amount of factor VIII R:Ag.

A number of approaches have been introduced to evaluate the multimeric composition of factor VIII/von Willebrand factor. The approaches include crossed immunoelectrophoresis and sodium dodecyl sulfate-agarose gel electrophoresis. The latter system makes use of an autoradiographic technique with ^{125}I-labeled antibodies.

Clinical Picture. von Willebrand's disease may be inherited or acquired. Autosomal recessive and autosomal dominant patterns of inheritance have been described (Table 2). Persons with the more common autosomal dominant form of the disease typically have a relatively mild bleeding tendency. Children often have mucosal bleeding, such as epistaxis and gingival bleeding, after tooth brushing. In addition, there may be excessive blood loss after minor surgical procedures, such as dental extraction and tonsillectomy. Easy bruising is also frequently found, although this complaint is more frequently voiced by female patients. In addition, female patients complain of abnormally heavy menstrual periods, and there may be excessive postpartum bleeding. The pattern of bleeding that is typical of hemophilia A (i.e., intramuscular hemorrhage and hemarthrosis) is rarely seen in the autosomal dominant form of von Willebrand's disease.

The biochemical abnormality in the type I form of von Willebrand's disease is strictly quantitative. In such patients, analysis of the multimeric structure of von Willebrand factor with crossed immunoelectrophoresis or sodium dodecyl sulfate-agarose gel electrophoresis is normal. There are concordant decreases in the levels of factor VIII R:RCo, factor VIII R:Ag and factor VIII:C. The quantity and multimeric composition of factor VIII/

Table 1
Ristocetin Agglutination of Platelet Rich Plasma*

Decreased Agglutination

  von Willebrand's disease (I, IIa, IIc and III)

  Idiopathic thrombocytopenic purpura

  Storage pool disease

  Bernard-Soulier syndrome

  Acute myeloblastic leukemia

  Aspirin ingestion

  Infectious mononucleosis

  Cirrhosis

  Black population

Increased Agglutination

  von Willebrand's disease (IIB)

  Pseudo-von Willebrand's disease

*This table refers to ristocetin induced agglutination of platelet rich plasma. This procedure is a screening procedure and may not identify some cases of mild von Willebrand's disease (VIII R:RCo > 30%; N 50–150%). This procedure should not be confused with the ristocetin cofactor assay which is a quantitative test that utilizes formalin-fixed, washed or lyophilized platelet preparations.

Table 2
Classification of von Willebrand's Disease

	Type I	Type IIA	Type IIB	Type IIC	Type III, Autosomal Recessive, Homozygous or Double Heterozygous
Genetic Transmission	Autosomal Dominant	Autosomal Dominant	Autosomal Dominant	Autosomal Recessive	
Bleeding time	Prolonged	Prolonged	Prolonged	Prolonged	Prolonged
Factor VIII:C	Decreased	Decreased or normal	Decreased or normal	Normal	Markedly decreased
Factor VIII R:Ag	Decreased	Decreased or normal	Decreased or normal	Normal	Absent or minute amounts
Factor VIII R:RCo	Decreased	Markedly decreased	Decreased or normal	Decreased	Absent
Ristocetin-induced platelet agglutination (PRP)	Decreased or normal	Absent or decreased	Increased	Decreased	Absent
Crossed immunoelectrophoresis	Normal	Abnormal	Abnormal	Abnormal double peak	Variable—usually abnormal
Plasma multimeric structure	Normal	Large and intermediate forms absent	Large multimers absent	Large multimers absent; doublet multimer structure	Variable to absent
Platelet multimeric structure	Normal and (quantity of factor VIII R:Ag normal)	Large and intermediate forms absent (quantity of factor VIII R:Ag normal)	Normal multimers in platelets (quantity normal)	Large multimers absent; doublet multimer structure	Absent
Response to 1-desamino-8-D-arginine vasopressin (DDAVP)	Restore hemostasis to normal	Although factor VIII R:Ag increases, multimeric abnormality is not corrected	Transient correction of multimeric abnormality; bleeding time may be corrected		
Possible pathophysiology	Abnormal release from sites of synthesis	Inability to form or stabilize large multimers	Intrinsic abnormality of von Willebrand factor increases tissue binding	Intrinsic abnormality with doublet	Reduced synthesis or rapid breakdown at sites of synthesis

von Willebrand factor in platelets are normal. Similarly, factor VIII/von Willebrand factor is qualitatively and quantitatively normal in endothelial cells.

Treatment. The objective in therapy is to correct the bleeding time defect and the abnormalities of blood coagulation. The most effective blood product is cryoprecipitate. Infusion of cryoprecipitate causes a delayed and disproportionate increase in the amount of factor VIII:C (Figure 2). After cryoprecipitate has been infused, factor VIII:C may continue to rise to a peak within about 12 to 24 hours. The response of factor VIII:C is in contrast to the responses of factor VIII R:RCo and factor VIII R:Ag, which decrease almost immediately after completion of infusion. Correction of the bleeding time defect is even more transient than correction of the levels of factor VIII R:RCo and factor VIII R:Ag.

Commercially prepared concentrates of factor VIII are not effective in the treatment of patients with von Willebrand's disease. They usually fail to correct the bleeding time defect. In addition, use of such concen-

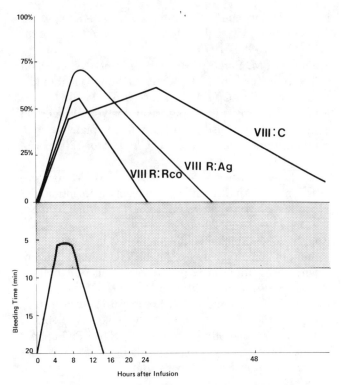

Figure 2. Hemostatic response of von Willebrand's disease to infusion of cryoprecipitate. The shaded area corresponds to the normal range of bleeding times.

trates increases the risk for the development of hepatitis as a complication since they are prepared from large pools of donor plasma (2000 to 20,000 donors).

A typical dose of cryoprecipitate is approximately 1 bag per 10 kg of body weight. This dose should raise the level of factor VIII:C and correct the bleeding time defect. Although the level of factor VIII:C may remain elevated for 24 hours, correction of the bleeding time defect is transient; consequently, cryoprecipitate should be administered twice a day.

1-Desamino-8-D-arginine vasopressin (DDAVP) has also been used in the management of von Willebrand's disease. It is most effective in treating patients with the type I form of the disease. After DDAVP has been infused, the hemostatic abnormality may be corrected for 4 to 6 hours. There is an atypical response in patients with the type IIA or type IIB form of the disease. In these variants, the level of factor VIII:C may be increased to within the normal range; however, the bleeding time defect may not be corrected. DDAVP is not recommended for treatment of the type IIA, B, C or Type III von Willebrand's disease patients.

ε-Aminocaproic acid is a useful adjuvant in dental surgery. In some cases, it may be possible to perform dental surgery without cryoprecipitate replacement therapy. The usual loading dose is 5 g, which is followed by 1 g every hour. This dosage schedule may be maintained for 5 to 7 days after dental procedures.

Bibliography

Variants of von Willebrand's Disease

Ardaillou N, Girma JP, Meyer D, et al: "Variants" of von Willebrand's disease. Demonstration of a decreased antigenic reactivity by immunoradiometric assay. *Thromb Res* 12(5):817–830, 1978.

Armitage H, Rizza CR: Two populations of factor VIII-related antigen in a family with von Willebrand's disease. *Brit J Haematol* 41:279–289, 1979.

Cramer AD, Melarango AJ, Phifer SJ, et al: von Willebrand's disease San Diego, a new variant. *Lancet* 2:12–14, 1976.

Fernandez MFL, Ginsberg MH, Ruggeri ZM, et al: Multimeric structure of factor VIII/von Willebrand factor: The presence of larger multimers and their reassociation with thrombin-stimulated platelets. *Blood* 60:1132–1138, 1982.

Gralnick HR, Coller BS, Sultan Y: Carbohydrate deficiency of the factor VIII/von Willebrand factor protein in von Willebrand's disease variants. *Science* 192:56–59, 1976.

Gralnick HR, Cregger MC, Williams SB: Characterization of the defect of the factor VIII/von Willebrand factor protein in von Willebrand's disease. *Blood* 59:542–548, 1982.

Gralnick HR, Jackson GM, Williams SB, et al: Factor VIII/von Willebrand factor protein: Sensitivity of periodic acid Schiff stain to carbohydrate deficiency. *Blood* 59:1310–1316, 1982.

Gralnick HR, Sultan Y, Coller BS: von Willebrand's disease, combined qualitative and quantitative abnormalities. *N Engl J Med* 296(18):1024–1030, 1977.

Gralnick HR, Williams SB, Shafer BC, et al: Factor VIII/von Willebrand factor binding to von Willebrand's disease patients. *Blood* 60:328–332, 1982.

Hanna W, McCarroll D, McDonald T, et al: Variant von Willebrand's disease and pregnancy. *Blood* 58:873–879, 1981.

Hill FGH, Chan MCK, Hardisty RM: von Willebrand's syndrome. Studies of a variant factor VIII. *Haemostasis* 5:276–284, 1976.

Howard MA, Hendrix L, Firkin BG: Further studies on the factor VIII of a patient with a variant form of von Willebrand's disease. *Thromb Res* 14:609–619, 1979.

Howard MA, Perkin J, Koutts J, et al: Quantitation of binding of factor VIII to concanavalin A. *Brit J Haematol* 47:607–615, 1981.

Howard MA, Salem HH, Thomas KB, et al: Variant von Willebrand's disease type B-revisited. *Blood* 60:1420–1428, 1982.

Hoyer LW: von Willebrand's disease. In Spaet TH (ed):

Progress in Hemostasis and Thrombosis. New York: Grune & Stratton, 1976, vol 3, pp 231–287.

Montgomery RR, Hathaway WE, Johnson J, et al: A variant of von Willebrand's disease with abnormal expression of factor VIII procoagulant activity. *Blood* 60:201–207, 1982.

Peake IR, Bloom AL, Giddings JC: Inherited variants of factor-VIII-related protein in von Willebrand's disease. *N Engl J Med* 291(3):113–117, 1974.

Peake IR, Bloom AL: Abnormal factor VIII related antigen (factor VIII R:Ag) in von Willebrand's disease (VWD): Decreased precipitation by concanavalin A. *Thromb Haemostasis* 37:361–362, 1977.

Ruggeri ZM, Lombardi R, Gatti L, et al: Type II B von Willebrand's disease: Differential clearance of endogenous versus transfused large multimer von Willebrand factor. *Blood* 60:1453–1456, 1982.

Ruggeri ZM, Pareti FI, Mannucci PM, et al: Heightened interaction between platelets and factor VIII/von Willebrand factor in a new subtype of von Willebrand's disease. *N Engl J Med* 302:1047–1051, 1980.

Ruggeri ZM, Zimmerman TS: Variant von Willebrand's disease. Characterization of two subtypes by analysis of multimeric composition of factor VIII/von Willebrand factor in plasma and platelets. *J Clin Invest* 65:1318–1326, 1980.

Thomson C, Forbes CD, Prentice CRM: Evidence for a qualitative defect in factor-VIII-related antigen in von Willebrand's disease. *Lancet* 1:594–596, 1974.

Weiss HJ, Ball AP, Mannucci PM: Incidence of severe von Willebrand's disease. (Letter to editor) *N Engl J Med* 307:127, 1982.

Review Articles

Buchanan GR: von Willebrand's disease—A confusing disorder. *Pediatr Ann* 22:22–46, 1980.

Nachman RL: von Willebrand's disease: A clinical and molecular enigma. *West J Med* 136:318–325, 1982.

Steuber CP: von Willebrand's disease—Update. *Tex Med* 75:45–49, 1979.

Weiss HJ, Phillips LL, Rosner W: Separation of subunits of antihemophilic factor (AHR) by agarose gel chromatography. *Thromb Diath Haemorrh* 27:212–219, 1972.

Zimmerman TS, Ruggeri ZM: von Willebrand's disease. *Clin Haematol* 12:175–200, 1983.

Techniques for Studying Factor VIII Complex

Fulcher CA, Ruggeri ZM, Zimmerman TS: Isoelectric focusing of human von Willebrand factor in urea-agarose gels. *Blood* 61:304–310, 1983.

Green D, Philip KJ: Variant von Willebrand's disease. A study emphasizing crossed immunoelectrophoresis. *Thromb Haemostasis* 43:2–5, 1980.

Head DR, Bowman RP, Marmer DJ, et al: An improved assay for von Willebrand factor. *Amer J Clin Pathol* 72(6):991–995, 1979.

Mannucci PM, Pareti FI, Holmberg L, et al: Studies on the prolonged bleeding time in von Willebrand's disease. *J Lab Clin Med* 88:662–667, 1976.

Ramsey R, Evatt BL: Rapid assay for von Willebrand factor activity using formalin-fixed platelets and microtitration technic. *Amer J Clin Pathol* 72(6):996–999, 1979.

Read MS, Shermer RW, Brinkhous KM: Venom co-agglutinin: An activator of platelet aggregation dependent on von Willebrand factor. *Proc Natl Acad Sci USA* 75:4514–4521, 1978.

Ruggeri ZM, Mannucci PM, Jeffcoate SL, et al: Immunoradiometric assay of factor VIII related antigen, with observations in 32 patients with von Willebrand's disease. *Brit J Haematol* 33:221–232, 1976.

Ruggeri ZM, Mannucci PM, Lombardi R, et al: Multimeric composition of factor VIII/von Willebrand factor following administration of DDAVP: Implications for pathophysiology and therapy of von Willebrand's disease subtypes. *Blood* 59:1272–1278, 1982.

Pseudo- (Platelet Type) von Willebrand's Disease

Nielsen EG, Svejgaard A: von Willebrand's disease associated with intermittent thrombocytopenia. *Lancet* II:966–968, 1967.

Miller JL, Buselli BD, Kupinski JM: In vivo interaction of von Willebrand factor with platelets following cryoprecipitate transfusion in platelet type von Willebrand's disease. *Blood* 63:226–230, 1984.

Miller JL, Castella A: Platelet type von Willebrand's disease: Characterization of a new bleeding disorder. *Blood* 60:790–794, 1982.

Miller JL, Kupinski JM, Castella A, et al: von Willebrand factor binds to platelets and induces aggregation in platelet type but not Type IIB. von Willebrand's disease. *J Clin Invest* 72:1532, 1983.

Rivard GE, Daviault MB, Brault N, et al: von Willebrand's disease associated with thrombocytopenia and a fast migrating factor VIII related antigen. *Thromb Res* 11:507–516, 1977.

Takahashi H, Nagayama R, Hattori A, et al: von Willebrand disease with familiar thrombocytopenia and increased ristocetin induced platelet aggregation. *Amer J Hematol* 10:89–99, 1981.

Takahashi H, Sakuragawa N, Shibata A: von Willebrand's disease with an increased ristocetin induced platelet aggregation and a qualitative abnormality of the factor VIII protein. *Amer J Hematol* 8:299–308, 1980.

Weiss HJ, Meyer D, Rabinowitz R, et al: Pseudo-von

Willebrand's disease. *N Engl J Med* 306:326–333, 1982.

Treatment

Korninger CH, Niessner H, Lechner K: Impaired fibrinolytic response to DDAVP and venous occlusion in a sub-group of patients with von Willebrand's disease. *Thromb Res* 23:365–374, 1981.

Takahashi H: Studies on the pathophysiology and treatment of von Willebrand's disease. V. Properties of factor VIII and DDAVP infusion in variant von Willebrand's disease. *Thromb Res* 21:357–361, 1981.

CASE
12

PATIENT: 30-year-old woman

CHIEF COMPLAINT: This patient was referred for evaluation of a possible abnormality of platelet function. She was originally evaluated at a neighboring hospital, where she was found to have a large number of bruises over the arms and legs.

MEDICAL HISTORY: The patient's medical history included a number of surgical procedures: tonsillectomy at 2½ years of age, appendectomy at 9 years, removal of a cyst of the right ovary at 19 years and left salpingo-oophorectomy and hysterectomy at 25 years. She reported no untoward bleeding during any of these surgical procedures. However, the patient did receive transfusions; the exact number of transfusions in the most recent surgical procedures was unknown to the patient. The patient also stated that she had bled profusely from various superficial wounds and that she had recurrent bouts of epistaxis during childhood.

FAMILY HISTORY: The mother and a maternal grandmother had bleeding problems after superficial injuries. There were three brothers, none of whom had any bleeding difficulty. The patient had two children, who were living and well, although the eldest child (8-year-old girl) had epistaxis and bleeding after tonsillectomy.

DRUG HISTORY: No medication

PHYSICAL EXAMINATION: The patient was a well-developed, well-nourished woman. A number of bruises were noted over the arms and legs, and there were several telangiectatic lesions. The largest lesion was located over the right flank and measured approximately 5 mm in greatest dimension. The other telangiectatic areas were pinpoint in size. Telangiectatic lesions were also noted on the oral mucosa.

Laboratory Results

A. Screening Procedures

	Patient	Normal
Prothrombin time	12 seconds	10–12 seconds
APTT	36 seconds	<42 seconds
Platelet count	315,000/μl	200,000–450,000/μl
Bleeding time (template)	13 minutes	1–8 minutes

Questions

1. What additional laboratory procedures are indicated?
2. Are telangiectatic lesions associated with any hereditary disorder of hemostasis?
3. Do patients with hereditary hemorrhagic telangiectasia have abnormal hemostasis?

Laboratory Results

B. Confirmatory Procedures

	Patient	Normal
Factor VIII:C	35%	50% to 150%
Factor VIII R:Ag	40%	50% to 150%
Factor VIII R:RCo	40%	50% to 150%

Platelet aggregation studies were performed with adenosine diphosphate, collagen and epinephrine. The aggregation responses to adenosine diphosphate and epinephrine were within normal limits, as was the aggregation response to collagen. Agglutination studies performed with ristocetin at a concentration of 1.5 mg/ml

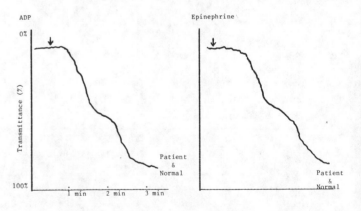

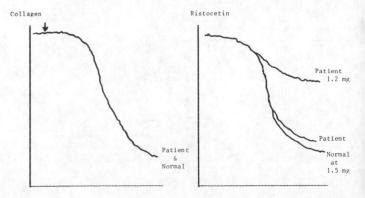

VON WILLEBRAND'S DISEASE (TYPE I), IN ASSOCIATION WITH HEREDITARY HEMORRHAGIC TELANGIECTASIA (OSLER-WEBER-RENDU DISEASE)

CLINICAL PICTURE

PHYSICAL PROPERTIES OF FACTOR VIII
See table, page 134.

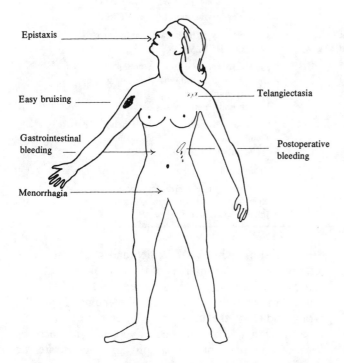

Epistaxis

Easy bruising

Telangiectasia

Gastrointestinal bleeding

Postoperative bleeding

Menorrhagia

Pattern of inheritance: Autosomal dominant for von Willebrand's disease and hereditary hemorrhagic telangiectasia

LABORATORY FINDINGS

A. Screening Procedures

Test	Patient's Result	Normal Range
Prothrombin time	Normal	10–12 seconds
APTT	Abnormal or normal	<42 seconds
Platelet count	Normal	130,000–400,000/μl
Bleeding time	Abnormal or normal	1–8 minutes

B. Confirmatory Procedures

Factor VIII:C	Abnormal	Normal
Factor VIII R:Ag	Abnormal	Normal
Factor VIII R:RCo	Abnormal	Normal
Platelet aggregation	Normal ADP, epinephrine, collagen, normal or abnormal ristocetin	

*Evaluation of the various properties of factor VIII may vary from time to time in a given patient. Typical findings are indicated. The crossed immunoelectrophoresis may be normal in multimetric distribution; however, the amount of VIII R:Ag is decreased in a Type I von Willebrand's disease.

TREATMENT

Cryoprecipitate, 1 bag per 10 kg of body weight twice a day
1-Desamino-8-D-arginine vasopressin (DDAVP)
ε-Aminocaproic acid (EACA) in dental surgery
Avoidance of aspirin containing compounds

Factor VIII Complex

Property	Factor VIII:C	von Willebrand Factor
Site of production	?, Perhaps liver	Megakaryocytes and endothelial cells
Gene control	Sex chromosome	Autosome
Molecular weight	285,000 (range, 85,000–270,000)	Series of multimers varying from 800,000 to 12,000,000 Individual multimers having three bands
Function in vivo	Secondary hemostasis (coagulation)	Primary hemostasis: platelet adhesion Carrier protein: stabilizes factor VIII:C Regulates production of factor VIII:C
Antigenic properties	Homologous or monoclonal antibodies to factor VIII:C:Ag	Heterologous or monoclonal antibodies to factor VIII R:Ag
Laboratory measurement of antigen	Radioimmunoassay or immunoradiometric assay	Laurell rocket immunoelectrophoresis Enzyme-linked immunosorbent assay Radioimmunoassay Immunoradiometric assay
Laboratory measurement of function	Factor VIII:C assay (modified APTT)	Screening: ristocetin + platelet rich plasma Confirmatory: risocetin cofactor assay (factor VIII R:RCo)
Evaluation in vivo	—	Bleeding time
Evaluation of variants	Radioimmunoassay for factor VIII:C:Ag	Crossed immunoelectrophoresis Agarose multimer analysis Immunoradiometric assay

were within normal limits; however, when ristocetin was used at a lower concentration, 1.2 mg/ml, there was a slight decrease in the agglutination response (see platelet aggregation tracings).

The two daughters were also evaluated and were found to have the following results:

	Daughter 1	Daughter 2	Normal
Prothrombin time	12 seconds	12 seconds	10–12 seconds
APTT	37.5 seconds	42 seconds	<42 seconds
Platelet count	355,000/μl	455,000/μl	200,000–450,000/μl
Bleeding time	>15 minutes	10 minutes and 50 seconds	1–8 minutes
Factor VIII:C	24%	65%	50 to 150%
Factor VIII R:Ag	40%	45%	50% to 150%
Factor VIII R:RCo	45%	50%	50% to 150%

In addition, physical examination of the daughters revealed similar telangiectatic lesions over the trunk and on the oral mucosa.

DIAGNOSIS: von Willebrand's disease (type I), in association with hereditary hemorrhagic telangiectasia (Osler-Weber-Rendu disease).

Discussion

This case is an example of classical type I von Willebrand's disease in association with hereditary hemorrhagic telangiectasia (Osler-Weber-Rendu disease). Both of these disorders are inherited in an autosomal dominant manner. It has recently been emphasized that some persons with von Willebrand's disease have arteriovenous malformations of the gastrointestinal tract and associated telangiectasia. Often, such patients present with intractible gastrointestinal bleeding. Typically, x-ray studies of the upper and lower segments of the gastrointestinal tract are negative, and it becomes necessary to perform angiography to demonstrate the arteriovenous malformations.

On electron microscopy, the dilated vessels appear to be small venules that lack supporting smooth muscle or elastic fibers. In addition, it has been demonstrated that there are defective junctions between endothelial cells.

Typically, patients with hereditary hemorrhagic telangiectasia do not show abnormalities on primary screening procedures unless there is an associated disorder, such as von Willebrand's disease.

Patients with von Willebrand's disease may have a number of associated abnormalities. These include: angiodysplasia, mitral valve prolapse, qualitative platelet defects, dysfibrinogenemia, and factor XII deficiency.

The clinical management of bleeding in this patient would be similar to that of any other patient with mild Type I von Willebrand's disease.

Bibliography

Cass AJ, Bliss BP, Bulton RP, et al: Gastrointestinal bleeding, angiodysplasia of the colon and acquired von Willebrand's disease. *Brit J Surg* 67:639–641, 1980.

CASE
13

PATIENT: 4-year-old girl

CHIEF COMPLAINT: This patient was hospitalized because of episodes of spontaneous epistaxis and the recent onset of hematemesis.

MEDICAL HISTORY: The patient had been hospitalized at 3 years of age because of epistaxis and spontaneous bruising. During that hospitalization, she was found to be anemic, with a hemoglobin level of 4.6 g/dl and a hematocrit of 12%. She was transfused with fresh-frozen plasma and washed, packed red cells. An extensive coagulation evaluation was not undertaken.

FAMILY HISTORY: A maternal grandmother also apparently experienced "easy bruising."

DRUG HISTORY: No medication

PHYSICAL EXAMINATION: The patient was a pale, obviously anemic girl. The pulse rate was 110 per minute, and the blood pressure was 90/50 mm Hg. No petechia or telangiectatic areas were noted.

Laboratory Results

A. Screening Procedures

	Patient	Normal
Prothrombin time	12 seconds	10–12 seconds
APTT	40 seconds	<42 seconds
Platelet count	262,000/μl	200,000–450,000/μl
Bleeding time	11 minutes	1–8 minutes

Questions

1. What is the differential diagnosis?
2. What additional laboratory procedures are indicated?

Laboratory Results

B. Confirmatory Procedures

	Patient	Normal
Factor VIII:C	60%	50% to 150%
Factor VIII R:Ag	80%	50% to 150%
Factor VIII R:RCo	10%	50% to 150%

Factor VIII Complex

Property	Factor VIII:C	von Willebrand Factor
Site of production	?, Perhaps liver	Megakaryocytes and endothelial cells
Gene control	Sex chromosome	Autosome
Molecular weight	285,000 (range, 85,000–270,000)	Series of multimers varying from 800,000 to 12,000,000 Individual multimers having three bands
Function in vivo	Secondary hemostasis (coagulation)	Primary hemostasis: platelet adhesion Carrier protein: stabilizes factor VIII:C Regulates production of factor VIII:C
Antigenic properties	Homologous or monoclonal antibodies to factor VIII:C:Ag	Heterologous or monoclonal antibodies to factor VIII R:Ag
Laboratory measurement of antigen	Radioimmunoassay or immunoradiometric assay	Laurell rocket immunoelectrophoresis Enzyme-linked immunosorbent assay Radioimmunoassay Immunoradiometric assay
Laboratory measurement of function	Factor VIII:C assay (modified APTT)	Screening: ristocetin + platelet rich plasma Confirmatory: ristocetin cofactor assay (factor VIII R:RCo)
Evaluation in vivo	—	Bleeding time
Evaluation of variants	Radioimmunoassay for factor VIII:C:Ag	Crossed immunoelectrophoresis Agarose multimer analysis Immunoradiometric assay

VON WILLEBRAND'S DISEASE (TYPE IIA)

CLINICAL PICTURE

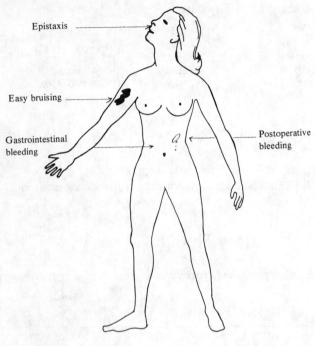

Epistaxis

Easy bruising

Gastrointestinal
bleeding

Postoperative
bleeding

Pattern of inheritance: Autosomal dominant

PHYSICAL PROPERTIES OF FACTOR VIII
See table, page 135.

LABORATORY FINDINGS

A. Screening Procedures

Test	Patient's Result	Normal Range
Prothrombin time	Normal	10–12 seconds
APTT	Normal	<42 seconds
Platelet count	Normal	130,000–400,000/μl
Bleeding time	Abnormal	1–8 minutes

B. Confirmatory Procedures

Factor VIII:C	Normal or abnormal	50% to 150%
Factor VIII R:Ag	Normal or abnormal	50% to 150%
Factor VIII R:RCo	Abnormal	50% to 150%
Crossed immunoelectro-phoresis	Abnormal	Normal
SDS-agarose gel	Abnormal large & intermediate multimers absent	All multimers present
Platelet aggregation	ADP, collagen, epinephrine normal, ristocetin abnormal	

TREATMENT

Cryoprecipitate, 1 bag per 10 kg of body weight twice a day
ε-Aminocaproic acid (EACA) in dental surgery
Avoidance of aspirin containing compounds

Platelet aggregation studies were performed using adenosine diphorplate, collagen, epinephrine and ristocetin. Aggregation in response to ADP, collagen and epinephrine was normal; however, the agglutination in response to ristocetin in a concentration of 1.2 mg/ml was decreased.

Because of the discrepancy between the factor VIII R:Ag and the factor VIII R:RCo, the factor VIII molecule was further evaluated by means of crossed immunoelectrophoresis. The pattern seen on crossed immunoelectrophoresis was abnormal. There appeared to be more rapid migration of the factor VIII molecule and an absence of the more cathodal portion of the pattern. The high-molecular-weight multimers typically migrate in this portion of the crossed immunoelectrophoretic arc. Further confirmation of the absence of the high-molecular-weight multimers was obtained by use of sodium dodecyl sulfate-agarose gel electrophoresis. The

Table 1
Classification of von Willebrand's Disease

	Type I	Type IIA	Type IIB	Type IIC	Type III, Autosomal Recessive, Homozygous or Doubly Heterozygous
Genetic Transmission	Autosomal Dominant	Autosomal Dominant	Autosomal Dominant	Autosomal Recessive	
Bleeding time	Prolonged	Prolonged	Prolonged	Prolonged	Prolonged
VIII:C	Decreased	Decreased or normal	Decreased or normal	Normal	Markedly decreased
VIII R:Ag	Decreased	Decreased or normal	Decreased or normal	Normal	Absent or minute amounts
VIII R:RCo	Decreased	Markedly decreased	Decreased or normal	Decreased	Absent
Ristocetin induced agglutination (platelet rich plasma)	Decreased or normal	Absent or decreased	Increased	Decreased	Absent
Crossed immunoelectrophoresis	Normal	Abnormal	Abnormal	Abnormal double peak	Variable—usually abnormal
Plasma multimeric structure	Normal	Large and intermediate forms absent	Large multimers absent	Large multimers absent Doublet multimer structure	Variable to absent
Platelet multimeric structure	Normal structure and quantity	Large and intermediate forms absent (quantity normal)	Normal multimer in platelets. Quantity normal	Large multimers absent. Doublet multimer structure	Absent
DDAVP Response	Restore hemostasis to normal	Although VIII R:Ag will increase, multimeric abnormality is not corrected	Transient correction of multimeric abnormality. Bleeding time usually corrected	—	—
Possible Pathophysiology	Abnormal release from production sites	Inability to form or stabilize large multimers	Intrinsic abnormality of von Willebrand factor increases tissue binding	Intrinsic abnormality with doublet	Reduce synthesis or rapid breakdown at site of synthesis

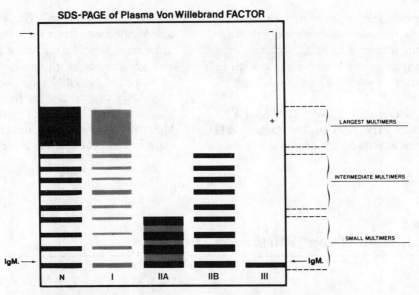

Figure 1. This schematic represents a multimeric analysis of human Factor VIII/von Willebrand factor. The technique utilizes SDS-agarose-acrylamide gel electrophoresis. In the illustration a discontinuous pH buffer system with 1% agarose was used. Following electrophoresis, the gels were reacted with affinity purified ^{125}I-anti-von Willebrand factor antibody. The gels were then developed utilizing autoradiography. The migration of IgM is indicated. A normal plasma sample is provided for reference in the lane indicated N (normal). The various forms of von Willebrand's disease are indicated below each lane (Type I, IIA, IIB, and III).

gels were then reacted with ^{125}I-labeled antibody to von Willebrand factor. The large and intermediate-size multimers were absent.

DIAGNOSIS: von Willebrand's disease (type IIA)

Discussion

This case is an example of a variant form of von Willebrand's disease, type IIA (Table 1). Although factor VIII R:Ag was present in normal amounts, the high-molecular-weight multimers were absent on crossed immunoelectrophoresis and sodium dodecyl sulfate-agarose gel electrophoresis with autoradiography (Figure 1). As this case illustrates, such patients typically have a prolonged bleeding time together with a decrease in factor VIII R:RCo.

In the differential diagnosis, it is necessary to rule out the possibility of a qualitative abnormality of platelet function. The platelet aggregation studies that were performed were within normal limits, with the exception of ristocetin-induced agglutination. Thus, in evaluating patients who present with a normal platelet count and a prolonged bleeding time, it is necessary to obtain a complete evaluation of the factor VIII molecule as well as platelet aggregation studies.

Biochemical Aspects. The type IIA form of von Willebrand's disease is characterized by an absence of the large and intermediate-size multimers of the factor VIII molecule. These multimers are absent from plasma and platelets. If such patients are given 1-desamino-8-D-arginine vasopressin (DDAVP), the factor VIII R:Ag level may increase; however, the multimeric abnormality will not be corrected.

Treatment. The treatment of choice is cryoprecipitate.

Bibliography

Ruggeri ZM, Mannucci PM, Federici AB, et al: Multimeric composition of factor VIII/von Willebrand factor following administration of DDAVP: Implications for pathophysiology and therapy of von Willebrand's disease subtypes. *Blood* 59:1272–1278, 1982.

Ruggeri ZM, Zimmerman TS: Variant von Willebrand's disease: Characterization of two subtypes of analysis of multimeric composition of factor VIII/von Willebrand factor in plasma and platelets. *J Clin Invest* 65:1318–1325, 1980.

Zimmerman TS, Ruggeri ZM, Fulcher CA: Factor VIII/von Willebrand factor. *Progress in Hematology* 13:279–309, 1983.

CASE
14

PATIENT: 32-year-old woman

CHIEF COMPLAINT: This patient was admitted for elective augmentive mammaplasty.

MEDICAL HISTORY: The patient had epistaxis during childhood and a lifelong history of easy bruising. In addition, the patient complained of abnormally heavy menstrual periods and had bled profusely after the birth of her first child. The patient had two children, and there were no problems with delivery of the second child.

FAMILY HISTORY: The patient had three brothers and one sister. The sister had a history similar to that of the patient. The patient's father had a history of abnormal bleeding after dental surgery and had also bled after tonsillectomy during childhood.

DRUG HISTORY: The patient was taking no medication at the time of admission.

PHYSICAL EXAMINATION: Several small ecchymotic areas were noted over the legs.

Laboratory Results

A. Screening Procedures

	Patient	Normal
Prothrombin time	12 seconds	10–12 seconds
APTT	38 seconds	<42 seconds
Platelet count	75,000/μl	130,000–400,000/μl
Bleeding time	10 minutes and 30 seconds	1–8 minutes

Questions

1. Would the mild thrombocytopenia in this patient explain the prolonged bleeding time?
2. The family history suggests an autosomal dominant pattern of inheritance. What abnormalities of coagulation or platelet function are associated with this pattern of inheritance?
3. What additional laboratory procedures are indicated?

Laboratory Results

B. Confirmatory Procedures

	Patient	Normal
Factor VIII:C	71%	50% to 150%
Factor VIII R:Ag	80%	50% to 150%
Factor VIII R:RCo	70%	50% to 150%
Platelet aggregation (see Figure 1)		

Platelet aggregation in response to adenosine diphosphate, collagen, and epinephrine was normal. However, ristocetin in a concentration of 1.2 mg/ml induced increased platelet agglutination. Lower concentrations of 1.0 mg/ml and 0.5 mg/ml of ristocetin also induced agglutination of the patient's plasma but had little effect on normal platelet rich plasma.

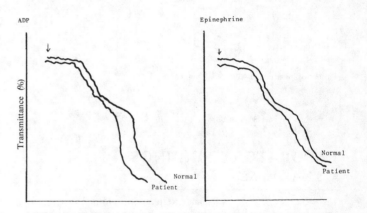
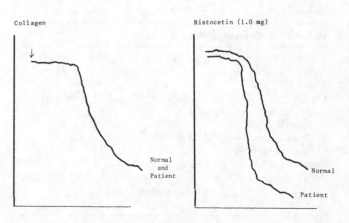

Figure 1

VON WILLEBRAND'S DISEASE (TYPE IIB)

CLINICAL PICTURE

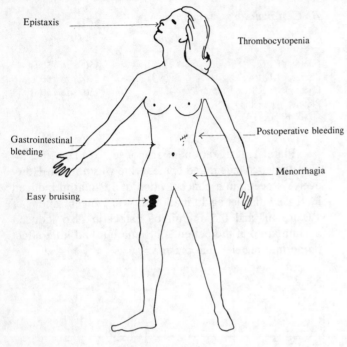

Epistaxis

Thrombocytopenia

Gastrointestinal bleeding

Postoperative bleeding

Menorrhagia

Easy bruising

Pattern of inheritance: Autosomal dominant

PHYSICAL PROPERTIES OF FACTOR VIII
See table, page 141.

LABORATORY FINDINGS

A. Screening Procedures

Test	Patient's Result	Normal Range
Prothrombin time	Normal	10–12 seconds
APTT	Normal or abnormal	<42 seconds
Platelet count	Normal or abnormal	130,000–400,000/μl
Bleeding time	Abnormal	1–8 minutes

B. Confirmatory Procedures

Factor VIII:C	Normal	50% to 150%
Factor VIII R:Ag	Normal	50% to 150%
Factor VIII R:RCo	Normal or abnormal	50% to 150%
Crossed immunoelectro-phoresis	Abnormal	Normal arc
SDS-agarose gel electrophoresis	Abnormal	Normal multimers
Platelet aggregation	Normal ADP, epinephrine, collagen, Increased response, ristocetin	

TREATMENT

Cryoprecipitate, 1 bag per 10 kg of body weight twice a day
DDAVP is contraindicated
Avoidance of aspirin containing compounds

Factor VIII Complex

Property	Factor VIII:C	von Willebrand Factor
Site of production	?, Perhaps liver	Megakaryocytes and endothelial cells
Gene control	Sex chromosome	Autosome
Molecular weight	285,000 (range, 85,000–270,000)	Series of multimers varying from 800,000 to 12,000,000 Individual multimers having three bands
Function in vivo	Secondary hemostasis (coagulation)	Primary hemostasis: platelet adhesion Carrier protein: stabilizes factor VIII:C Regulates production of factor VIII:C
Antigenic properties	Homologous or monoclonal antibodies to factor VIII:C:Ag	Heterologous or monoclonal antibodies to factor VIII R:Ag
Laboratory measurement of antigen	Radioimmunoassay or immunoradiometric assay	Laurell rocket immunoelectrophoresis Enzyme-linked immunosorbent assay Radioimmunoassay Immunoradiometric assay
Laboratory measurement of function	Factor VIII:C assay (modified APTT)	Screening: ristocetin + platelet rich plasma Confirmatory: ristocetin cofactor assay (factor VIII R:RCo)
Evaluation in vivo	—	Bleeding time
Evaluation of variants	Radioimmunoassay for factor VIII:C:Ag	Crossed immunoelectrophoresis Agarose multimer analysis Immunoradiometric assay

Crossed immunoelectrophoresis of the factor VIII molecule was also undertaken. On crossed immunoelectrophoresis, the more cathodal portion of the arc was absent, and there appeared to be more rapid migration of the factor VIII molecule.

Because the family history was positive, the sister was also evaluated. The sister was found to have a factor VIII:C of 55%, a factor VIII R:Ag of 70% and a factor VIII R:RCo of 60%. The pattern exhibited by factor VIII on crossed immunoelectrophoresis was similar to that of the patient.

Subsequently, multimeric analysis was undertaken, and the largest multimers were found to be absent from the patient's plasma. The small and intermediate-size multimers of factor VIII were present in normal to slightly increased amounts.

DIAGNOSIS: von Willebrand's disease (type IIB)

Discussion

In the type II form of von Willebrand's disease, the large multimers of factor VIII are absent from plasma, as determined by sodium dodecyl sulfate-agarose gel electrophoresis or crossed immunoelectrophoresis. Such patients can be subdivided on the basis of functional differences and differences in the multimeric structure of von Willebrand factor in plasma and platelets. The type IIA and IIB forms of von Willebrand's disease are inherited in an autosomal dominant manner; type IIC is inherited in an autosomal recessive manner.

The diagnosis of type IIB von Willebrand's disease in this patient was established by the positive family history, which indicated an autosomal dominant pattern of inheritance, together with the absence of the large multimers of factor VIII, as demonstrated by crossed immunoelectrophoresis and sodium dodecyl sulfate-agarose gel electrophoresis. (See Case 13, Figure 1.) Ristocetin-induced platelet agglutination was also abnormal. At a concentration of 1 mg/ml, ristocetin induced platelet agglutination was increased as compared to a relatively weak pattern, in the control. It is important to emphasize that results of the typical screening tests for von Willebrand's disease (factor VIII:C, factor VIII R:Ag and factor VIII R:RCo) were normal. Consequently, the prolonged bleeding time and the autosomal dominant pattern of inheritance were the only initial results that may have alerted a clinician to the possibility of von Willebrand's disease.

As has been noted, patients with the type IIB form of von Willebrand's disease show an absence of the large multimers of factor VIII from the plasma; however, when factor VIII from platelets is examined, it is found to have a normal multimeric distribution on sodium dodecyl sulfate-agarose gel electrophoresis. von Willebrand factor from platelets and plasma shows a hyperresponsiveness to ristocetin. Experimental studies have demonstrated that binding of von Willebrand factor from patients with type IIB disease to platelets is increased in the presence of low concentrations of ristocetin and also in vivo after administration of 1-desamino-8-D-arginine vasopressin (DDAVP). After administration of DDAVP, there is a transient correction of the multimeric abnormality in von Willebrand plasma, and there may also be correction of the ristocetin cofactor activity; however, the bleeding time usually is not corrected.

The increased binding of the abnormal multimer of factor VIII in the type IIB form of von Willebrand's disease must be differentiated from the recently described abnormality called pseudo-von Willebrand's disease, or platelet von Willebrand's disease. Addition of normal platelet-poor plasma or factor VIII concentrates to platelet-rich plasma of patients with pseudo-von Willebrand's disease causes platelet aggregation, but no such response is seen in patients with the type IIB form of the disease. The defect in pseudo-von Willebrand's disease is assumed to reside in platelet membranes, which show increased affinity for normal factor VIII/von Willebrand factor.

Clinical Picture. The clinical picture in patients with the type IIB form of von Willebrand's disease is typical of other forms of the disease. However, one important difference is that some patients have thrombocytopenia. The thrombocytopenia may be intermittent and has recently been demonstrated to be exacerbated by administration of DDAVP. This effect of DDAVP is thought to be due to the appearance in plasma of large multimers of factor VIII/von Willebrand factor. The large multimers that appear in plasma would preferentially cause platelet aggregation in vivo, leading to sequestration and destruction of the aggregated platelets. It has also been possible to demonstrate circulating platelet aggregates in patients with the type IIB form of von Willebrand's disease who have been treated with DDAVP.

Some patients with the type IIB form of the disease also demonstrate fluctuating or spontaneous thrombocytopenia. A potential explanation for the thrombocytopenia in such patients would be related to the fact that factor VIII/von Willebrand factor is an acute-phase reactant that may increase in response to many nonspecific stimuli, such as exercise and stress or other acute reactive processes. The rise in the level of factor VIII/von Willebrand factor in such a situation would be analogous to the rise that occurs after administration of DDAVP and would result in platelet aggregation and a shortened platelet life span.

Treatment. Because DDAVP has been shown to induce platelet aggregation in vivo and a shortened life span without correcting the bleeding time, use of this agent is contraindicated in the type IIB form of von Willebrand's disease (Table 1). Thus, although DDAVP has been effective in the type I form of the disease, it is important to identify the type of von Willebrand's disease before administering this agent. For patients with the type IIB form of the disease, cryoprecipitate remains the treatment of choice. Because the abnormality in type IIB von Willebrand's disease resides in the structure of the factor VIII/von Willebrand factor, platelets are normal.

Table 1
Response of VIII/von Willebrand Factor to DDAVP

| Before DDAVP* | Normal | von Willebrand's Disease | | |
		Type I	Type IIa	Type IIb
Multimer analysis	Normal	All present in decreased amounts	Large and intermediate forms absent	Large multimers absent
After DDAVP				
Multimer analysis	All forms increased; large forms appear	All forms increased; large forms appear	Minimal change; no large forms appear	Rapid appearance and disappearance of large forms
Bleeding time	Normal	Corrected in some patients	Shortened but not corrected	Shortened but not corrected
Factor VIII R:Ag	Increased	Corrected in some patients	Markedly increased	Increased
Factor VIII R:RCo	Increased	Corrected in some patients	Moderately increased	Increased

*1-Desamino-8-D-arginine vasopressin.

Thus, administration of cryoprecipitate with high-molecular-weight multimers of factor VIII/von Willebrand factor would not be expected to cause platelet aggregation in vivo. Cryoprecipitate should correct the bleeding abnormality and at least transiently correct the bleeding time as well.

Bibliography

Corder MP, Culp MW, Barrett O: Familial occurrence of von Willebrand's disease, thrombocytopenia, and severe gastrointestinal bleeding. *Amer J Med Sci* 265:219–223, 1973.

Holmberg L, Nilsson IM, Borge L, et al: Platelet aggregation induced by 1-desamino-8-D-arginine vasopressin (DDAVP) in type IIb von Willebrand's disease. *N Engl J Med* 309:816–821, 1983.

Rivard GE, Daviault MB, Brault N, et al: von Willebrand's disease associated with thrombocytopenia and a fast migrating factor VIII related antigen. *Thromb Res* 11:507–516, 1977.

Ruggeri ZM, Lombardi R, Gatti L, et al: Type IIb von Willebrand's disease: Differential clearance of endogenous versus transfused large multimer von Willebrand factor. *Blood* 60:1453–1456, 1982.

Ruggeri ZM, Mannucci PM, Lombardi R, et al: Multimeric composition of factor VIII/von Willebrand factor following administration of DDAVP: Implications for pathophysiology and therapy of von Willebrand's disease subtypes. *Blood* 59:1272–1278, 1982.

Takahashi H, Nagayama R, Hattori A, et al: von Willebrand disease associated with familial thrombocytopenia and increased ristocetin-induced platelet aggregation. *Amer J Hematol* 10:89–99, 1981.

Ruggeri ZM, Pareti FI, Mannucci PM, et al: Heightened interaction between platelets and factor VIII/von Willebrand factor in a new subtype of von Willebrand's disease. *N Engl J Med* 302:1047–1051, 1980.

Ruggeri ZM, Zimmerman TS: Variant von Willebrand's disease: Characterization of two subtypes by analysis of multimeric composition of factor VIII/von Willebrand factor in plasma and platelets. *J Clin Invest* 65:1318–1325, 1980.

Takahashi H, Handa M, Watanabe, K et al: Further Characterization of Platelet-Type von Willebrand's Disease in Japan. *Blood* 64:1254–1262, 1984.

Takahashi H, Handa M, Watanabe, K et al: Further brand's disease with an increased platelet aggregation and a qualitative abnormality of the factor VIII protein. *Amer J Hematol* 8:299–308, 1980.

Zimmerman TR, Ruggeri ZM: von Willebrand's disease. *Prog Hemostasis Thromb* 6:203–236, 1982.

CASE
15

PATIENT: Newborn baby boy

CHIEF COMPLAINT: This infant was the product of a term gestation. No difficulty was encountered during gestation or at the time of delivery. However, because of a family history of bleeding, a decision was made not to perform circumcision. The intern who was involved with the delivery contacted the coagulation laboratory and discussed the case with a consultant. After the discussion, venous blood samples were obtained for evaluation of a possible coagulopathy.

FAMILY HISTORY: The patient's mother had a history of spontaneous bruising together with abnormally heavy menstrual periods that occasionally lasted 7 days. The mother had not previously undergone a surgical procedure and had never required transfusion.

The maternal uncle and the maternal grandfather had similar histories of easy bruising and abnormal bleeding after minor cuts (see Figure 1). The maternal grandfather had serious bleeding after dental extractions in 1955 while he was serving in the United States Army.

The patient's father reported no history of abnormal bleeding, with the exception of bouts of epistaxis that were associated with seasonal changes.

The paternal grandmother had a history of easy bruising and abnormally heavy menstrual periods that often lasted 8 to 10 days.

DRUG HISTORY: No medication

PHYSICAL EXAMINATION: A number of bruises were noted over the chest and arms.

Laboratory Results (Patient and Family)

A. Screening Procedures

	Patient	Mother	Father	Maternal Grandfather	Maternal Uncle	Maternal Grandmother
Prothrombin time	15 seconds	11 seconds	10 seconds	13.5 seconds	11 seconds	12 seconds
APTT	70 seconds	38.5 seconds	29 seconds	32.5 seconds	37 seconds	27 seconds
Platelet count	250,000/μl	274,000/μl	314,000/μl	354,000/μl	288,000/μl	300,000/μl
Bleeding time	Not done	>15 minutes	5 minutes and 15 seconds	12 minutes	10 minutes	4 minutes and 30 seconds

Questions

1. Is the patient's prothrombin time abnormal?
2. What additional laboratory procedures are indicated?
3. What is the normal range for the various components of factor VIII in newborn infants?

Laboratory Results

B. Confirmatory Procedures

	Patient	Mother	Father	Maternal Grandfather	Maternal Uncle	Maternal Grandmother
Factor VIII:C	3%	50%	85%	62%	62%	68%
Factor VIII R:Ag	0%	33%	68%	28%	35%	39%
Factor VIII R:RCo	0%	36%	52%	16%	35%	35%
Factor IX:C	27.5%					

VON WILLEBRAND'S DISEASE (TYPE III)

CLINICAL PICTURE

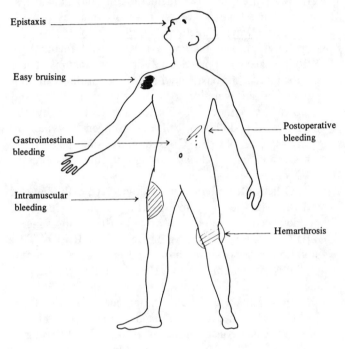

Epistaxis

Easy bruising

Gastrointestinal bleeding

Intramuscular bleeding

Postoperative bleeding

Hemarthrosis

Pattern of inheritance: Autosomal recessive or doubly heterozygous, autosomal dominant

PHYSICAL PROPERTIES OF FACTOR VIII
See table, page 141.

LABORATORY FINDINGS

A. Screening Procedures

Test	Patient's Result	Normal Range
Prothrombin time	Normal	10–12 seconds
APTT	Abnormal	<42 seconds
Platelet count	Normal	130,000–400,000/μl
Bleeding time	Abnormal	1–8 minutes

B. Confirmatory Procedures

Factor VIII:C	Abnormal	Normal
Factor VIII R:Ag	Abnormal	Normal
Factor VIII R:RCo	Abnormal	Normal
Crossed immunoelectro-phoresis	Abnormal	Normal
SDS-agarose gel electrophoresis	Abnormal	Normal multimers composition
Platelet aggregation	Normal ADP, epinephrine, collagen, abnormal ristocetin	

TREATMENT

Cryoprecipitate, 1 bag per 10 kg of body weight twice a day

ε-Aminocaproic acid (EACA) in dental surgery

Avoidance of aspirin containing compounds and other medications that inhibit platelets

On sodium dodecyl sulfate-glyoxal-agarose gel electrophoresis, the patient was found to lack all the large and intermediate-size multimers of factor VIII. The maternal grandfather was found to lack the large multimers of factor VIII.

DIAGNOSIS: von Willebrand's disease (type III)

Discussion

This case is an example of severe von Willebrand's disease that has been inherited from the mother and the father, resulting in a double heterozygous state in the offspring. It is likely that this patient will have severe clinical bleeding. In many instances, patients with the autosomal recessive form of von Willebrand's disease, or the double-heterozygous form, have a clinical picture that closely resembles that of severe hemophilia A. Consequently, in addition to the mucous membrane type of bleeding that is classically associated with the milder forms of von Willebrand's disease, there is bleeding into the major muscle masses of the body as well as hemarthroses.

The prothrombin time that was measured with cord blood was within normal limits for a newborn infant; however, the activated partial thromboplastin time (APTT) was prolonged. The various components of the factor VIII molecule were all markedly abnormal. In normal cord blood, factor VIII:C, factor VIII R:Ag and factor VIII R:RCo are within the normal adult range.

Biochemical Aspects. In patients with the autosomal recessive form of von Willebrand's disease, or the double-heterozygous form, factor VIII R:RCo and factor VIII R:Ag are typically undetectable. In most instances, the bleeding time is greater than 30 minutes. Factor VIII:C is always detectable, ranging from 1% to 5%. Typically, platelet factor VIII R:Ag and factor VIII R:RCo is absent or present only in trace amounts. Thus, it appears that the basic biochemical abnormality in such persons is an inability to synthesize von Willebrand factor. This concept is further substantiated by the absence of endothelial cell plasminogen activator in many affected persons. Consequently, such patients do not respond to 1-desamino-8-D-arginine vasopressin (DDAVP).

Other affected family members typically have a mild clinical bleeding picture. Many such patients may be identified on the basis of an increased ratio of factor VIII:C to factor VIII R:Ag or factor VIII R:RCo. This situation is opposite to that found in carriers of hemophilia A, in whom factor VIII:C is reduced, whereas factor VIII R:Ag is normal.

In patients with the autosomal recessive form of von Willebrand's disease, there usually is no family history of the disease; consanguinity is an occasional finding.

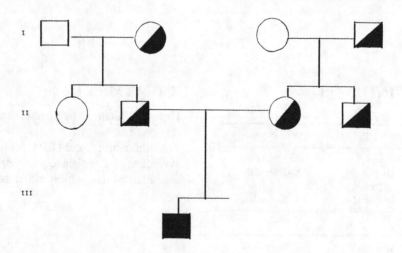

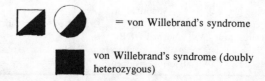

= von Willebrand's syndrome

von Willebrand's syndrome (doubly heterozygous)

Figure 1

Treatment. Because of the severe nature of the defect in such patients, replacement therapy is frequently necessary. The treatment of choice is cryoprecipitate. However, it should be noted that in patients with the recessive form of von Willebrand's disease, antibodies to von Willebrand factor may arise. As has been noted above, such patients do not respond to DDAVP.

Bibliography

Holmberg L, Mannucci PM, Turesson I, et al: Factor VIII antigen in the vessel walls in von Willebrand's disease and haemophilia. *Scand J Haematol* 13:33–38, 1974.

Peake IR, Bloom AL: Immunoradiometric assay of procoagulant factor VIII antigen in plasma and serum and its reduction in haemophilia—Preliminary studies on adult and fetal blood. *Lancet* 1:473–475, 1978.

Zimmerman TS, Abildgaard C, Meyer D: The factor VIII abnormality in severe von Willebrand's disease. *N Engl J Med* 301:1307–1310, 1979.

CASE
16

PATIENT: 30-year-old woman

CHIEF COMPLAINT: This patient was referred for evaluation of a possible hemostatic abnormality. She had a lifelong history of easy bruising, epistaxis and abnormally heavy menstrual periods.

PAST MEDICAL HISTORY: She had three children, and with each delivery, there had been abnormally heavy postpartum bleeding. After the birth of the patient's first child, her postpartum bleeding was of such severity that it necessitated administration of 2 units of whole blood. The patient's medical history also included several episodes of joint swelling and discoloration involving the knees, right ankle and left elbow. In most instances, the joint swelling and pain had not been associated with a specific traumatic event. Past surgical procedures included extraction of a wisdom tooth about 6 years before this evaluation. After the extraction, the patient bled profusely for 5 days. However, she received no transfusion.

FAMILY HISTORY: The patient had five sisters and six brothers. One of the brothers was deceased; the patient was uncertain as to the circumstances surrounding this brother's death. Three siblings had a history of bleeding problems similar to that of the patient. However, none of them had been evaluated.

The mother and father were living and well and apparently had no hemorrhagic problems.

DRUG HISTORY: The patient was taking no medication at the time of evaluation.

PHYSICAL EXAMINATION: A number of large ecchymotic areas were noted over the left arm. There also was discoloration and swelling of the right ankle.

Laboratory Results

A. Screening Procedures

	Patient	Normal
Prothrombin time	29 seconds	10–12 seconds
APTT	34 seconds	<42 seconds
Platelet count	310,000/μl	130,000–400,000/μl
Bleeding time	4 minutes	1–8 minutes

Questions

1. What is the most likely diagnosis?
2. Is the family history helpful in establishing this diagnosis?
3. What is the treatment of choice?

Laboratory Results

B. Confirmatory Procedures

	Patient	Normal
Prothrombin time (50% patient plasma/50% pooled normal plasma)	12 seconds	10–12 seconds
Factor VII:C activity	3%	50% to 150%

DIAGNOSIS: Hereditary deficiency of factor VII

Discussion

This case is an example of hereditary deficiency of factor VII. The results of the screening procedures were typical (abnormal prothrombin time, normal activated partial thromboplastin time). The results of these screening procedures suggested deficiency of factor VII or a circulating anticoagulant. Mixing procedures were performed, and there was complete correction of the prothrombin time when the patient's plasma was mixed with pooled normal plasma. The factor VII assay confirmed the diagnosis of hereditary deficiency of factor VII.

Deficiency of factor VII is inherited in an autosomal recessive manner. Thus, severe deficiency of factor VII clotting activity occurs in homozygotes and minor deficiency occurs in heterozygotes. The frequency of homozygous deficiency of factor VII has been estimated to be one case in 500,000 people.

Biochemical Aspects. Factor VII is a single-chain molecule with a molecular weight of approximately 47,000 (on sodium dodecyl sulfate-agarose gel electrophoresis). It may be converted to a two-chain molecule by factor Xa, factor IXa, thrombin and factor XIIa (Figure 1).

Factor VII is unique among the zymogens of coagulation. The single-chain form appears to possess

HEREDITARY DEFICIENCY OF FACTOR VII

CLINICAL PICTURE

Epistaxis

Central nervous system hemorrhage

Easy bruising

Postoperative bleeding

Hemarthrosis

Menorrhagia

Deep-vein thrombosis

Pattern of inheritance: Autosomal recessive

PHYSICAL PROPERTIES OF FACTOR VII

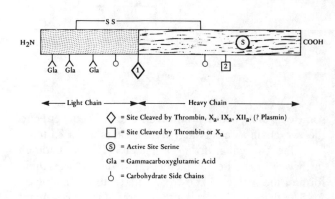

◇ = Site Cleaved by Thrombin, X_a, IX_a, XII_a, (? Plasmin)

□ = Site Cleaved by Thrombin or X_a

Ⓢ = Active Site Serine

Gla = Gammacarboxyglutamic Acid

⭘ = Carbohydrate Side Chains

LABORATORY FINDINGS

A. Screening Procedures

Test	Patient's Result	Normal Range
Prothrombin time	Abnormal	10–12 seconds
APTT	Normal	<42 seconds
Platelet count	Normal	130,000–400,000/μl
Bleeding time	Normal	1–8 minutes

B. Confirmatory Procedures

Prothrombin time, patient plasma/ pooled normal plasma	Normal	10–12 seconds
Factor VII:C activity	Abnormal	50% to 150%

TREATMENT

Fresh-frozen plasma
Prothrombin complex concentrates in life-threatening bleeding
Factor VII concentrate available in Europe
DDAVP (?)
Avoidance of aspirin containing compounds

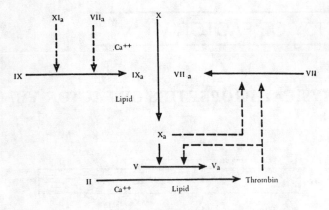

Figure 1

some coagulant activity; however, when it is converted to the two-chain form, its activity increases up to 85-fold.

The two-chain form of factor VII can undergo further cleavage (i.e., by factor Xa) to yield a three-chain form of the molecule known as beta-factor VIIa (Figure 2). The three-chain form of the molecule lacks coagulant activity; nevertheless, it is still able to hydrolyze small ester substrates. Unlike other activated bovine coagulation factors, factor VIIa is not appreciably inhibited by antithrombin III.

Clinical Picture. The correlation between clinical bleeding and the factor VII activity assay is poor. Recent studies have demonstrated a marked heterogeneity among patients with factor VII deficiency (Table 1). Early studies in which rabbit serum that contained antibodies to factor VII was used in an antibody neutralization assay demonstrated cross-reacting material (CRM) in some patients with a deficiency of factor VII. Such patients were designated CRM+. Other patients were found to have reduced amounts of CRM, with some discrepancy between factor VII antigen and factor VII coagulant activity. Such patients were designated CRM^R.

Further discrepancies have also been noted when various investigators have examined patients with a deficiency of factor VII by using thromboplastins of differing origins (e.g., human, ox and rabbit). One variant, factor VII Padua, is CRM+, as demonstrated by use of an antibody neutralization assay. Patients with this variant were also found to have reduced factor VII coagulant activity with rabbit brain and rabbit brain-lung thromboplastins but normal factor VII coagulant activity with an ox brain thromboplastin. The nature of this defect has not been further defined, although it has been suggested that there may be different sites for activation of factor VII by different thromboplastins. Further heterogeneity of hereditary deficiency of factor VII has been identified by a group of Israeli investigators. They have found an association between hereditary deficiency of factor VII and Dubin-Johnson syndrome. In addition, there has been speculation that deficiency of factor VII is associated with Rotor's syndrome and Gilbert's disease.

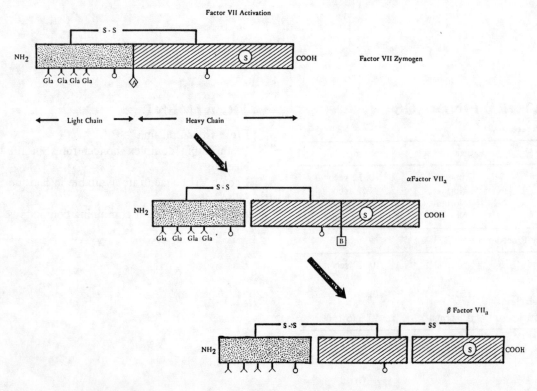

Figure 2

Table 1
Classification of Factor VII Deficiency

Congenital

    Homozygous

    Heterozygous

    Combined deficiency of factors II, VII, IX and X

Associated with other disease states (congenital)

    Qualitative abnormalities of platelets

    Dubin-Johnson syndrome

    Deficiency of factors VII and X with carotid body tumor

    Hemophilia A

    Hemophilia B

Acquired

    Vitamin K-deficient diet

    Malabsorption form gastrointestinal tract

    Sterilization of gastrointestinal tract due to antibiotic therapy

    Liver disease

    Oral anticoagulant therapy

    Newborn

        Lack of intestinal flora

        Low body stores of vitamin K

        Immature liver function

    Hodgkin's disease

    Nephrotic syndrome

    Inhibitor of factor VII with bronchogenic carcinoma

Deficiency of factor VII has also been reported in association with deficiency of factor IX.

Most persons with a hereditary deficiency of factor VII have bleeding episodes before they reach adulthood. A subgroup of affected persons manifests bleeding in the first few days of life. Such persons have a high incidence of central nervous system bleeding. Later in life, hemarthrosis, easy bruising and menorrhagia may be seen.

Patients with a severe deficiency of factor VII may undergo surgical procedures with little bleeding intraoperatively or postoperatively. This observation is difficult to reconcile. In addition, a number of patients have been described with a deficiency of factor VII and thrombotic disease, including pulmonary embolism and thrombosis of the inferior vena cava.

Treatment. Patients should receive prophylaxis before undergoing dental extraction or other surgical procedures. The biologic half-life of factor VII has been reported to be between 2 and 5 hours. A factor VII level of 20% is thought to be adequate to ensure hemostasis.

Available blood products include fresh-frozen plasma, prothrombin complex concentrates and a factor VII concentrate that is available in Europe. Fresh-frozen plasma is preferred because of its ready availability and its low incidence of side effects. Prothrombin complex concentrates may be thrombotic and also, of course, have a high potential for causing posttransfusion hepatitis. A loading dose of fresh-frozen plasma (10 to 20 ml/kg of body weight), followed every 12 hours by dose of 3 to 6 ml/kg of body weight, is usually satisfactory.

Bibliography

Biochemical Aspects

Broze GJ: Binding of human factor VII and VIIIa to monocytes. *J Clin Invest* 70:526–529, 1982.

Broze GJ, Majerus PW: Human factor VII. *Methods Enzymol* 80:228–231, 1982.

Gjonnaless H: Cold promoted activation of factor VII. *Thromb Diath Haemorrh* 28:155–168, 1972.

Jesty J: The inhibition of activated bovine coagulation factors X and VII by antithrombin III. *Arch Biochem Biophys* 185:165–173, 1978.

Jesty J, Nemerson Y: The tissue pathway of coagulation. In Ogston D, Bennett B (eds): *Haemostasis: Biochemistry, Physiology and Pathology*. London: John Wiley & Sons, 1977, pp 95–104.

Kisiel W, Davie EW: Isolation and characterization of bovine factor VII. *Biochemistry* 14:4928–4934, 1975.

Laake K, Osterud B: Activation of purified plasma factor VII by human plasmin, plasma kallikrein and activated components of the human intrinsic blood coagulation system. *Thromb Res* 5:759–772, 1974.

Marlar RA, Kleiss AJ, Griffin JH: An alternative extrinsic pathway of human blood coagulation. *Blood* 60:1353–1358, 1982.

Nemerson Y, Jackson CM, Aronson DL: Nomenclature recommendations for factor VII. *Thromb Haemostasis* 43:175–179, 1980.

Radcliffe R, Bagdasarian A, Colman R, et al: Activation of bovine factor VII by Hageman factor fragments. *Blood* 50:611–617, 1977.

Radcliffe R, Nemerson Y: Bovine factor VII. *Methods Enzymol* 45:49–56, 1976.

Radcliffe R, Nemerson Y: Mechanism of activation of bovine factor VII. *J Biol Chem* 251:4797–4802, 1976.

Seligsohn N, Osterud B, Brown SF, et al: Activation of factor VII in plasma and purified systems. *J Clin Invest* 64:1056–1065, 1979.

Seligsohn U, Osterud B, Griffin JH, et al: Evidence for the participation of both activated factor XII and activated factor IX in cold-promoted activation of factor VII. *Thromb Res* 13:1049–1055, 1978.

Zur M, Nemerson Y: The esterase activity of coagulation factor VII. Evidence for intrinsic activity of the zymogen. *J Biol Chem* 253:2203–2209, 1978.

Clinical Picture

Barberio G, Cordaro V, Gemelli M, et al: Isolated congenital deficiency of factor VII, clinical study. *Minerva Pediatr* 29:843–845, 1977.

Braun MW, Triplett DA: Factor VII deficiency in an obstetrical patient. *J Indiana State Med Ass* 72:900–902, 1979.

Britten AFH, Salzman EW: Surgery in congenital disorders of blood coagulation. *Surg Gynecol Obstet* 123:1333–1358, 1966.

Cartmill TB, Castaldi PA, Halliday EJ: Cardiac valve surgery in factor VII deficiency. *Lancet* 1:752–753, 1968.

Cleton FJ, Loeliger EA: Two typical hereditary charts of congenital factor VII deficiency. *Thromb Diath Haemorrh* 5:87–92, 1960–61.

Dische FE, Benfield V: Congenital factor VII deficiency. Hematological and genetic aspects. *Acta Haematol* 21:257–271, 1959.

Falter ML, Kaufman MF: Congenital factor VII deficiency. *J Pediatr* 79:298–304, 1971.

Fernandez PM, Torre Blanca J, Cuesta Garcia MV, et al: Congenital factor VII deficiency. *An Esp Pediatr* 13:611–618, 1980.

Galbraith PA: A case report of idiopathic factor VII deficiency. *Med Serv J Can* 15:445–449, 1959.

Girolami A, Cattarori Y, Mengarda G, et al: Congenital factor VII deficiency: A case report. *Blut* 27:236–244, 1973.

Glueck HI, Sutherland JM: Inherited factor VII defect in a Negro family. *Pediatrics* 27:204–213, 1961.

Hall CA, Rapaport SI, Ames SB, et al: A clinical and family study of hereditary proconvertin (factor VII) deficiency. *Amer J Med* 37:172–178, 1964.

Heikenheimo R, Reinikainen M: Congenital factor VII deficiency: Two cases in children of cousins. *Thromb Diath Hameorrh* 21:245–251, 1969.

Jain SC, Quadri MI, Garewal G, et al: Congenital deficiency of factor VII. Case reports of non-identical twins. *Indian Pediatr* 16:809–813, 1979.

Lopez CG, Thiruselvam A, Hutton RA: Factor VII deficiency in an East Indian family. *Clin Lab Haematol* 4:411–415, 1982.

Matthay KK, Koerper MA, Ablin AR: Intracranial hemorrhage in congenital factor VII deficiency. *J Clin Invest* 94:413–415, 1979.

Owens CA, Amundsen MA, Thompson JH, et al: Congenital deficiency of factor VII. *Amer J Med* 37:71–91, 1964.

Schricker KT: Congenital factor VII deficiency. *Med Klin (Munich)* 76:24–26, 1981.

Takamatsu J, Hayashi K, Ogata K, et al: A family of congenital factor VII deficiency. *Rinsho Ketsueki* 21:834–839, 1980.

Zimmerman R, Ehlers G, Ehlers W, et al: Congenital factor VII deficiency. A report of four new cases. *Blut* 32:119–125, 1979.

Variants of Factor VII

Brandt JT, Triplett DA, Schaeffer J: Functional variation in hereditary factor VII deficiency. (Abstract) *Blood* 58:211a, 1981.

Girolami A: The congenital factor VII abnormalities (dysproconvertinemias). The genetic plot thickens. *Folia Haematol (Leipzig)* 107:131–136, 1980.

Hall CA, London AR, Moynihan AC, et al: Hereditary factor VII and IX deficiency in a large kindred. *Brit J Haematol* 29:319–327, 1975.

Levanon M, Rimon S, Shari M, et al: Active and inactive factor VII in Dubin Johnson syndrome with factor VII deficiency and on coumadin administration. *Brit J Haematol* 23:669–674, 1972.

Mazzucconi MG, Bertina RM, Romoli D, et al: Factor VII activity and antigen in haemophilia B variants. *Thromb Haemostasis* 43:16–19, 1980.

Nenci GC, Agnelli G, DeRegis FM: Factor VII coagulant kinetics in factor VII-CRM+ and factor VII−CRM− deficiencies. *Brit J Haematol* 46:307–309, 1980.

Seligsohn U, Shani M, Ramot B: Gilbert syndrome and factor VII deficiency. *Lancet* 1:1398–1402, 1970.

Seligsohn U, Shani M, Ramot B, et al: Dubin-Johnson syndrome in Israel. II. Association with factor VII deficiency. *Q J Med [NS]* 39:569–584, 1970.

Laboratory Tests for Factor VII

Garner R, Conning DM: The assay of human factor VII by means of modified factor VII deficient dog plasma. *Brit J Haematol* 18:57–66, 1970.

Grant J, Biggs R: Experiments on the standardization of factor VII assay. *Thromb Diath Haemorrh Suppl* 26:407–411, 1967.

Hall DE: Sensitivity of different thromboplastin reagents to factor VII deficiency in the blood of beagle dogs. *Lab Anim* 4:55, 1970.

Mazzucconi MG, Orlando M, Hassan HJ, et al: Factor VII activity and cross reacting material in normal individuals. *Thromb Res* 14:241–244, 1979.

Nemerson Y, Clyne LP: An assay for coagulation factor VII using factor VII-depleted bovine plasma. *J Lab Clin Med* 83:301–303, 1974.

Poller L, Thompson JM, Bodzenta A, et al: An assessment of an amidolytic assay for factor VII in the laboratory control of oral anticoagulants. *Brit J Haematol* 49:69–75, 1981.

Seghatchian MJ: An agarose gel method for evaluating factor VII procoagulant electrophoretic distribution. *Ann NY Acad Sci* 370:236–240, 1981.

Treatment

Dike GWR, Griffiths D, Bidwell E, et al: A factor VII concentrate for therapeutic use. *Brit J Haematol* 45:107–118, 1980.

Dodds WJ, Packham MA, Rowsell HC, et al: Factor VII survival and turnover in dogs. *Amer J Physiol* 213:36–42, 1967.

Mariani G, Mannucci PM, Mazzucconi MG, et al: Treatment of congenital factor VII deficiency with a new concentrate. *Thromb Haemostasis* 39:675–682, 1978.

Yorke AJ, Mant MJ: Factor VII deficiency and surgery. Is preoperative replacement therapy necessary? *J Amer Med Ass* 238:424–432, 1977.

CASE
17

PATIENT: 25-year-old woman

CHIEF COMPLAINT: This patient presented to the hemophilia clinic for a yearly evaluation. She had a lifelong history of bleeding problems.

MEDICAL HISTORY: The patient was delivered without complications. Approximately 3 weeks after birth, bright red blood was noted in the stools. A coagulation evaluation obtained at that time was thought to be unremarkable. The Lee and White clotting time and platelet count were the only procedures performed. About 3 months later, she again bled from a superficial ulceration noted on the buccal mucosa. At 10 months of age, the patient had a large hematoma of the left arm as a result of a fall. Under similar circumstances at 12 months of age, she had a massive hematoma of the left gastrocnemius muscle.

The patient bled with the eruption of every deciduous tooth and on one occasion required a transfusion. When 18 months of age, she suffered a cerebral hemorrhage that caused convulsions and temporary paralysis of the left side of the body. The patient recovered from this episode with only minimal hemiparesis. She continued to have recurrent intramuscular hematomas and other bleeding episodes from the gastrointestinal mucosa. Eventually, she was placed on transfusions of plasma approximately every 2 weeks. During adolescence, the patient sustained a number of hemarthroses that necessitated confinement to a wheelchair. Epistaxis was not a problem; however, there were episodes of marked menorrhagia.

At the time of her clinic visit, the patient was confined to a wheelchair and was receiving fresh-frozen plasma as a prophylactic measure on a biweekly basis.

FAMILY HISTORY: No family member had a history of bleeding problems.

DRUG HISTORY: The patient had originally been evaluated by Dr. Armand Quick and had been instructed to avoid all aspirin and aspirin-containing compounds. Because of the recurrent hemarthrosis and intramuscular hematomas, she used acetaminophen frequently. Oral contraceptives had also been given in an attempt to control the menorrhagia.

PHYSICAL EXAMINATION: There was no evidence of the left hemiparesis that had originally resulted from the cerebral hemorrhage at 18 months of age. However, there was muscular atrophy of the legs and limited motion of the knees as a result of recurrent hemarthroses. Slight contractures were noted in the arms. The veins of the arms were sclerotic as a result of frequent transfusions and blood-drawing procedures.

Laboratory Results

A. Screening Procedures

	Patient	Normal
Prothrombin time	35 seconds	10–12 seconds
APTT	36 seconds	<42 seconds
Platelet count	300,000/μl	130,000–400,000/μl
Bleeding time	6 minutes	1–8 minutes

Questions

1. What is the provisional differential diagnosis?
2. Is this clinical picture typical?

Laboratory Results

B. Confirmatory Procedures

	Patient	Normal
Prothrombin time (50% patient plasma/ 50% pooled normal plasma)	12 seconds	10–12 seconds
Factor VII:C activity	4%	50% to 150%

DIAGNOSIS: Hereditary deficiency of factor VII

Discussion

This case is an example of hereditary deficiency of factor VII in which the patient has striking clinical bleeding. In fact, the degree of bleeding in this patient is comparable to that of a patient with a severe deficiency of factors VIII or IX. Most patients with a deficiency of factor VII present with mild clinical bleeding, although it has been emphasized that patients with a deficiency of factor VII may have a high incidence of cerebral bleeding shortly after birth. In this patient, the cerebral hemorrhage did not occur until 18 months of age.

HEREDITARY DEFICIENCY OF FACTOR VII

CLINICAL PICTURE

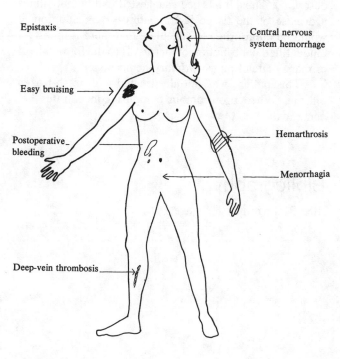

Epistaxis

Central nervous system hemorrhage

Easy bruising

Postoperative bleeding

Hemarthrosis

Menorrhagia

Deep-vein thrombosis

Pattern of inheritance: Autosomal recessive

PHYSICAL PROPERTIES OF FACTOR VII

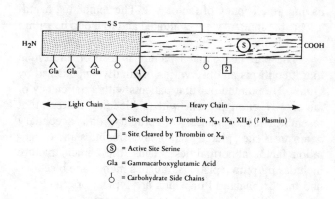

◇ = Site Cleaved by Thrombin, X_a, IX_a, XII_a, (? Plasmin)

□ = Site Cleaved by Thrombin or X_a

Ⓢ = Active Site Serine

Gla = Gammacarboxyglutamic Acid

⌀ = Carbohydrate Side Chains

LABORATORY FINDINGS

A. Screening Procedures

Test	Patient's Result	Normal Range
Prothrombin time	Abnormal	10–12 seconds
APTT	Normal	<42 seconds
Platelet count	Normal	130,000–400,000/μl
Bleeding time	Normal	1–8 minutes

B. Confirmatory Procedures

Prothrombin time: 50% patient/50% pooled normal plasma	Normal	10–12 seconds
Factor VII:C activity	Abnormal	50% to 150%

TREATMENT

Fresh-frozen plasma

Prothrombin complex concentrates in life-threatening bleeding

Avoidance of aspirin containing compounds.

The patient's subsequent clinical course of recurrent hemarthrosis and intramuscular hematomas is unusual. As would be expected, the initial evaluation of this patient in 1952 was negative because only the intrinsic system was evaluated with a relatively insensitive test, the Lee and White clotting technique. Subsequently, the patient was found to have a markedly prolonged prothrombin time and was diagnosed as having a deficiency of factor VII. The remaining hematologic parameters were evaluated and found to be within normal limits.

The patient's clinical picture is also of interest in that it confirms an observation originally emphasized by Quick. He pointed out that patients with a deficiency of factor VII often present with a bleeding pattern that resembles abnormalities of primary and secondary hemostasis (i.e., platelet factor abnormalities and coagulation factor abnormalities). Thus, the clinical picture includes purpura, epistaxis, mucous membrane bleeding, and menorrhagia, all of which are typical of platelet or vascular disorders, together with hemarthrosis and intramuscular hematomas which are characteristic of abnormalities of coagulation proteins. This type of clinical picture suggests that factor VII does not participate solely in the extrinsic system of coagulation. Factor VII plays a part in the intrinsic system of coagulation by virtue of its ability to activate factor IX. Reciprocal activation of factor VII by factor IXa has also been described. Thus, it has been suggested that hemophilia is a disease of the tissue factor pathways. In addition, it would be appropriate to speculate that there is an as yet unidentified contribution of factor VII to the formation of primary platelet plugs (primary hemostasis).

This patient was initially treated with fresh-frozen plasma. When prothrombin complex concentrates became available, they were used.

Bibliography

(See Bibliography for Case 16)

CASE
18

PATIENT: 12-year-old boy

CHIEF COMPLAINT: This patient originally presented to his dentist with pain in the left lower mandibular region. After examination of the oral cavity, the diagnosis of an impacted left mandibular molar was made. The patient was referred to an oral surgeon for consultation and extraction of the molar.

On February 23, the impacted left mandibular molar was extracted in the office of the oral surgeon. After the extraction, the patient did well until the evening of February 25, when he bled from the extraction site. Bleeding was controlled after 1 to 2 hours with pressure and a gauze packing. On February 27, he was seen as an outpatient in the emergency room because of recurrence of spontaneous bleeding from the extraction site. After ruling out the possibility of retained bone fragments, the extraction site was repacked, and the patient was referred to the coagulation laboratory at Ball Memorial Hospital for hemostatic evaluation.

MEDICAL HISTORY: The patient had a history of minimal bleeding problems. Delivery, circumcision and umbilical cord separation were achieved without hemostatic difficulties. When 4 years of age, the patient had swelling in the left knee and ankle, and a pediatrician made a diagnosis of juvenile rheumatoid arthritis. Subsequently, the patient was placed on aspirin, which caused several episodes of epistaxis and gastrointestinal hemorrhage. After these bleeding complications, the aspirin was discontinued, and the patient had no subsequent problems with "arthritis."

The parents and patient reported a tendency to bruise easily, particularly over the legs. The bruising often was associated with prominent hematoma formation. At the time of the patient's initial evaluation, he could recall no recent episode of viral illness. He was a physically active boy who participated in a number of sports, including basketball, cross-country, track and baseball.

FAMILY HISTORY: The patient had a sister (15 years of age) and a brother (16 years of age), neither of whom had bleeding difficulties. The mother and father were well and admitted to no bleeding problems. The maternal grandmother reportedly had epistaxis, although she had never been evaluated for a bleeding diathesis.

DRUG HISTORY: No medication

PHYSICAL EXAMINATION: A hematoma was noted over the left mandibular region. There was no evidence of splenomegaly, hepatomegaly or petechiae.

Laboratory Results

A. Screening Procedures

	Patient	Normal
Prothrombin time	30 seconds	10–12 seconds
APTT	76 seconds	<42 seconds
Platelet count	399,000/μl	130,000–400,000/μl
Bleeding time	7 minutes and 30 seconds	1–8 minutes

HOSPITAL COURSE: After the patient had been evaluated in the coagulation laboratory on March 2, a hematoma developed under his surgical flap medial to the left mandible. It was drained, and a continuous, slow oozing from the surgical site was noted later that afternoon. On the following day, a hematoma was again noted under the flap and was again drained. The contents of the hematoma were noted to be unclotted blood. The boy was admitted to the hospital, and 2 units of fresh-frozen plasma were administered. The patient responded immediately. On March 5, 1 additional unit of fresh-frozen plasma was infused. Inspection of the surgical site indicated normal healing. The patient was discharged from the hospital on a regimen of Amicar ([aminocaproic acid], 100 mg/kg every 6 hours) and penicillin.

Questions

1. What is the provisional differential diagnosis?
2. What additional laboratory procedures are indicated?

Laboratory Results

B. Confirmatory Procedures

	Patient	Normal
APTT (50% patient plasma/50% pooled normal plasma)	34 seconds	<42 seconds
Prothrombin time (50% patient plasma/50% pooled normal plasma)	12 seconds	10–12 seconds
Stypven time	25 seconds	6–10 seconds
Factor X assay	3%	50% to 150%

HEREDITARY DEFICIENCY OF FACTOR X

CLINICAL PICTURE

PHYSICAL PROPERTIES OF FACTOR X

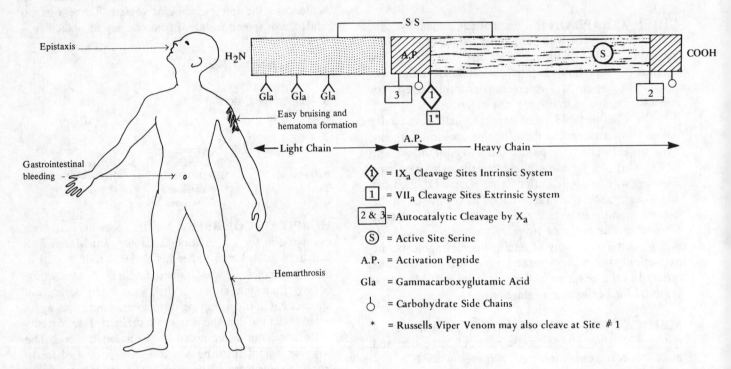

Epistaxis

Easy bruising and hematoma formation

Gastrointestinal bleeding

Hemarthrosis

Pattern of inheritance: Autosomal recessive

H_2N — Gla Gla Gla — Light Chain — A.P. — Heavy Chain — COOH

S S

A.P.

① = IX_a Cleavage Sites Intrinsic System

1 = VII_a Cleavage Sites Extrinsic System

2 & 3 = Autocatalytic Cleavage by X_a

Ⓢ = Active Site Serine

A.P. = Activation Peptide

Gla = Gammacarboxyglutamic Acid

○ = Carbohydrate Side Chains

* = Russells Viper Venom may also cleave at Site #1

LABORATORY FINDINGS

A. Screening Procedures

Test	Patient's Result	Normal Range
Prothrombin time	Abnormal	10–12 seconds
APTT	Abnormal	<42 seconds
Platelet count	Normal	130,000–400,000/μl
Bleeding time	Normal	1–8 minutes

B. Confirmatory Procedures

Mixing APTT	Normal	<42 seconds
Mixing prothrombin time	Normal	10–12 seconds
Stypven time	Abnormal	6–10 seconds
Factor X assay	Abnormal	50% to 150%

TREATMENT

Fresh-frozen plasma
Prothrombin complex concentrates in severe cases
Avoidance of aspirin and aspirin containing compounds

Table 1
Differential Diagnosis of Classical Deficiency of Factors VII and X

Test	Factor VII	Factor X
Prothrombin time	Abnormal	Abnormal
Thromboplastin generation time	Normal	Abnormal
Stypven time	Normal	Abnormal*
Activated partial thromboplastin time	Normal	Abnormal

*Except in patients with the Friuli variant of factor X deficiency.

DIAGNOSIS: Hereditary deficiency of factor X

Discussion

In 1956, groups from Oxford, England and Chapel Hill, North Carolina simultaneously reported a "new" coagulation defect. This new coagulation factor was distinguished from factor VII by abnormal results on a thromboplastin generation test (Table 1). Subsequently, the missing factor was designated factor X, or Stuart-Prower factor, after the surnames of the affected persons.

During the 5 years after the initial case reports, a number of patients with a deficiency of factor X were studied. Several extensive family studies were undertaken, and it was established that the Stuart-Prower defect is inherited as a highly penetrant, incompletely recessive, autosomal trait. On the basis of these studies, it was postulated that the frequency of heterozygotes for deficiency of factor X is approximately 2 in 1000 people. Approximately 58 cases of hereditary deficiency of factor X have been reported. Several variant states of factor X deficiency (e.g., Friuli) also have been reported.

A number of acquired states of isolated factor X deficiency also have been identified. Most such cases have been seen in association with primary systemic amyloidosis, although other conditions, such as primary atypical pneumonia, have been described (Table 2).

Biochemical Aspects. Factor X is a vitamin K-dependent clotting factor, as are factors IX, II and VII and the recently described proteins C and S. Vitamin K is required for the formation of a unique amino acid, γ-carboxyglutamic acid. This amino acid is found in each vitamin K-dependent clotting factor and is thought to be responsible for the calcium-binding properties of all such factors. The molecular relevance of the calcium-binding sites in the vitamin K-dependent proteins has only recently been appreciated.

Table 2
Classification of Factor X Deficiency

Hereditary deficiency
    Cross-reacting material negative
    Cross-reacting material positive (Friuli variant, etc.)
Acquired deficiency
    Primary systemic amyloidosis
    Transient
        Atypical pneumonia
        Fungicide exposure
        Miscellaneous
Combined deficiency of factors II, VII, IX and X
Combined deficiency of factors VII and X associated with carotid body tumors

Rapid activation of vitamin K-dependent proteins requires a lipid-water interface. Adsorption to such an interface is necessary for achieving a high reactant concentration for overcoming the effects of plasma protease inhibitors (i.e., antithrombin III). This interaction requires calcium ions, which apparently bridge the negatively charged groups in the proteins and bind to phospholipid surfaces. The phospholipid surfaces that are necessary for these reactions are supplied by activated platelets. Deficiency of vitamin K or administration of oral anticoagulants prevents the conversion of glutamic acid to γ-carboxyglutamic acid. Consequently, although vitamin K-dependent proteins are present antigenically, they are unable to bind calcium and are inactive in coagulation. Recent work on the synthesis of prothrombin has shown that vitamin K is involved in modification of the glutamic acid residues in a post-translational reaction (i.e., after ribosomal assembly of proteins).

There is appreciable sequence similarity between vitamin K-dependent coagulation factors and other serine proteases. Partial amino acid sequence analysis has shown that the amino-terminal sequences of prothrombin, factors IX and X and pancreatic trypsin are homologous. The amino-terminal region of vitamin K-dependent proteins contains the calcium-binding sites.

Factor X is a glycoprotein that is found in plasma at a concentration of 4 to 5 μg/ml with a molecular weight of approximately 54,000. It is composed of two polypeptide chains that are linked by one or more disulfide bonds. Factor X and protein C are unique among the zymogens of the coagulation system because they are recovered from plasma as disulfide-bonded, two-chain proteins. There is controversy regarding the molecular weights of the light and heavy chains of factor X; however, there is a consensus regarding the exclusive location of the carbohydrate moieties in the heavy chain.

The light chain of factor X contains the γ-carboxyglutamic acid residues and is responsible for the calcium-mediated binding of factor Xa to phospholipid surfaces. The active serine residue is located in the heavy chain.

Factor X is activated by factors IXa and VIII or by factor VII and a tissue factor. In addition, factor X can be activated by trypsin or Russell's viper venom. Activation of factor X by each of these systems involves cleavage of an Arg 51-Ile 52 peptide bond in the heavy chain; this cleavage gives rise to the formation of a glycoprotein with a molecular weight of approximately 44,000 and an activation peptide with a molecular weight of approximately 11,000. The resultant protease is called alpha-factor Xa. A carboxy-terminal peptide is autolytically cleaved from the enzyme's heavy chain in

vitro without discernible biochemical effect. This species is termed beta-factor Xa.

Protein substrates for factor Xa include prothrombin and factors VII, V, VIII and IX. Factor Xa also has esterase activity toward synthetic esters and synthetic substrates, such as S-2222 and S-2337 (supplied by Kabi-Helena).

Factor Xa is inhibited by a number of different serine protease inhibitors, including antithrombin III and soybean trypsin inhibitor, and by diisopropyl fluorophosphate, which binds to the active serine residue in the molecule's heavy chain. Other inhibitors of factor X have been described and include phenylmethylsulfonyl fluoride.

Table 3

Variants of Factor X Deficiency*

Case	Prothrombin Time	Activated Partial Thromboplastin Time	Russell's Viper Venom Time	Chromogenic Substrate Assay	Factor X Antigen	Clinical Picture	Comments
Stuart	Abnormal	Abnormal	Abnormal	Abnormal	Very low, in parallel with factor X coagulation activity (radioimmunoassay)	Hemarthrosis, hematoma, epistaxis	
Prower	Abnormal	Abnormal	Abnormal		73% to 85% (antibody neutralization technique)	Bleeding after dental extraction, menorrhagia	Precipitin line of identity with normal factor X (Ouchterlony technique)
Friuli defect	Abnormal	Abnormal	Normal	Abnormal S2222 assay with Russell's viper venom	Normal (antibody neutralization and radioimmunoassay)	Mild epistaxis, posttraumatic, hemarthrosis, bleeding after dental extraction	Crossed electrophoresis normal
Case of Parkin et al.	Normal	Abnormal	Normal		Normal (antibody neutralization technique)	No bleeding tendency	
Case of Bertina et al.	Abnormal	Normal	50% activity	44% activity (S2337)	50% (Laurell technique)	No bleeding tendency	Crossed immunoelectrophoresis normal; adsorbed from plasma by Al(OH)₃
Case of Denson et al.	Abnormal	Slightly abnormal			Slightly abnormal (antibody neutralization technique)		
Factor X, Vorarlberg	112 seconds (control, 17 seconds)	54 seconds (control, 40 seconds)	13.7 seconds (control, 11.5 seconds)		20% (antibody neutralization technique)	Mild bleeding tendency	Factor X assays, 1% (prothrombin time), 12% (Russell's viper venom time) or 32% (activated partial thromboplastin time)

*This table is based on a review of the literature. Recently, Dr. D. S. Fair has reported a more comprehensive classification of factor X variants that is based on antigen measured by radioimmunoassay and on activity measured by prothrombin time, activated partial thromboplastin time and Russell's viper venom time. With these assays, he has identified 10 classes and subclasses of abnormal factor X molecules.

† From Triplett DA: Thrombosis and Hemostasis Check Sample Program. Chicago: A.S.C.P.

Clinical Picture. Inherited deficiency of factor X is among the most rare disorders of blood coagulation. If one includes the variant forms of factor X deficiency, approximately 70 cases have been reported. Deficiency of factor X also has been reported in cocker spaniel dogs.

The bleeding history of patients with a deficiency of factor X is not clinically distinguishable from that of patients with a deficiency of factor VII. Neonatal bleeding may occur intracranially or from the gastrointestinal tract or vagina. The most common complaint in later life is easy bruising and hematoma formation after minor surgical procedures. The nature of the clinical bleeding varies with the severity of the deficiency. Hemarthrosis, exsanguinating postoperative bleeding and central nervous system hemorrhage have been reported in the most severely affected patients; mildly affected patients suffer from easy bruisability or mucous membrane bleeding. Menstruation may be severe, even life-threatening. Several patients have been treated with radiation to the ovaries or hysterectomy to control the menorrhagia.

Patients with a deficiency of factor X typically have an abnormal prothrombin time and an abnormal activated partial thromboplastin time (APTT). The Russell's viper venom time (Stypven time) is also abnormal (except in patients with the Friuli variant). A specific assay for factor X may be based on the prothrombin time or the APTT, with an appropriate factor X-deficient plasma used as a substrate. It recently has become evident, however, that there are variant forms of factor X deficiency in which the abnormal factor X molecule behaves normally in one assay system (i.e., based on the prothrombin time or APTT) and abnormally in a second assay system.

With the introduction of synthetic chromogenic and fluorogenic substrates, it is now possible to assay factor X without using factor X-deficient plasma as a substrate. Specific substrates (S-2222 and S-2337) have been developed for factor X. These substrates are tetrapeptides that have been designed to mimic the amino acid sequence around the factor Xa cleavage sites in prothrombin. It should be emphasized, however, that discrepant results have been reported, with variant molecules, (e.g., Friuli) using these substrate assays.

In addition to assays that are based on the coagulant activity of factor X, immunologic assays have been designed. Initially, such assays made use of an antibody that was raised in rabbits. The assay techniques included an antibody neutralization procedure, as well as crossed electrophoresis and immunodiffusion. More recently, a specific radioimmunoassay for factor X has been described. With this assay system, together with the Stypven time and factor X assays based on the prothrombin time and APTT, a number of variant forms of factor X deficiency have been described (Table 3).

Treatment. The need for factor replacement depends on the severity of the deficiency. The half-life of transfused factor X is in the range of 24 to 40 hours and has a bimodal survival curve. The initial decay may be partially due to extravascular diffusion of factor X, but it can also be related to other mechanisms, such as endothelial adsorption, denaturation and neutralization. The second phase of disappearance may be attributed to catabolism.

Plasma is the preferred therapeutic agent. In patients with life-threatening bleeding and those with a severe deficiency of factor X, prothrombin complex concentrates are indicated. The primary hazard associated with use of prothrombin complex concentrates is the high risk of hepatitis and thromboembolic phenomena. Also, recent reports have raised the possibility that administration of such concentrates may be associated with the development of acquired immune deficiency syndrome.

A factor level of 10% to 40% is considered adequate for ensuring hemostasis. Consequently, infusions of plasma every 12 hours prove satisfactory in most instances. The usual loading dose is 10 to 20 mg of plasma per kilogram of body weight, followed by 3 to 6 mg/kg every 12 hours.

In addition to the use of plasma and prothrombin complex concentrates, hormone therapy reportedly affects the level of factor X. In one case, a patient with a congenital deficiency of factor X showed dramatic improvement during pregnancy; she subsequently was treated with progesterone, which diminished the clinical signs and shortened the abnormal prothrombin time. This finding, however, has not been subsequently confirmed.

Bibliography

Aurell L, Friberger P, Karlsson G, et al: A new sensitive and highly specific chromogenic peptide substrate for factor Xa. *Thromb Res* 11:595–609, 1977.

Bachmann FF, Duckert F, Fluckiger P, et al: Uber einen neuartigen kongenitalen Gerinnungsdefects (Mangel an Stuart Faktor). *Thromb Diath Haemorrh* 1:87–93, 1957.

Bachmann F, Duckert F, Koller F: The Stuart-Prower factor assay and its clinical significance. *Thromb Diath Haemorrh* 2:14, 1958.

Bajaj S, Mann KG: Simultaneous purification of bovine prothrombin and factor X. Activation of prothrombin by trypsin activated X. *J Biol Chem* 248:7720–7741 1973.

Biggs R, Denson KW: The fate of prothrombin and factors VIII, IX, and X transfused to patients deficient in these factors. *Brit J Haematol* 9:532–547, 1963.

Brody JI, Finch SC: Improvement of factor X deficiency during pregnancy. *N Engl J Med* 263:996–999, 1960.

Denson KW: Electrophoretic studies of the Prower factor; a blood coagulation factor which differs from factor VII. *Brit J Haematol* 4:313, 1958.

Denson KW: The specific assay of Prower-Stuart factor and factor VII. *Acta Haematol* 25:105–120, 1961.

Denson KW, Lurie A, DeCatalodo F, et al: The factor X defect: Recognition of abnormal forms of factor X. *Brit J Haematol* 18:317–327, 1970.

Dodds WJ: Canine factor X (Stuart-Prower factor) deficiency. *J Lab Clin Med* 82:560–566, 1973.

Dorantes S, Soto R, Castrejon O: Defecto de coagulation "Prower-Stuart" algunas caracteristicas del factor. *Bol Med Hosp Infant Mex* (*Span Ed*) 17:139–156, 1960.

Fair DS, Edgington TS: Group analysis of abnormal factor X molecules. (Abstract) *Thromb Haemostasis* 46:297, 1981.

Fair DS, Plow EF, Edgington TS: Combined functional and immunochemical analysis of normal and abnormal human factor X. *J Clin Invest* 64:884–894, 1979.

Fujikawa K, Coan MH, Legaz ME, et al: The mechanism of activation of bovine factor X (Stuart factor) by extrinsic and intrinsic pathways. *Biochem J* 13:5290–5299, 1974.

Fujikawa K, Legaz ME, Davie EW: Bovine factors X, and X_2 (Stuart factor). Isolation and characterization. *Biochem J* 11:4882–4891, 1972.

Girolami A, Molaro C, Lazzarin M, et al: Congenital hemorrhagic condition similar but not identical to factor X deficiency. *A hemorrhagic state due to an abnormal factor X. Scand J Haematol* 7:91–99, 1970.

Girolami A, Molaro C, Lazzarin M, et al: A "new" congenital hemorrhagic condition due to the presence of an abnormal factor X (factor X Friuli). Study of a large kindred. *Brit J Haematol* 19:179–192, 1970.

Girolami A, Saggin L, Boeri G: Factor X assays using chromogenic substrate 2222. *Amer J Clin Pathol* 73:400–402, 1980.

Gitel SM, Owen WG, Esmon CT, et al: A polypeptide region of bovine prothrombin specific for binding to phospholipids. *Proc Natl Acad Sci USA* 70:1344–1348, 1973.

Gonyea LM, Krivit W: Congenital coagulation deficiency of Stuart factor activity. *J Lab Clin Med* 51:398–409, 1958.

Graham JB, Barrow EM, Hougie C: Stuart clotting defect. II. Genetic aspects of a new hemorrhagic state. *J Clin Invest* 36:497–501, 1957.

Haber S: Norethynodrel in the treatment of factor X deficiency. *Arch Intern Med* 114:89–94, 1964.

Hartley BS: Homologies in serine proteases. *Philos Trans R Soc London* 257:77–89, 1970.

Hellemans J, Vorlat M, Verstraete M: Survival time of prothrombin and factors VII, IX, and X after completely synthesis blocking doses of coumarin derivatives. *Brit J Haematol* 9:506–512, 1963.

Hougie C, Barrow HM, Graham JB: Stuart clotting defect. I. Segregation of a hereditary hemorrhagic state from the heterozygous group heretofore called 'stable factor' (SPCA, proconvertin, factor VII) deficiency. *J Clin Invest* 36:485–496, 1957.

Jackson CM: Characterization of two glycoprotein variants of bovine factor X and demonstration that the factor X zymogen contains two polypeptide chains. *Biochem J* 11:4873–4883, 1972.

MacFarlane RG: The coagulant action of Russell's viper venom: The use of antivenom in defining its reaction with a serum factor. *Brit J Haematol* 7:496–511, 1961.

Parkin JD, Madaras F, Sweet B, et al: A further inherited variant of coagulation factor X. *Aust NZ J Med* 4:561–564, 1974.

Rabiner SF, Kretchmer N: The Stuart-Prower factor: Utilization of clotting factors obtained by starch-block electrophoresis for genetic evaluation. *Brit J Haematol* 7:99–111, 1961.

Roos J, Van Arkel C, Verloop MC, et al: A "new" family with Stuart-Prower deficiency. *Thromb Diath Haemorrh* 3:59–76, 1959.

Silverberg SA, Nemerson Y, Zur M: Kinetics of the activation of bovine coagulation factor X by components of the extrinsic system. *J Biol Chem* 252:8481–8488, 1977.

Suttie JW: Vitamin K and prothrombin synthesis. *Nutr Rev* 31:105–109, 1970.

Suttie JW: Metabolism and properties of a liver precursor to prothrombin. *Vitam Horm* (*NY*) 32:463–481, 1974.

Telfer TP, Denson KW, Wright DR: A "new" coagulation defect. *Brit J Haematol* 2:308–316, 1956.

Triplett DA: Diagnostic dilemmas in hemostasis. ASCP Workshop, Fall ASCP/CAP meeting, 1982, Miami Beach, Florida.

CASE
19

PATIENT: 26-year-old woman

CHIEF COMPLAINT: This patient was seen in consultation for further evaluation of a lifelong history of bleeding.

MEDICAL HISTORY: The patient's mother first observed that the woman had bruising and frequent nosebleeds when she was 3 years of age. At 5 years of age, the patient underwent tonsillectomy and postoperatively was noted to have increased bleeding from the tonsillar fossae. However, she did not receive blood products at that time. The patient continued to have bouts of epistaxis and bruising and was admitted to a local hospital when she was 7 years of age. The patient was seen in consultation by a pediatrician who thought that she might have acute lymphoblastic leukemia on the basis of her symptoms, and she was referred to the University of Michigan at Ann Arbor. She was seen in Ann Arbor by Dr. John Penner. The laboratory work from this original evaluation was not available. When 12 years of age, the patient began menstruating and had periods that lasted approximately 3 weeks. She was then placed on oral contraceptives in an attempt to control the menstrual bleeding. Nevertheless, the patient required fresh-frozen plasma to control the bleeding. After several years, the menorrhagia appeared to diminish and was reasonably controlled with oral contraceptives alone.

In 1968, the patient was involved in an automobile accident and sustained minor injuries, although she received a number of units of fresh-frozen plasma at that time. In 1974, her upper and lower wisdom teeth were extracted by a dentist under the cover of fresh-frozen plasma, and the patient had only slight postoperative bleeding difficulties.

In 1974, the patient was hospitalized because of recurrent urinary tract infection. Cystoscopy was performed, and abdominal hemorrhage developed after the procedure. She was transfused with a number of units of fresh-frozen plasma, and exploratory laparotomy was undertaken. A large hematoma was found in the pelvis. Postoperatively, as a result of administration of the numerous units of fresh-frozen plasma, congestive heart failure developed due to volume overload.

In 1975, the patient was admitted to the obstetrical service. At that time, she was 38 weeks gravid. For the 2 days before delivery, she received 4 units of fresh-frozen plasma daily; for the 7 days after delivery, she received 1 unit of fresh-frozen plasma daily. She delivered a healthy male infant.

FAMILY HISTORY: The patient's parents were living and well, as were her brother and sister. There was no family history of bleeding.

DRUG HISTORY: At the time of evaluation, the patient was taking no medication. She had been instructed to avoid aspirin and aspirin-containing medications.

PHYSICAL EXAMINATION: There were a number of ecchymotic areas over the arms and legs and a surgical scar over the lower portion of the abdomen.

Laboratory Results

A. Screening Procedures

	Patient	Normal
Prothrombin time	23 seconds	10–12 seconds
APTT	>300 seconds	<42 seconds
Platelet count	250,000/μl	130,000–400,000/μl
Bleeding time	7 minutes	1–8 minutes

Questions

1. What is the differential diagnosis?
2. What additional laboratory procedures are indicated?
3. What is the treatment of choice?

Laboratory Results

B. Confirmatory Procedures

	Patient	Normal
APTT (50% patient plasma/50% pooled normal plasma)	40 seconds	<42 seconds
Prothrombin time (50% patient plasma/50% pooled normal plasma)	12 seconds	10–12 seconds
Prothrombin time (patient plasma plus adsorbed plasma)	12 seconds	10–12 seconds
Thrombin time	21 seconds	<24 seconds
Factor V assay	<1%	50% to 150%

DIAGNOSIS: Hereditary deficiency of factor V, severe

HEREDITARY DEFICIENCY OF FACTOR V, SEVERE

CLINICAL PICTURE

PHYSICAL PROPERTIES OF FACTOR V

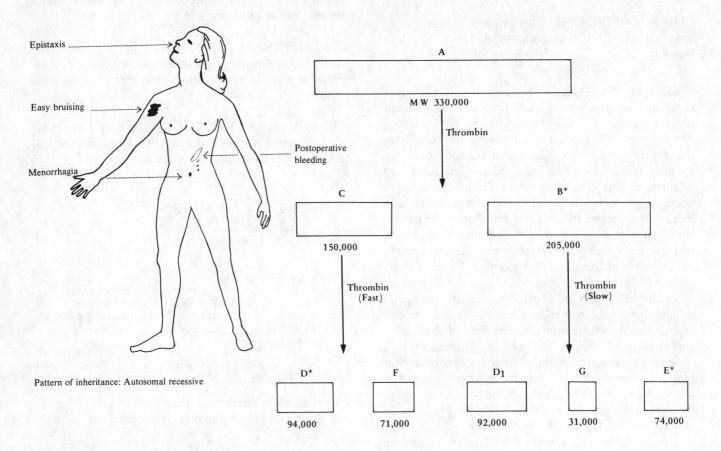

Epistaxis

Easy bruising

Menorrhagia

Postoperative bleeding

Pattern of inheritance: Autosomal recessive

A

M W 330,000

Thrombin

C
150,000

B*
205,000

Thrombin (Fast)

Thrombin (Slow)

D*
94,000

F
71,000

D₁
92,000

G
31,000

E*
74,000

LABORATORY FINDINGS

A. Screening Procedures

Test	Patient's Result	Normal Range
Prothrombin time	Abnormal	10–12 seconds
APTT	Abnormal	<42 seconds
Platelet count	Normal	130,000–400,000/μl
Bleeding time	Normal*	1–8 minutes

B. Confirmatory Procedures

Prothrombin time (50% patient plasma/50% pooled normal plasma)	Normal	10–12 seconds
Prothrombin time, adsorbed plasma	Normal	10–12 seconds
Factor V assay	Abnormal	50% to 150%

*One-third of patients may have a prolonged bleeding time.

TREATMENT

Fresh-frozen plasma
Platelet concentrates
Avoidance of aspirin containing compounds

Discussion

This case is typical of severe deficiency of factor V. Deficiency of factor V is inherited in an autosomal recessive manner. Consanguineous marriages are a frequent finding in the family history of patients with abnormalities inherited in an autosomal recessive manner. As would be expected, the prothrombin time and activated partial thromboplastin time (APTT) were prolonged due to an abnormality in the final common pathway of coagulation. Mixing studies identified the abnormality as a factor deficiency. The normal thrombin time would rule out an abnormality of fibrinogen and the correction of the prothrombin time by adsorbed plasma would rule out an abnormality of prothrombin or factor X; thus, by exclusion, the diagnosis is deficiency of factor V. A specific assay for factor V was markedly abnormal, with factor V activity being less than 1%. Special studies in this patient indicated that platelet factor V (alpha granules) was absent.

Biochemical Aspects. Factor V was found in early studies to be extremely unstable; consequently, it was termed "labile factor." This instability led to difficulties in isolating factor V; therefore, homogenous preparations have been reported only in the last 3 years. Factor V is an asymmetric, high-molecular-weight, single-chain protein with no complex subunit structure. It appears to have a molecular weight of approximately 330,000. In plasma, factor V corresponds to a procofactor that may be proteolytically cleaved to generate the cofactor molecule that participates in activation of prothrombin by factor Xa.

Activation of the procofactor to the cofactor involves thrombin. Factor V is cleaved by thrombin to yield two initial components; however, there is no measurable increase in activity. The initial two components are component C, which has a molecular weight of approximately 150,000, and component B, which has a molecular weight of approximately 205,000. Cleavage of component C leads to the appearance of component D, which has a molecular weight of approximately 94,000. At this point, the cofactor activity of factor V is expressed. Component B is cleaved at a slower rate with minimal increases in activity. Studies of the inactivation of factor Va by activated protein C have revealed that loss of activity is associated with cleavage of component D. The full activity of factor Va requires a complex of components D and E. Association of factor Va polypeptide chains is dependent on the presence of a tightly bound calcium ion. Treatment of factor Va with chelators results in loss of activity and allows components D and E, the peptides required for activation, to be resolved chromatographically.

Clinical Picture. Deficiency of factor V is inherited as an autosomal recessive trait. Homozygous persons are affected, whereas heterozygous persons are asymptomatic, having a level of factor V activity of approximately 50%. Initial studies performed with heterologous antibodies were unable to demonstrate factor V antigen in patients with a deficiency of factor V. However, more recent studies performed with monoclonal antibodies have demonstrated cross-reacting material (CRM) in some patients with a deficiency of factor V. Consequently, there appears to be a degree of heterogeneity in hereditary deficiency of factor V. This finding is similar to the heterogeneity reported in other hereditary factor deficiency states.

A combined deficiency of factors V and VIII has been reported. Factor V and factor VIII activities as low as 8% and 4%, respectively, have been observed, but in most instances, the activity is approximately 15% for both factors. The inheritance pattern in combined deficiency of factors V and VIII appears to be autosomal recessive. Factor V- and factor VIII-related antigens have been found in such patients.

Marlar and Griffin have reported that plasma of patients with a combined deficiency of factors V and VIII lacks protein C inhibitory activity. Consequently, they have postulated that the uninhibited activity of protein C may account for the clinical state of combined deficiency of factors V and VIII. However, more recent studies by Suzuki et al have disproved this theory. The specific plasma inhibitor of activated protein C was found to be normal. Consequently, the pathophysiology of the paradoxical association of factor V and VIII deficiency remains unresolved.

The hemorrhagic manifestations associated with deficiency of factor V include ecchymosis, epistaxis and menorrhagia. Hemarthrosis is relatively uncommon, even in severely affected persons. There also may be bleeding from the gingiva and gastrointestinal tract, and central nervous system hemorrhage has occasionally been reported. The degree of bleeding in affected persons appears to be associated with the level of factor V activity found within platelets rather than with the plasma level of factor V.

The differential diagnosis of hereditary deficiency of factor V includes combined deficiency of factors V and VIII and acquired deficiency of factor V. Acquired deficiency of factor V usually is due to specific antibodies to factor V, which may be associated with a variety of underlying disease states. A history of streptomycin use has been reported in a number of such cases. Acquired deficiency of factor V may also be seen in severe liver disease and disseminated intravascular coagulation, but in these clinical settings, other coagulation factors are decreased and the clinical picture usually is sufficiently characteristic to allow the clinician to rule out hereditary deficiency of factor V.

Treatment. Patients with a deficiency of factor V should be treated with fresh-frozen or fresh plasma (factor V concentrates have been prepared experimentally by use of monoclonal antibodies to factor V). In general, the factor V level is raised to 25% to 30% in patients who are undergoing surgical procedures. The half-life of transfused factor V has been variably reported to range from 4½ to 36 hours. However, the average half-life is approximately 12 hours. It has been suggested that platelet concentrates may also be of value in treating factor V deficiency. They have been used successfully to treat patients with factor V antibodies.

Bibliography

Biochemical Aspects

Chiu HC, Whitaker E, Colman RW: Detection of factor V antigen in congenital factor V deficiencies using monoclonal and polyclonal antibodies. (Abstract) *Blood* 58:213a, 1981.

Nesheim ME, Mann KG: Isolation and properties of inter-mediates involved in thrombin-catalyzed conversion of bovine factor V to factor Va. (Abstract) *Thromb Haemostasis* 46:88, 1981.

Tracy PB, Eide LH, Bowie EJW, et al: Radioimmunoassay of factor V in human plasma and platelets. *Blood* 60:59–63, 1982.

Clinical Picture

Brink AJ, Kingsley CS: A familiar disorder of blood coagulation due to deficiency of labile factor. *Q J Med* 21:19–31, 1952.

DeVries SI: Hemorrhagische diathese doore tekoit aan factor V (proacceierine). *Ned Tijdschr Geneeskd* 112:741–745, 1968.

Friedman I: Hereditary labile factor (factor V) deficiency. *J Amer Med Ass* 175:370–378, 1961.

Melliger EJ, Duckert F: Major surgery in a subject with factor V deficiency: Cholecystectomy in a parahaemophiliac woman. Review of the literature. *Thromb Diath Haemorrh* 25:438–446, 1971.

Miller SP: Coagulation dynamics in factor V deficiency: A family study, with a note on the occurrence of thrombophlebitis. *Thromb Diath Haemorrh* 13:500–517, 1965.

Mitterstieler G, Muller W, Geir W: Congenital factor V deficiency: A family study. *Scand J Haematol* 21:9–13, 1978.

O'Brien JR: Factor V in blood coagulation in vitro and a report of a case of factor V deficiency. *Brit J Haematol* 4:210–217, 1958.

Oeri J, Matter M, Isenschmed H, et al: Angeborener Mangel an Factor V (Parahaemophilie) verbunden mit echter Haemophilie A bei Zwei Brudern. *Mod Probl Paediatr* 1:575–592, 1954.

Seeler RA: Parahemophilia (factor V deficiency). *Med Clin North Amer* 56:119–125, 1972.

Factor V Inhibitors

Chediak J, Ashenhurst JB, Garlick I, et al: Successful management of bleeding in a patient with factor V inhibitor by platelet transfusions. *Blood* 56:835–841, 1980.

Coots MC, Muhleman AF, Gluelic HI: A factor V inhibitor in vitro; interference by calcium. *Amer J Hematol* 7:173–180, 1979.

Feinstein DI, Rapaport SI, McGehee WG, et al: Factor V anticoagulants: Clinical, biochemical and immunologic observations. *J Clin Invest* 49:1578–1588, 1970.

Combined Deficiency of Factors V and VIII

Giddings JC, Sugrue A, Bloom AL: Quantitation of coagulant antigens and inhibition of activated protein C in combined V/VIII deficiency. *Br J Haematol* 52:495–502, 1982.

Iverson T, Bastrup-Madsen P: Congenital familial deficiency of factor V (parahaemophilic) combined with deficiency of antihemophilic globulin. *Brit J Haematol* 2:265–271, 1956.

Marlar RA, Griffin JH: Deficiency of protein C inhibitor in combined factor V/VIII deficiency disease. *J Clin Invest* 66:1186–1189, 1980.

Mazzone D, Fichera A, Practico G, et al: Combined congenital deficiency of factor V and factor VIII. *Acta Haematol* 68:337–338, 1982.

Suzuki K, Nishioka J, Hashimoto S, et al: Normal titer of functional and immunoreactive protein C inhibitor in plasma of patients with congenital combined deficiency of factor V and factor VIII. *Blood* 62:1266–1270, 1984.

CASE
20

PATIENT: 22-year-old man

CHIEF COMPLAINT: This patient was referred for evaluation of a lifelong history of bruising and other bleeding problems.

MEDICAL HISTORY: At birth, the patient was noted to have a large cephalhematoma. Nevertheless, circumcision was undertaken, and there was profound bleeding. He was transfused with an unknown volume of fresh whole blood. The transfusions were successful in controlling the bleeding, and the patient was discharged. As a child, the patient was noted to have spontaneous bruising, and he had several episodes of gastrointestinal bleeding that necessitated multiple transfusions. At 10 years of age, he was admitted to a hospital, and exploratory laparotomy was performed because of recurrent gastrointestinal bleeding. At that time, partial gastrectomy was done. There was bleeding associated with the surgical procedure, and the patient received a number of units of fresh whole blood. Despite the gastroectomy, he continued to have recurrent bouts of gastrointestinal bleeding but did not undergo further surgical intervention.

When 16 years of age, the patient had a large staphylococcal abscess of the left hip; the abscess was drained surgically after transfusions of fresh-frozen plasma. When 21 years of age, several molars were extracted, and he again received fresh-frozen plasma preoperatively and postoperatively.

Immediately prior to his referral, the patient complained of swelling of the knees and ankles and bilateral calf pain. The swelling made walking difficult.

FAMILY HISTORY: There was no family history of bleeding problems. The patient had five brothers and one sister. The patient was married and had a 2-year-old son who had no bleeding difficulties.

DRUG HISTORY: No medication

PHYSICAL EXAMINATION: There was a large keloid at the site of the abdominal incision. The ankles were slightly swollen, and there was limited range of motion. There was also a large, unsightly scar over the forehead. This scar had resulted from surgical drainage of a large hematoma.

Laboratory Results

A. Screening Procedures

	Patient	Normal
Prothrombin time	No end point	10–12 seconds
APTT	No end point	<42 seconds
Platelet count	310,000/μl	130,000–400,000/μl
Bleeding time	9 minutes	1–8 minutes

Questions

1. What is the most likely diagnosis?
2. Does the patient have abnormalities of both primary and secondary hemostasis?
3. What additional laboratory procedures are indicated?

Laboratory Results

B. Confirmatory Procedures

	Patient	Normal
APTT (50% patient plasma/50% pooled normal plasma)	40 seconds	<42 seconds
Prothrombin time (50% patient plasma/50% pooled normal plasma)	12 seconds	10–12 seconds
Fibrinogen (clottable)	0 mg/dl	170–410 mg/dl
Fibrinogen (immunologic)	0 mg/dl	170–410 mg/dl
Platelet Aggregation Studies (Figure 1)		
Adenosine diphosphate	No response	Biphasic aggregation
Epinephrine	No response	Biphasic aggregation
Collagen	Weak response	Monophasic aggregation

DIAGNOSIS: Congenital afibrinogenemia

Discussion

This case is an example of hereditary afibrinogenemia. Hereditary afibrinogenemia is inherited in an autosomal

AFIBRINOGENEMIA

CLINICAL PICTURE

PHYSICAL PROPERTIES OF FIBRINOGEN

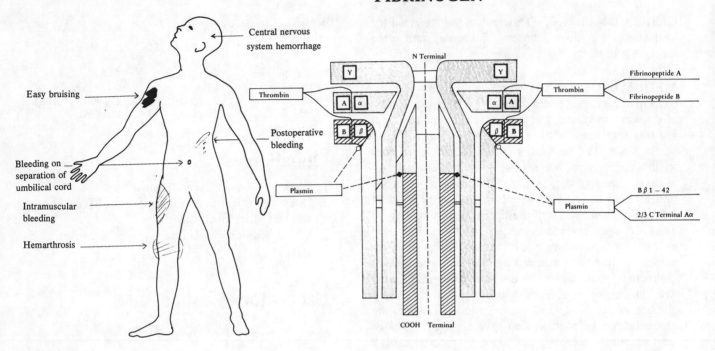

Central nervous system hemorrhage

Easy bruising

Postoperative bleeding

Bleeding on separation of umbilical cord

Intramuscular bleeding

Hemarthrosis

N Terminal

Thrombin

Plasmin

Thrombin — Fibrinopeptide A / Fibrinopeptide B

Plasmin — Bβ 1 – 42 / 2/3 C Terminal Aα

COOH Terminal

Pattern of inheritance: Autosomal recessive

LABORATORY FINDINGS

A. Screening Procedures

Test	Patient's Result	Normal Range
Prothrombin time	Abnormal	10–12 seconds
APTT	Abnormal	<42 seconds
Platelet count	Normal	130,000–400,000/μl
Bleeding time	Normal or abnormal	1–8 minutes

B. Confirmatory Procedures

Mixing prothrombin time	Normal	10–12 seconds
Clottable Fibrinogen	Absent or trace	170–410 mg/dl
Immunologic fibrinogen	Absent or trace	170–410 mg/dl

TREATMENT

Cryoprecipitate
Avoidance of aspirin containing compounds

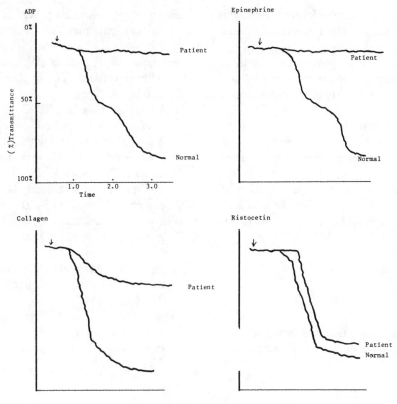

Figure 1

recessive manner; consequently, the absence of a family history of the disorder is typical. Patient with afibrinogenemia may have a clinical picture that is consistent with abnormalities of primary and secondary hemostasis. In this patient, the recurrent gastrointestinal hemorrhage suggests an abnormality of primary hemostasis, whereas the recurrent hemarthrosis of the ankles would be compatible with an abnormality of secondary hemostasis.

Because no end point was demonstrable with the prothrombin time or the activated partial thromboplastin time (APTT), the differential diagnosis would include afibrinogenemia and a circulating inhibitor. Mixing studies in this patient demonstrated correction of the prothrombin time and the APTT when pooled normal plasma was mixed 1:1 with the patient's plasma. A quantitative assay of fibrinogen detected no fibrinogen.

Biochemical Aspects. The diagnosis of afibrinogenemia is established definitively by quantitative determination of fibrinogen. In a true case of afibrinogenemia, no clottable fibrinogen is demonstrable. In addition, there is no antigenic fibrinogen or fibrinogen quantitated by precipitation or chemical techniques.

There appears to be some heterogeneity among patients with afibrinogenemia. Some patients have a total absence of fibrinogen in plasma and platelet alpha granules. Other patients, however, have trace (normal) amounts of fibrinogen within the alpha granules but lack plasma fibrinogen. These discrepancies between plasma and platelet fibrinogen are in many ways analogous to the situation in patients with von Willebrand's disease.

Clinical Picture. Most patients with congenital afibrinogenemia have a history of mild to moderate spontaneous bleeding. Frequently, there is bleeding at the time of separation of the umbilical cord and also at the time of circumcision, as occurred in this patient. In addition, spontaneous hematoma formation, melena and hematemesis are frequently noted. Severe bleeding may occur after trauma or surgical procedures. Menstrual bleeding may be marked, and a few patients with afibrinogenemia have died of cerebral hemorrhage.

Ironically, several patients with afibrinogenemia have died of pulmonary embolism. These patients were found to have thrombi and emboli that did not contain fibrin. The thrombi and emboli consisted of platelets and other cellular elements.

Treatment. The treatment of choice is cryoprecipitate. A single bag of cryoprecipitate contains approximately 250 mg of fibrinogen. It should, however, be stressed that the amount of fibrinogen in cryoprecipitate varies depending on the technique of preparation. Normal hemostasis can be achieved by elevating the level of fibrinogen to between 50 and 100 mg/dl. The half-life of infused fibrinogen is approximately 3 to 5 days.

This patient was placed on prophylactic infusions of cryoprecipitate as an outpatient. He responded well and has had few difficulties with recurrent hemarthroses of the ankles.

It has been noted that after infusion of cryoprecipitate, some patients do well for a considerable period even though fibrinogen is present in plasma in only trace amounts.

The primary complication of transfusion therapy is formation of antibodies to fibrinogen. Also, patients may experience allergic reactions, and hepatitis may develop.

Bibliography

Alexander B, et al: Congenital afibrinogenemia: A study of some basic aspects of coagulation. *Blood* 9:843–865, 1954.

Bommer W, Kuenzer W, Schroeer H: Kongenitale Afibrinogenamie Teil I. *Ann Paediatr* 200:46–59, 1963.

Bommer W, Kuenzer W, Schroeer H: Kongenitale Afibrinogenamie Teil II. *Ann Paediatr* 200:180–183, 1963.

deVries A, Rosenberg T, Kochwa S, et al: Precipitating antifibrinogen antibody appearing after fibrinogen infusions in a patient with congenital afibrinogenemia. *Amer J Med* 30:486–494, 1961.

Egbring R, Andrassy K, Egli H, et al: Diagnostische und therapeutische Probleme bei congenitaler Afibrinogenamie. *Blut* 22:175–201, 1971.

Girolami A, Zacchelo G, D'Elia R: Cogenital afibrinogenemia. *Thromb Diath Haemorrh* 25:460–468, 1971.

Ingram GIC, McBrain DJ, Spencer H: Fatal pulmonary embolus in congenital fibrinopenia. *Acta Haematol* 35:56–59, 1966.

Weiss HJ, Rogers J: Fibrinogen and platelets in the primary arrest of bleeding. Studies in two patients with congenital afibrinogenemia. *N Engl J Med* 285:369–374, 1971.

CASE
21

PATIENT: 42-year-old woman

CHIEF COMPLAINT: This patient was admitted for dilation and curettage. The admitting diagnosis was dysfunctional uterine bleeding.

MEDICAL HISTORY: When 10 years of age, the patient had undergone tonsillectomy as an outpatient, and severe hemorrhage developed postoperatively. This surgical procedure had been performed in the office of a surgeon; consequently, she was rushed to the hospital where a number of units of whole blood were given. The transfusions were apparently successful in controlling the hemorrhage, and after several days of hospitalization, the patient was discharged.

While in high school, the patient had a series of teeth extracted. The dentist had been careful to pack each socket and had tried to be as gentle as possible in performing the extractions. The patient had oozing after the extractions but required no blood transfusions.

At the time of delivery of each of her three children, the patient had profuse vaginal bleeding and received multiple units of whole blood on each occasion.

FAMILY HISTORY: The patient's parents were deceased, each having died of coronary artery disease. One brother had died at 6 days of age. There were two living siblings, a brother (36 years of age) who had a myocardial infarction at 29 years of age and a sister (46 years of age) who was living and well. Neither sibling had bleeding problems (Figure 1).

DRUG HISTORY: No medication

PHYSICAL EXAMINATION: A few minor ecchymotic areas were noted over the arms.

Laboratory Results

A. Screening Procedures

	Patient	Normal
Prothrombin time	13 seconds	10–12 seconds
APTT	30 seconds	<42 seconds
Platelet count	250,000/μl	130,000–400,000/μl
Bleeding time	4 minutes and 50 seconds	1–8 minutes

Questions

1. What additional laboratory procedures are necessary to exclude a disorder of hemostasis?
2. What hereditary bleeding abnormalities may present with normal results on screening tests?

Laboratory Results

B. Confirmatory Procedures

	Patient	Normal
Thrombin time	42.5 seconds	<24 seconds
Fibrinogen (clottable)	74 mg/dl	170–410 mg/dl
Fibrinogen (immunologic)	78 mg/dl	170–410 mg/dl

Immunoelectrophoresis revealed a normal migration pattern for fibrinogen, although the quantity was decreased.

DIAGNOSIS: Hereditary hypofibrinogenemia

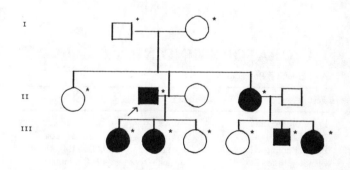

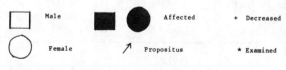

	Male		Affected	+	Decreased
	Female		Propositus	*	Examined

Figure 1

HEREDITARY HYPOFIBRINOGENEMIA

CLINICAL PICTURE

PHYSICAL PROPERTIES OF FIBRINOGEN

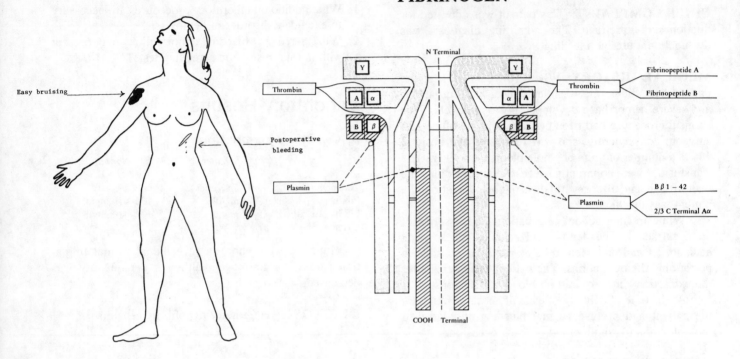

Pattern of inheritance: Autosomal dominant

LABORATORY FINDINGS

A. Screening Procedures

Test	Patient's Result	Normal Range
Prothrombin time	Normal	10–12 seconds
APTT	Normal	<42 seconds
Platelet count	Normal	130,000–400,000/μl
Bleeding time	Normal	1–8 minutes

B. Confirmatory Procedures

Thrombin time	Abnormal	<24 seconds
Fibrinogen, clottable	Abnormal	170–410 mg/dl
Fibrinogen, immunologic	Abnormal	170–410 mg/dl

TREATMENT

Cryoprecipitate
Avoidance of aspirin containing compounds

**Table 1
Hemostatic Disorders in Which Results of
Primary Screening Procedures
May Be Normal**

von Willebrand's disease

Mild deficiencies of coagulation factors

Deficiency of factor XIII

Dysfibrinogenemia

Hypofibrinogenemia

Qualitative abnormalities of platelets

Deficiency of α_2-antiplasmin

Increased release of plasminogen activators

Discussion

Screening tests of this patient were within normal limits, with the exception of the prothrombin time, which was 13 seconds. There are a number of diagnostic possibilities in a patient with a history of bleeding and normal results on screening procedures (Table 1). They include factor deficiency states, such as mild hemophilia A and B, α_2 antiplasmin deficiency and mild von Willebrand's disease. In addition, abnormalities of fibrinogen (quantitative or qualitative) as well as deficiency of factor XIII must be considered. In this patient, the confirmatory procedures included a thrombin time, which was abnormal. Subsequently, the clottable and immunologic fibrinogen were found to be decreased, thus establishing the diagnosis of hypofibrinogenemia. The parallel decreases in the clottable and immunologic fibrinogen would, in most instances, rule out the possibility of dysfibrinogenemia. Patients with dysfibrinogenemia typically have decreased clottable fibrinogen but normal immunologic fibrinogen. Hereditary hypodysfibrinogenemia has rarely been reported.

In hereditary hypofibrinogenemia, the fibrinogen level usually is less than 100 mg/dl. Patients with this disorder may have a mild tendency to bleed, as was the case in this patient. The inheritance pattern is autosomal recessive in some cases and autosomal dominant in others. In this case, subsequent evaluation of the patient's children established that two of them had fibrinogen levels comparable to that of the patient; consequently, this family has an autosomal dominant pattern of inheritance. The question as to whether such patients may be carriers of afibrinogenemia has not been resolved.

If patients who have dysfibrinogenemia are evaluated by clotting techniques alone, they may be mistakenly diagnosed as having hypofibrinogenemia. It is important in evaluating patients with disorders of fibrinogen to perform a clottable fibrinogen assay as well as an immunologic, or precipitating, type of assay to identify dysfibrinogenemic states and distinguish them from hypofibrinogenemia.

Treatment. The treatment of choice is cryoprecipitate. A unit of cryoprecipitate typically contains approximately 250 mg of fibrinogen.

Bibliography

Barbui T, Porciello PI, Dini E: Coagulation studies in a case of severe congenital hypofibrinogenemia. *Thromb Diath Haemorrh* 28:129–134, 1972.

Beck EA: Congenital abnormalities of fibrinogen. *Clin Haematol* 8:169–181, 1979.

Hahn L, Lundberg PA: Congenital hypofibrinogenemia and recurrent abortions. Case report. *Brit J Obstet Gynaecol* 85:790–793, 1978.

Hasselback R, Marion RB, Thomas JW: Congenital hypofibrinogenemia in 5 members of a family. *Can Med Ass J* 88:19–22, 1963.

Risak E: Die Fibrinopenie. *Klin Med (Vienna)* 128:605–629, 1935.

CASE
22

PATIENT: 43-year-old woman

CHIEF COMPLAINT: This patient was admitted for elective septoplasty and bilateral antrostomy.

MEDICAL HISTORY: The patient had a history of excessive bleeding associated with childbirth. On one occasion, blood transfusions were given immediately after delivery. There was no history of previous surgeries.

FAMILY HISTORY: The patient's mother died at the time of delivery. Reportedly, she had uncontrollable hemorrhage. The patient had one sister, who also bled profusely at the time of delivery. In addition, the patient's daughter bled abnormally after extraction of a lower molar.

DRUG HISTORY: The patient was taking no medication at the time of evaluation.

PHYSICAL EXAMINATION: Noncontributary

Laboratory Results

A. Screening Procedures

	Patient	Normal
Prothrombin time	14 seconds	10–12 seconds
APTT	49 seconds	<42 seconds
Platelet count	190,000/μl	130,000–400,000/μl
Bleeding time	6 minutes	1–8 minutes

Questions

1. What additional laboratory procedures are indicated?
2. When the prothrombin time and APTT are prolonged, what are the differential diagnostic possibilities?

Laboratory Results

B. Confirmatory Procedures

	Patient	Normal
APTT (50% patient plasma/50% pooled normal plasma)	41 seconds	<42 seconds

	Patient	Normal
Thrombin time	72 seconds	<24 seconds
Reptilase time	40 seconds	18–22 seconds
Fibrinogen (clottable)	49 mg/dl	170–410 mg/dl
Fibrinogen (immunologic)	426 mg/dl	170–410 mg/dl
Prothrombin assay	100%	50% to 150%
Factor X assay	100%	50% to 150%
Factor V assay	100%	50% to 150%

DIAGNOSIS: Hereditary dysfibrinogenemia

Discussion

The patient had a lifelong history of bleeding problems together with a family history of bleeding. Indeed, the patient's mother bled to death at the time of childbirth. This degree of bleeding is uncommon in patients with hereditary dysfibrinogenemia.

The differential diagnosis in this case would include circulating inhibitors of the final common pathway of coagulation as well as isolated deficiency (or structural abnormality) of any coagulation factor in the final common pathway. Mixing stuides did not demonstrate an inhibitor. Specific assays for factors II, V and X were within normal limits. The markedly prolonged thrombin time together with abnormalities of the prothrombin time and APTT suggest hypofibrinogenemia or dysfibrinogenemia. The discrepancy between the clottable and immunologic fibrinogen establishes the diagnosis of dysfibrinogenemia.

Biochemical Aspects. Congenital dysfibrinogenemia is inherited in an autosomal dominant manner, thus affecting both sexes. The physiochemical properties of abnormal fibrinogens have been extensively investigated in many cases. In some instances, abnormal electrophoretic mobility has been described, although most abnormal fibrinogens have normal electrophoretic mobilities. There have been reports of abnormalities of all three phases of fibrin formation (i.e., proteolytic, polymerization and stabilization phases). In some instances, specific amino acid substitutions have been identified within one of the three constituent chains of fibrinogen. For instance, in fibrinogens Metz and Zurich I, the arginine in position 16 of the A alpha chain is replaced by cystine. In fibrinogen Manchester, a histidine residue is substituted for the arginine in position 16. Abnormalities of the amino acid in position 19 of the A alpha chain have

DYSFIBRINOGENEMIA

CLINICAL PICTURE

Majority of patients
with dysfibrinogenemia
are asymptomatic

PHYSICAL PROPERTIES OF FIBRINOGEN

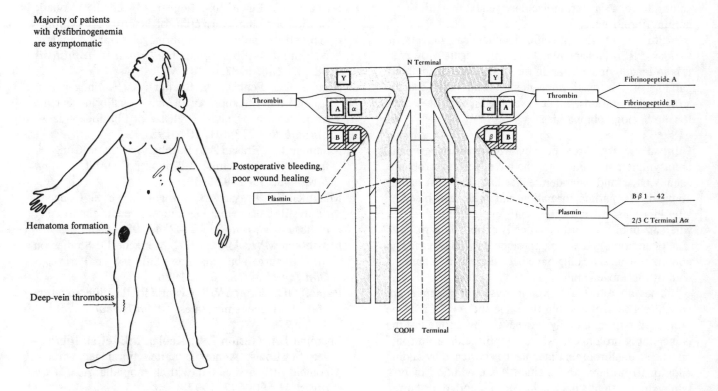

Postoperative bleeding,
poor wound healing

Hematoma formation

Deep-vein thrombosis

Pattern of inheritance: Autosomal dominant

LABORATORY FINDINGS

A. Screening Procedures

Test	Patient's Result	Normal Range
Prothrombin time	Abnormal	10–12 seconds
APTT	Abnormal	<42 seconds
Platelet count	Normal	130,000–400,000/μl
Bleeding time	Normal	1–8 minutes

B. Confirmatory Procedures

Test	Patient's Result	Normal Range
APTT (50% patient plasma/50% pooled normal plasma)	Normal	<42 seconds
Thrombin time	Abnormal	<24 seconds
Reptilase time	Abnormal	18–22 seconds
Fibrinogen, clottable	Abnormal	170–410 mg/dl
Fibrinogen, immunologic	Normal	170–410 mg/dl

TREATMENT

Cryoprecipitate in instances of bleeding
Heparin—oral anticoagulants—in cases of thrombosis

also been described. In fibrinogen Detroit, the arginine in position 19 is replaced by serine. Amino acid substitutions on the beta and gamma chains of abnormal fibrinogens have yet to be described, although some abnormal fibrinogens are characterized by delayed cleavage of fibrinopeptide B.

In fibrinogen Paris I, an abnormal gamma chain has been postulated. In this dysfibrinogenemia, the gamma chains have a higher molecular weight than those of normal fibrinogen.

Studies of the specific biochemical defects in various dysfibrinogenemias have only begun. However, it is to be anticipated that in the near future, a complete catalog of the dysfibrinogenemias and their specific structural alterations will be assembled, as has been done for the hemoglobinopathies.

Clinical Picture. Most patients with dysfibrinogenemia are asymptomatic. Patients who have bleeding problems usually have mild to moderate bleeding. This case is thus atypical. Hematoma formation and prolonged bleeding after injury are the most frequently encountered findings, whereas umbilical cord bleeding is extremely rare.

In addition to bleeding, thromboembolic disease and abnormal wound healing have been described in patients with dysfibrinogenemia.

The laboratory findings in dysfibrinogenemia are variable. The prothrombin time and the APTT may be prolonged only minimally. However, the thrombin time is inevitably prolonged, as is the reptilase time. In some instances, the thrombin time may be shortened by adding additional thrombin or calcium. Also, addition of protamine to a patient's plasma has been reported to shorten the thrombin time in some instances. Laboratory diagnosis relies most importantly on demonstration of a discrepancy between the level of clottable fibrinogen and the level of fibrinogen measured immunologically or chemically.

Treatment. In general, patients with dysfibrinogenemia do not have life-threatening bleeding. If medical intervention is indicated for hemorrhage, cryoprecipitate is the treatment of choice. Usually, it is sufficient to keep the level of clottable fibrinogen slightly above 100 mg/dl.

Patients with thromboembolic disease are appropriately treated with anticoagulants.

Bibliography

Clinical Picture

Al-Mondhiry H, Bilezikian SB, Nossel HL: Fibrinogen "New York"—An abnormal fibrinogen associated with thromboembolism: Functional evaluation. *Blood* 45:607–619, 1975.

Andes WA, Chavin SI, Beltran G, et al: Fibrinogen New Orleans: Hereditary dysfibrinogenemia with an Aα chain abnormality. *Thromb Res* 25:41–50, 1982.

Bove JR: Fibrinogen—Is the benefit worth the risk? *Transfusion* 18:129–136, 1978.

Higgins DL, Lewis SD, Penner JA, et al: A kinetic method for characterization of heterogenous fibrinogen and its application to fibrinogen Grand Rapids, a congenital dysfibrinogenemia. *Thromb Haemostasis* 48:182–186, 1982.

Higgins DL, Penner JA, Shafter JA: Fibrinogen Petoskey: Identification of a new dysfibrinogenemia characterized by altered release of fibrinopeptide A. *Thromb Res* 213:491–504, 1981.

Mammen EF, Prasad AS, Barnhart MI, et al: Congenital dysfibrinogenemia: Fibrinogen Detroit. *J Clin Invest* 48:235–249, 1969.

Mammen EF, Prasad AS, Barnhart MI, et al: Congenital dysfibrinogenemia Detroit: Molecular abnormality of fibrinogen. *Blut* 33:229–234, 1976.

Mossesson MW, Amrani DL, Menache D: Studies on the structural abnormalities of fibrinogen Paris I. *J Clin Invest* 57:782–790, 1976.

Ratnoff OD, Forman WB: Criteria for the differentiation of dysfibrinogenemic states. *Semin Hematol* 13:141–157, 1976.

Sherman LA, Gaston LW, Kaplan ME, et al: Fibrinogen St. Louis: A new inherited fibrinogen variant, coincidently associated with hemophilia A. *J Clin Invest* 51:590–597, 1972.

Review Articles

Beck EA: Congenital abnormalities of fibrinogen. *Clin Hematol* 8:169–181, 1979.

Crum ED: Abnormal fibrinogens. In Ogston D, Bennett B (eds): *Hemostasis: Biochemistry, Physiology and Pathology*. New York: John Wiley & Sons, 1977, pp 424–445.

Flute PT: Disorders of plasma fibrinogen synthesis. *Brit Med Bull* 33:253–259, 1977.

Gralnick HR: Congenital disorders of fibrinogen. In Williams WJ, Beutler E, Erslev AJ, et al (eds): *Hematology* (2nd edition). New York: McGraw-Hill, 1977, pp 1423–1431.

Gralnick HR, Finlayson JS: Congenital dysfibrinogenemias. *Ann Intern Med* 77(3):471–473, 1972.

Mammen EF: Congenital abnormalities of the fibrinogen molecule. *Semin Thromb Hemostasis* 1:184–201, 1974.

Marder VJ: The functional defects of hereditary dysfibrinogens. *Thromb Haemostasis* 36:1–8, 1976.

Menache D: Congenital abnormal fibrinogens. In

Menache D, Surgenor DMacN, Anderson H (eds): *Hemophilia and Hemostasis*. New York: Alan R. Liss, 1981, pp 205–220.

Morse EE: The fibrinogenopathies. *Ann Clin Lab Sci* 8:234–238, 1978.

Samama M, Soria J, Soria C: Congenital and acquired dysfibrinogenemia. In Pollar L (ed): *Recent Advances in Blood Coagulation* (2nd edition). Edinburgh: Churchill Livingstone, 1977, pp 313–335.

CASE
23

PATIENT: 22-year-old woman

CHIEF COMPLAINT: This patient had no history of bleeding problems. She was a laboratory employee who had agreed to participate in a study conducted to establish a new normal range for the activated partial thromboplastin time (APTT). Her APTT was determined with a BioData CP-8 Coagulation Profiler. The APTT result was 36 seconds, with normal being less than 42 seconds; however, the Thrombokinetic® curve was abnormal. The amplitude of the curve was strikingly diminished, and the slope was markedly decreased. As a result of these findings, further evaluation was undertaken.

MEDICAL HISTORY: No history of bleeding problems

FAMILY HISTORY: No history of bleeding problems

DRUG HISTORY: No medication

PHYSICAL EXAMINATION: Noncontributary

Laboratory Results

A. Screening Procedures

	Patient	Normal
Prothrombin time	12 seconds	10–12 seconds
APTT	36 seconds	<42 seconds
Platelet count	190,000/μl	130,000–400,000/μl
Bleeding time	6 minutes	1–8 minutes

Questions

1. What additional laboratory procedures are indicated?
2. Is it necessary to evaluate fibrinogen completely?

Laboratory Results

B. Confirmatory Procedures

	Patient	Normal
Thrombin time	60 seconds	<24 seconds
Reptilase time	31 seconds	18–22 seconds

	Patient	Normal
Fibrinogen (clottable)	75 mg/dl	170–410 mg/dl
Fibrinogen (immunologic)	85 mg/dl	170–410 mg/dl

Platelet aggregation studies were undertaken. The responses to adenosine diphosphate, epinephrine, collagen and ristocetin were within normal limits (Figure 1).

On the basis of the initial evaluation of the patient, it was thought that she had hereditary hypofibrinogenemia. However, to rule out the possibility of dysfibrinogenemia, additional tests were done. One unit of plasma was obtained from the patient, and the fibrinogen was purified. The thrombin and reptilase times were determined using the purified fibrinogen, which was adjusted to a concentration of 300 mg/dl. Both times were abnormal. In addition, sodium dodecyl sulfate-agarose gel electrophoresis was performed, and it appeared that the alpha, beta and gamma chains of fibrinogen migrated abnormally. Immunoelectrophoretic studies were performed with the fibrinogen, and there was abnormally slow migration.

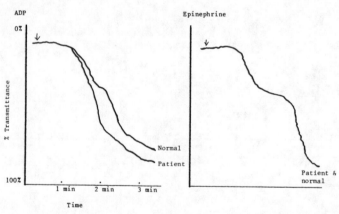

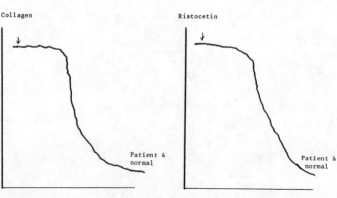

Figure 1

HEREDITARY HYPODYSFIBRINOGENEMIA

CLINICAL PICTURE

Clinical symptoms: None

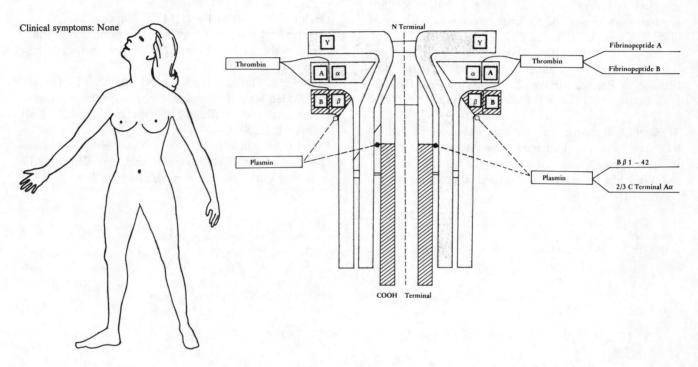

Pattern of inheritance: Autosomal dominant

PHYSICAL PROPERTIES OF FIBRINOGEN

LABORATORY FINDINGS

A. Screening Procedures

Test	Patient's Result	Normal Range
Prothrombin time	Abnormal	10–12 seconds
APTT	Abnormal	<42 seconds
Platelet count	Normal	130,000–400,000/μl
Bleeding time	Normal	1–8 minutes

B. Confirmatory Procedures

Test	Patient's Result	Normal Range
Thrombin time	Abnormal	<24 seconds
Reptilase time	Abnormal	18–22 seconds
Fibrinogen, clottable	Abnormal	170–410 mg/dl
Fibrinogen, immunologic	Abnormal	170–410 mg/dl

TREATMENT

Cryoprecipitate in instances of bleeding

DIAGNOSIS: Hereditary hypodysfibrinogenemia

Biochemical Aspects. The patient was found to have hypofibrinogenemia. Subsequent studies demonstrated not only hypofibrinogenemia but also an apparent dysfibrinogenemia. The simultaneous association of hypofibrinogenemia and dysfibrinogenemia has been reported on several occasions. One explanation for the apparent association of hypofibrinogenemia with dysfibrinogenemia is increased clearance of the dysfibrinogenemic protein from the plasma. There have been at least nine reported variants of hypodysfibrinogenemia: fibrinogens Parma, Mitaka, St. Louis, Leuven, Chapel Hill, Bethesdas II and III, Philadelphia and New York.

Treatment. Because the patient was asymptomatic, treatment was not indicated. She had no history of surgical intervention; consequently, it is anticipated that she might bleed abnormally if a surgical procedure were performed.

Bibliography

Euraki H: Fibrinogen "Mitaka"—A hereditary hypodysfibrinogenemia. Abstracts of the Sixteenth Proceedings of the International Congress on Hematology, Kyoto, 1976, p 310.

Gralnick HR, Coller BS, Frantantoni JC, et al: Fibrinogen Bethesda III: A hypodysfibrinogenemia. *Blood* 53(1):28–46, 1979.

Gralnick HR, Givelber HM, Finlayson JS: A new congenital abnormality of human fibrinogen. Fibrinogen Bethesda II. *Thromb Diath Haemorrh* 20:562–567, 1963.

Martinez J, Holburn RR, Shapiro SS, et al: Fibrinogen Philadelphia, a hereditary hypodysfibrinogenemia characterized by fibrinogen hypercatabolism. *J Clin Invest* 53:600–611, 1974.

Owen CA, Bowie EW, Fass DN, et al: Hypofibrinogenemia—Dysfibrinogenemia and von Willebrand's disease in the same family. *Mayo Clin Proc* 54:375–380, 1979.

CASE
24

PATIENT: 35-year-old man

CHIEF COMPLAINT: This patient was admitted for evaluation of a lifelong tendency to ooze from superficial wounds. In addition to the oozing, he reported a history of easy bruising and occasional formation of large, unsightly hematomas.

MEDICAL HISTORY: The patient had a lifelong history of abnormal bleeding from superficial wounds. He had no history of surgical intervention or transfusion.

FAMILY HISTORY: There was a family history of bruising and abnormal bleeding from superficial wounds. In addition, the patient reported that several family members had died of head injuries. In each instance, the trauma associated with the head injury was relatively minor.

DRUG HISTORY: No medication

PHYSICAL EXAMINATION: Several large ecchymotic areas were noted over the legs together with hematomas over the thighs and upper left arm.

Laboratory Results

A. Screening Procedures

	Patient	Normal
Prothrombin time	12 seconds	10–12 seconds
APTT	35 seconds	<42 seconds
Platelet count	230,000/μl	130,000–400,000/μl
Bleeding time	7 minutes	1–8 minutes

Questions

1. What additional laboratory procedures are indicated?
2. What hereditary bleeding disorders are frequently associated with intracranial bleeding?

Laboratory Results

B. Confirmatory Procedures

	Patient	Normal
Thrombin time	20 seconds	20–24 seconds
Fibrinogen level (clottable)	350 mg/dl	170–410 mg/dl
Platelet Aggregation Studies		
ADP	Biphasic response	Biphasic aggregation
Epinephrine	Biphasic response	Biphasic aggregation
Collagen	Full-range monophasic response	Full-range monophasic aggregation
Ristocetin	Full-range monophasic agglutination	Full-range monophasic agglutination or biphasic agglutination

Because of the history of oozing and the family history of intracranial bleeding, a clot solubility test in 5 molar urea solution was ordered. The clot was soluble.

DIAGNOSIS: Hereditary deficiency of factor XIII (fibrin-stabilizing factor)

Discussion

This patient had a history typical of patients with a deficiency of factor XIII. The family history of intracranial hemorrhage together with the clinical picture of bruising and abnormal oozing from superficial wounds suggest deficiency of factor XIII. Deficiency of factor XIII and hereditary afibrinogenemia are associated with an increased risk for intracranial hemorrhage. Recently, it has been appreciated that deficiency of factor VII is associated with central nervous system hemorrhage.

Biochemical Aspects. Factor XIII is the only enzyme in the coagulation system that is not a serine protease. It functions as a transamidase and has an active sulfhydryl group. Activated factor XIII is essential for normal hemostasis and appears to have an important function in certain physiologic and pathologic processes, such as thrombosis, and in wound healing. In its activated form, factor XIII catalyzes the formation of covalent bonds between the gamma chains and alpha chains of fibrin.

HEREDITARY DEFICIENCY OF FACTOR XIII
(FIBRIN-STABILIZING FACTOR)

CLINICAL PICTURE

PHYSICAL PROPERTIES OF FACTOR XIII

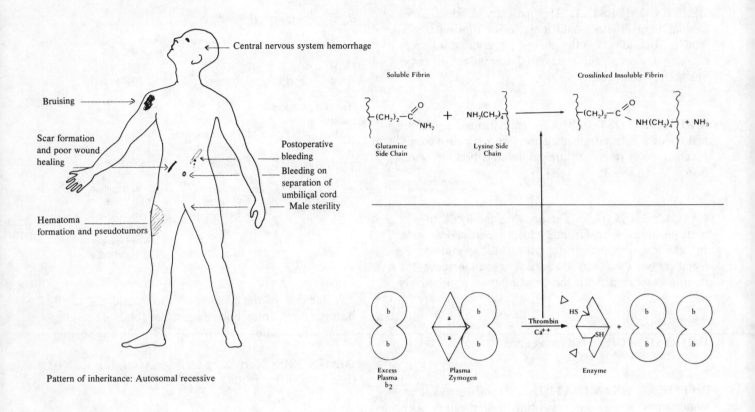

Pattern of inheritance: Autosomal recessive

LABORATORY FINDINGS

A. Screening Procedures

Test	Patient's Result	Normal Range
Prothrombin time	Normal	10–12 seconds
APTT	Normal	<42 seconds
Platelet count	Normal	130,000–400,000/μl
Bleeding time	Normal	1–8 minutes

B. Confirmatory Procedures

Test	Patient's Result	Normal Range
Thrombin time	Normal	20–24 seconds
Clot solubility, 5 molar urea	Soluble	Insoluble
Immunologic a chain	No a chain	Normal a chain

TREATMENT

Cryoprecipitate or fresh-frozen plasma as a prophylactic measure

Factor XIII concentrates (available in Europe)

The consequences of cross-linking are increased mechanical stability of fibrin clots and relative resistance to digestion by plasmin.

Factor XIII has two nonidentical polypeptide subunits, the a chain and the b chain, that form a tetrameric molecular complex that consists of two a chains and two b chains. The interaction between the a and b chains is noncovalent. The molecular weight of the complex is approximately 320,000, with the a chain having a molecular weight of 75,000 and the b chain having a weight 80,000. No disulfide bond is found in the a chains; however, the b chains contain 16 or 17 intrachain disulfide bridges that have no free sulfhydryl groups.

In normal plasma, the number of b chains exceeds the number of a chains; consequently, there are free b chains in the circulation. The plasma concentration of factor XIII is approximately 4 to 8 μg/ml. The plasma concentration of free b chains is approximately 4 μg/ml.

Platelets also contain factor XIII; however, platelet factor XIII is composed of a chains only, which have a molecular weight of approximately 160,000. It has been estimated that approximately 50% of the potential factor XIII activity in blood is distributed in platelets, with more than 90% being localized in the soluble fraction of platelets. Platelet factor XIII is not released during the platelet release reaction.

Plasma factor XIII and platelet factor XIII require proteolytic modification by thrombin and conformational alteration by calcium ions to exhibit enzymatic activity. The a chains contain the thrombin cleavage site and the tight calcium-binding site. In proteolytic activation, thrombin cleaves the arginine-glycine bond between residues 37 and 38 from the amino terminal of the a chain to release an activation peptide with a molecular weight of 4500. Binding of calcium may occur with the zymogen or the thrombin-cleaved intermediate. Thus, calcium binding may occur before cleavage by thrombin or after modification by thrombin. Once activation by thrombin and calcium occurs, the active cysteine residue on the a chains is exposed, and the activated enzyme is formed.

Once the active center of plasma factor XIII is generated, there is dissociation of the b chain dimer from the complex. Obviously, in the case of platelet factor XIII, the sequence of activation is identical, except for dissociation of the b dimer, which is not present in platelet factor XIII.

Other enzymes have been reported to be capable of activating factor XIII; such enzymes include trypsin and papain. Low-grade activation of factor XIII has been reported for the serine proteases Xa and kallikrein. Plasmin neither activates nor degrades factor XIII.

Factor XIIIa catalyzes the cross-linking of fibrin. This reaction involves the gamma and alpha chains of fibrin. Glutamine acts as an electron acceptor, or acyl donor, whereas lysine acts as an electron donor, or acyl acceptor. The result is the formation of an ε (γ-glutamyl) lysyl bond. Several synthetic primary amino compounds (monodansylcadaverine, putrescine and histamine) can substitute for lysine and have been used for in vitro quantification of factor XIII activity. With the formation of the covalently cross-linked fibrin, clot stabilization and release of ammonia occur. In the activation of factor XIII, the rate-limiting step is dissociation of the b dimer from the thrombin-modified complex. It may be that the b chains have a protective, or carrier, function for the plasma a chains.

Factor XIII has also been identified in the placenta, uterus, prostate and liver. All the tissue zymogens are immunochemically identical to the platelet zymogen. It would appear that the a chains are produced in the megakaryocytes and liver and that the b chains are synthesized only in the liver. On the basis of observations in patients with a congenital deficiency of factor XIII, it has been concluded that the a chains have a controlling effect on the plasma concentration of the b chain. Patients with a deficiency of factor XIII have no detectable a chain and approximately 50% of the normal plasma b chain level. Heterozygous members of the same family have approximately 50% of the normal a chain level and 80% of the normal b chain level. The half-life of plasma factor XIII is approximately 12 to 14 days.

Factor XIIIa cross-linking of fibrin monomers involves formation of two sets of cross-links between the gamma chains to yield gamma dimers. In addition, cross-links are formed between the alpha chains to yield large alpha polymers. Cross-linking of the gamma chains occurs at the carboxy-terminal end of the chain. This cross-linking occurs in an antiparallel fashion and is rapid, with completion taking 2 to 5 minutes in vitro. Cross-linking of the alpha chains to form alpha polymers is more complex. The sites of cross-linking are thought to be in the carboxy-terminal portion of the alpha chains, although the exact locations have not been identified. Cross-linking of the alpha chains occurs more slowly than formation of the gamma dimers, both in vivo and in vitro.

In addition to the cross-linking of fibrin, factor XIII may cross-link fibrinogen, fibronectin and collagen. Fibronectin (cold-insoluble globulin) is a large dimeric plasma protein that may be cross-linked to fibrin. This cross-linking results in the formation of soluble fibrin and appears to occur between the alpha but not the gamma chains of fibrin. In addition to these cross-linking abilities, factor XIII may cross-link fibrin to platelet actin and myosin and cross-link α_2-antiplasmin to fibrin.

Clinical Picture. Patients with a hereidtary deficiency

of factor XIII have an almost total lack of factor XIII activity. Typically, such patients bleed into and around fascial planes and into soft tissues. Often, the bleeding is insidious and is characterized by slow, progressive formation of hematomas that have the appearance of large hemorrhagic cysts or pseudotumors.

Bleeding often is not seen postoperatively in such patients because plasma or whole blood frequently is given during major surgery; consequently, the deficiency is masked. Umbilical cord hemorrhage is a frequent complication in the neonatal period and strongly suggests a diagnosis of hereditary deficiency of factor XIII. In the differential diagnosis, the possibility of afibrinogenemia must be considered. A common finding in such patients is delayed wound healing, resulting in the formation of large, unsightly scars at the site of minor trauma or surgical procedures. In addition, there is a high degree of fetal wastage and male sterility.

The pattern of inheritance appears to be autosomal recessive. As in other recessively transmitted diseases, consanguinity is often present.

The laboratory diagnosis of deficiency of factor XIII is not difficult once the possibility has been identified on the basis of the history and normal results on screening tests. The screening procedure of choice is clot solubility in a 5 molar urea solution. In patients with a deficiency of factor XIII, 5 molar urea disrupts fibrin monomer clots within 2 hours after initiation of the test. In patients with normal coagulation, the clots usually do not dissolve in 5 molar urea. Another satisfactory screening procedure is clot solubility in 1% monochloroacetic acid. More specific assays that are performed with synthetic substrates have been developed. An immunologic assay that makes use of antibodies to the a and b chains is also available. As has been noted above, patients with a deficiency of factor XIII lack the a chains and have roughly 50% of the b chain antigenicity normally present in plasma.

Treatment. Deficiency of factor XIII is easily managed in a prophylactic manner. This disorder is easy to manage because only a small amount of the factor assures normal physiologic action (i.e., roughly 2% to 3% of normal activity) and because factor XIII has a relatively long half-life, approximately 7 days. Patients may be treated prophylactically with cryoprecipitate or fresh-frozen plasma. Factor XIII concentrates are available in Europe.

Bibliography

Clinical Picture

Barbui T, Rodeghiero F, Dini E, et al: Subunits A and S inheritance in four families with congenital factor XIII deficiency. *Brit J Haematol* 38:267–271, 1978.

Beck E, Duckert F, Ernst M: The influence of fibrin stabilizing factor on the growth of fibroblasts in vitro and wound healing. *Thromb Diath Haemorrh* 6:485–491, 1961.

Bharucha C, Cherian M, Bauman JH: Congenital deficiency of factor XIII in an Indian kindred. *Scand J Haematol* 7:325–329, 1970.

Castle S, Board PG, Anderson RAM: Genetic heterogeneity of factor XIII deficiency: First description of unstable A subunits. *Brit J Haematol* 48:337–342, 1981.

Duckert F: Fibrin stabilizing factor (factor XIII): Consequence of its deficiency. *Thromb Diath Haemorrh Suppl* 13:115–119, 1964.

Duckert F: The fibrin stabilizing factor (FSF). *Ser Haematol* 7:58–62, 1965.

Duckert F: Documentation of the plasma factor XIII deficiency in man. *Ann NY Acad Sci* 202:190–199, 1972.

Duckert F, Jung E, Shmerling DH: A hitherto undescribed congenital hemorrhagic diathesis probably due to fibrin stabilizing factor deficiency. *Thromb Diath Haemorrh* 5:179–186, 1960.

Fisher S, Rikover M, Naor S: Factor XIII deficiency with severe hemorrhagic diathesis. *Blood* 28:34–39, 1966.

Francis JL, Todd PJ: Factor XIII deficiency, a family study by measurement of factor XIII subunits A and S. *Acta Hameatol* 62:167–172, 1979.

Girolami A, Burul A, Fabris F, et al: Studies on factor XIII antigen in congenital factor XIII deficiency. A tentative classification of the disease in two groups. *Folia Haematol (Lepizig)* 105:131–141, 1978.

Girolami A, Burul A, Sticchi A: Congenital deficiency of factor XIII with normal subunit S and lack of subunit A, report of a new family. *Acta Haematol* 58:17–26, 1977.

McDonagh J, McDonagh RP Jr, Duckert F: Genetic aspects of factor XIII deficiency. *Ann Hum Genet* 35:197–206, 1971.

Rodeghiero F, Barbui T: Fibrin cross-linking in congenital factor XIII deficiency. *J Clin Pathol* 33:434–437, 1980.

Walls WD, Losowsky MS: Congenital deficiency of fibrin-stabilizing factor. *Coagulation* 1:111–121, 1968.

Laboratory Evaluation

Lorand L, Urayama T, de Kiewiet JWC, et al: Diagnostic and genetic studies on fibrin-stabilizing factor with a new assay based on amine incorporation. *J Clin Invest* 48:1054–1064, 1969.

Treatment

Ikkala E: Transfusion therapy in factor XIII (FSF) deficiency. *Scand J Haematol* 1:308–312, 1964.

Ikkala E: Transfusion therapy in congenital deficiencies of plasma factor XIII. *Ann NY Acad Sci* 202:200–203, 1972.

Miloszewski K, Losowsky MS: The half-life of factor XIII in vivo. *Brit J Haematol* 19:685–690, 1970.

Miloszewski K, Losowsky MS: Factor XIII concentrate in the long term management of congenital factor XIII deficiency. *Thromb Diath Haemorrh* 34:323–324, 1975.

CASE
25

PATIENT: 45-year-old woman

CHIEF COMPLAINT: This patient was admitted because of massive hemoptysis. At the time of admission, she was receiving Coumadin (sodium warfarin) for superficial thrombophlebitis. The patient's prothrombin time was 21 seconds, although she had not taken Coumadin since the day preceding admission.

MEDICAL HISTORY: The patient's medical history was complex. The first episode of thrombophlebitis occurred in 1964 after the birth of her second daughter. Three days after childbirth, she experienced left calf pain. She consulted her physician, who made a diagnosis of thrombophlebitis. The patient was readmitted 10 days after delivery and placed an oral anticoagulants. However, she did not respond to the oral anticoagulants, and a few days later, a diagnosis of left femoral vein thrombophlebitis was established on the basis of a venogram. The patient was placed on subcutaneous heparin, which was then followed by oral anticoagulants. From October 1964 until March 1965, she was taking Coumadin as an outpatient.

Uneventful pregnancies followed in 1966 and 1968. After a spontaneous abortion in 1969, the patient was placed on oral contraceptives. In 1972, she experienced superficial left calf vein thrombophlebitis. In June 1974, she had bilateral superficial thrombophlebitis, and the oral contraceptives were discontinued. In November 1978, the patient underwent breast biopsy and elective tubal ligation. After this surgical procedure, thrombophlebitis developed in the left calf. She was placed on continuous intravenous infusion of heparin and subsequently switched to Coumadin. Coincident with the onset of left calf pain thrombophlebitis, thrombophlebitis developed in the right antecubital fossa. A venogram obtained during this hospital stay showed old femoral vein occlusion on the left side and an abnormally draining saphenous vein. In 1979 and 1980, there were several bouts of superficial thrombophlebitis, which were often associated with minor trauma. In 1981, there were two episodes of thrombophlebitis of the legs that were not associated with trauma. In January 1982, thrombophlebitis of the left leg developed as a result of a minor bruise.

FAMILY HISTORY: The paternal grandfather, who died at 32 years of age, had a history of "swollen legs" (Figure 1). The patient's father had a pulmonary embolism at 27 years of age after appendectomy. At 33 years of age, thrombophlebitis developed in his left leg, and he died suddenly at 42 years of age after an attack of thrombophlebitis of the left leg. There were no autopsy studies to substantiate the clinical impression of pulmonary embolism. A paternal uncle died of gastrointestinal hemorrhage at 32 years of age. Also, a cousin died at 39 years of age after several episodes of thrombophlebitis. Another cousin, 63 years of age, had a number of problems with thrombotic disease, including a history of arterial embolism that necessitated amputation of the left leg at the knee.

DRUG HISTORY: At the time of the initial evaluation, the patient was taking Inderal (propranolol hydrochloride), Dyazide (Hydrochbrothiazide), Serax (oxazepam) and Coumadin.

PHYSICAL EXAMINATION: Superficial varices were noted over the legs.

Laboratory Results

A. Screening Procedures

	Patient	Normal
Prothrombin time	21 seconds	10–12 seconds
APTT	43 seconds	<42 seconds
Platelet count	315,000/μl	130,000–400,000/μl
Bleeding time	7 minutes and 30 seconds	1–8 minutes

Questions

1. What additional laboratory procedures are indicated?
2. What hereditary abnormalities have been identified as predisposing patients to recurrent deep-vein thrombosis?
3. Should family members be evaluated for a thrombotic tendency?

Laboratory Results

B. Confirmatory Procedures

	Patient	Normal
Antithrombin III (activity)	62.1%	85% to 115%
Antithrombin III (immunologic)	19 mg/dl	23–40 mg/dl
Protein C (immunologic)	85%	68–150%
Protein S (immunologic)	90%	61–130%

HEREDITARY DEFICIENCY OF ANTITHROMBIN III

CLINICAL PICTURE

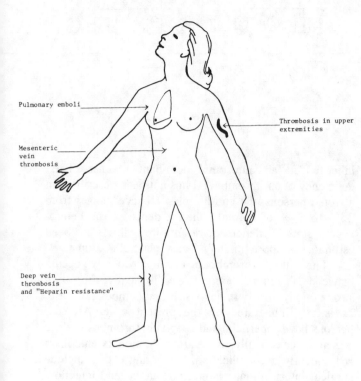

Pulmonary emboli

Thrombosis in upper extremities

Mesenteric vein thrombosis

Deep vein thrombosis and "Heparin resistance"

Pattern of inheritance: Autosomal dominant

ANTICOAGULANT PROPERTIES OF ANTITHROMBIN III

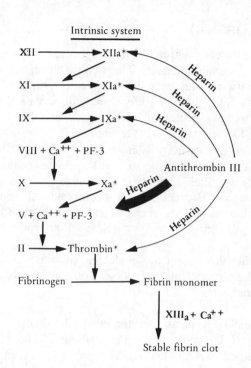

Intrinsic system

$$XII \longrightarrow XIIa^*$$
$$XI \longrightarrow XIa^*$$
$$IX \longrightarrow IXa^*$$
$$VIII + Ca^{++} + PF\text{-}3$$
$$X \longrightarrow Xa^*$$
$$V + Ca^{++} + PF\text{-}3$$
$$II \longrightarrow Thrombin^*$$
$$Fibrinogen \longrightarrow Fibrin\ monomer$$
$$XIII_a + Ca^{++}$$
$$Stable\ fibrin\ clot$$

Heparin
Heparin
Heparin
Antithrombin III
Heparin
Heparin

BORATORY FINDINGS

creening Procedures

	Patient's Result	Normal Range
rombin time	Normal	10–12 seconds
T	Normal	<42 seconds
let count	Normal	130,000–400,000/μl
ing time	Normal	1–8 minutes

onfirmatory Procedures

hrombin III, nunologic	Abnormal or normal	85% to 115%
hrombin III, ivity	Abnormal	23–40 mg/dl
in C unologic)	Normal	68%–150%
in S munologic)	Normal	61%–130%

TREATMENT

Long-term oral anticoagulants
?Anabolic steroids
Fresh-frozen plasma or antithrombin III concentrates for short-term replacement therapy

Crossed immunoelectrophoresis of antithrombin III ◄ was also performed. This study revealed a decreased amount of antithrombin III immunologically and a second abnormal antithrombin III component.

DIAGNOSIS: Hereditary deficiency of antithrombin III

Discussion

Deficiency of antithrombin III is inherited in an autosomal dominant manner. The family history of this patient clearly illustrates this mode of inheritance. The patient's four children were evaluated, and each was found to have decreased immunologic and functional levels of antithrombin III (see Figure 1).

Several hereditary abnormalities have now been identified as being associated with a predisposition to thrombosis. Such abnormalities include deficiency of antithrombin III, deficiencies of proteins C and S, dysfibrinogenemia, dysplasminogemia and an abnormality of plasminogen activator release from endothelial cells.

After this patient was evaluated, she was continued on oral anticoagulants and was seen on a regular basis as an outpatient.

Biochemial Aspects. Antithrombin III (heparin cofactor) is the most important inhibitor of the serine proteases of coagulation. Antithrombin III consists of a single polypeptide chain with a molecular weight of approximately 65,000. The plasma concentration has been reported as varying from 20 to 40 mg/dl. Antithrombin III inhibits not only thrombin but also the other serine proteases of coagulation, including factors XIIa, XIa, IXa Xa and, perhaps very weakly, VIIa. Plasma kallikrein and plasmin are also inhibited by antithrombin III in vitro.

Antithrombin III is unique because it is the only plasma protein whose inhibitory activity is strikingly accelerated in the presence of heparin. The reaction between antithrombin III and thrombin, or factor Xa, is enhanced at least 1000-fold by heparin. Antithrombin III forms a 1:1 stoichiometric complex with serine proteases. The active serine residue of the enzyme interacts with an arginyl residue in the antithrombin molecule to form a covalent bond.

It appears that heparin interacts with the antithrombin III molecule at a lysyl residue (positively charged). Also, it has been recently demonstrated that heparin directly interacts with thrombin. The effect of the heparin-thrombin interaction on the inhibition of thrombin remains unclear.

Clinical Picture. Deficiency of antithrombin III is

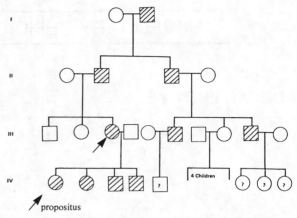

Figure 1

propositus

inherited in an autosomal dominant manner. Total deficiency of antithrombin III has not been described. In affected persons, the antithrombin III level ranges from 25% to 50% of normal. The incidence of the heterozygous state for deficiency of antithrombin III has been estimated at approximately 1 case per 5000 people.

The initial thrombotic event frequently occurs between 10 and 30 years of age. Typically, there is a strong family history of venous thromboembolic disease, as is well illustrated by the present case. Affected persons have superficial and deep-vein thrombosis of the legs and, occasionally, of the arms. Pulmonary embolism is frequently a complication. Triggering events include surgical intervention, trauma, pregnancy and infection. Often, patients appear to be resistant to heparin anticoagulation. Consequently, administration of oral anticoagulants is the treatment of choice.

There appears to be heterogeneity in persons with a deficiency of antithrombin III (see Table 1). In most cases, the immunologic and functional levels of the protein show parallel decreases. However, some families have a normal level of antithrombin III antigen but a decrease in functional activity. In such cases, crossed immunoelectrophoresis demonstrates two distinct peaks, reflecting the presence of normal and abnormal antithrombin III in the plasma.

Treatment. Oral anticoagulant therapy is the treatment of choice. As has been noted, such patients often appear to be resistant to heparin anticoagulation. Anabolic steroids may also be helpful in treating patients with a hereditary deficiency of antithrombin III.

When rapid anticoagulation is needed, fresh-frozen plasma may be used as a source of antithrombin III. After replacement of antithrombin III, patients respond appropriately to heparin. Antithrombin III concentrates are available in Europe. These concentrates have been used in the treatment of patients with hereditary deficiency of antithrombin III as well as in the treatment

Table 1
Variants of Antithrombin III Deficiency

Type	Concentration of Antigen	Heparin-Independent Inhibition	Heparin-Dependent Inhibition		Crossed Immunoelectrophoresis
			Factor Xa	Factor IIa	
I	Abnormal or decreased	Abnormal or decreased	Abnormal or decreased	Abnormal or decreased	Abnormal or decreased
II	Abnormal or decreased	Abnormal or decreased	Abnormal or decreased	Abnormal or decreased	Abnormal or decreased
III	Normal	Normal*	Normal	Abnormal or decreased	Normal
IV	Normal	Abnormal or decreased	Abnormal or decreased	Abnormal or decreased	Abnormal or decreased

*Normal with factor Xa; decreased with factor IIa.

of those with an acquired deficiency (e.g., eclampsia, disseminated intravascular coagulation or deep-vein thrombosis).

Bibliography

Abildgaard U: Highly purified antithrombin III with heparin cofactor activity prepared by disc electrophoresis. *Scand J Clin Lab Invest* 21:89–91, 1968.

Banerjee RN, Sahni AL, Kumar V, et al: Antithrombin III deficiency in maturity onset diabetes mellitus and atherosclerosis. *Thromb Diath Haemorrh* 31:339–345, 1974.

Buller H, Weeink AH, Treffers P, et al: Severe antithrombin III deficiency in a patient with pre-eclampsia: Observations on the effect of human AT III concentrate transfusion. *Scand J Haematol* 25:81–86, 1980.

Chan V, Chan TK, Wong V, et al: The determination of antithrombin III by radioimmunoassay and its clinical application. *Brit J Haematol* 41:563–572, 1979.

Chockly M, Penner J: An improved clinical assay for antithrombin III (heparin cofactor). *Amer J Clin Pathol* 74:213–217, 1980.

Collen D, Schetz J, Cook J, et al: Metabolism of antithrombin III (heparin-cofactor) in man: Effects of venous thrombosis and of heparin administration. *Eur J Clin Invest* 7:27–35, 1977.

Duckert F: Behavior of antithrombin III in liver disease. *Scand J Gastroenterol* 8:109–112, 1973.

Egeberg O: Inherited antithrombin deficiency causing thrombophilia. *Thromb Diath Haemorrh* 13:516–530, 1965.

Fagerhol MK, Abildgaard U: Immunological studies on human antithrombin III. *Scand J Haematol* 7:10–17, 1970.

Hedner U, Nilsson IM: Antithrombin III in clinical material. *Thromb Res* 3:631–641, 1973.

Jorgenson KA, Stofferson E: Antithrombin III and the nephrotic syndrome. *Scand J Haematol* 22:442–448, 1979.

Jorgenson KA, Stofferson E, Sorensen PJ, et al: Alterations in plasma antithrombin III following total hip replacement and elective cholecystecomy. *Scand J Haematol* 24:101–104, 1980.

Marciniak E, Gockerman J: Heparin-induced decrease in circulating antithrombin III. *Lancet* 2:581–584, 1977.

Penner JA, Hunter MJ: Antithrombins: Clinical aspects, chemical and biological properties. In *Trace Components of Plasma: Isolation and Clinical Significance*. New York: Alan R. Liss, 1976, pp 277–300.

Petersen TE, Dudek-Wojciechowska G, Sottrup-Jensen L, et al: The primary structure of antithrombin III. *Thromb Haemostasis* 38:201–212, 1977.

Rosenberg RD, Damus PS: The purification and mechanism of action of human antithrombin heparin cofactor. *J Biol Chem* 248:6490–6505, 1973.

Sorensen PJ, Dyerberg J, Stofferson E, et al: Familial functional antithrombin III deficiency. *Scand J Haematol* 24:105–109, 1980.

von Kaulaa E, Droegmueller W, Aoki N, et al: Antithrombin III depression and thrombin generation acceleration in women taking oral contraceptives. *Amer J Obstet Gynecol* 109:868–873, 1971.

von Kaulla E, von Kaulla K: Antithrombin III and diseases. *Amer J Clin Pathol* 48:69–80, 1967.

von Kaulla E, von Kaulla KN: Oral contraceptives and low antithrombin III activity. *Lancet* 1:36, 1970.

CASE
26

PATIENT: 35-year-old woman

CHIEF COMPLAINT: This patient was referred for an evaluation of a possible von Willebrand's disease. She had been seen at another hospital, where she was found to have a prolonged bleeding time. This finding, coupled with her medical history, suggested a diagnosis of von Willebrand's disease to the referring physician.

MEDICAL HISTORY: The patient had a lifelong history of an increased bleeding tendency. When 7 years of age, she had bled profusely after tonsillectomy. Transfusions were necessary to control the postoperative bleeding. In addition, she had serious bleeding as a teenager when two molars were extracted. Repeated packings were necessary, although at that time, transfusions were not given. She also had a history of abnormally heavy menstrual periods and profuse bleeding after breast biopsy for fibrocystic disease.

FAMILY HISTORY: A paternal uncle had a questionable bleeding tendency.

DRUG HISTORY: Noncontributory

PHYSICAL EXAMINATION: Within normal limits

Laboratory Results

A. Screening Procedures

	Patient	Normal
Prothrombin time	12 seconds	10–12 seconds
APTT	39 seconds	<42 seconds
Platelet count	250,000/μl	130,000–400,000/μl
Bleeding time	6 minutes	1–8 minutes

Questions

1. Does the normal bleeding time rule out the possibility of von Willebrand's disease?
2. What additional laboratory procedures are indicated?

Laboratory Results

B. Confirmatory Procedures

	Patient	Normal
Factor VIII:C	80%	50% to 150%
Factor VIII R:Ag	75%	50% to 150%
Factor VIII R:RCo	70%	50% to 150%
Factor IX	80%	50% to 150%
Factor XI	95%	50% to 150%
Clot solubility in 5 molar urea	Insoluble	Insoluble
Euglobulin clot lysis	Complete lysis within 30 minutes	>60 minutes lysis time
Fibrin split products	<10 μg/ml	<10 μg/ml
α_2-Antiplasmin (functional)	<10%	50% to 130%
α_2-Antiplasmin (immunologic)	0.1 mg/dl	5.2–6.9 mg/dl
Platelet Aggregation Studies ADP	Biphasic response	Biphasic aggregation
Epinephrine	Biphasic aggregation	Biphasic aggregation
Collagen	Full-range monophasic aggregation	Full-range monophasic aggregation
Ristocetin	Full-range monophasic agglutination	Full-range monophasic agglutination or biphasic agglutination

DIAGNOSIS: Hereditary deficiency of α_2-antiplasmin (Miyasato's disease)

Discussion

This patient had an extremely rare hereditary abnormality of α_2-antiplasmin. The clinical history of the patient suggested a serious bleeding abnormality that dated to early childhood. The family history suggested an autosomal recessive pattern of inheritance.

Results of screening tests were within normal limits, although prolonged bleeding time had been documented previously. Presumably, the abnormal bleeding time was secondary to ingestion of aspirin, which the patient admitted to on careful questioning. The combination of a history of serious bleeding and normal results on screening tests suggests a few abnormalities, including von Willebrand's disease, mild deficiency of factor VIII, IX or XI, a qualitative abnormality of platelet function,

HEREDITARY DEFICIENCY OF α-ANTIPLASMIN
(MIYASATO DISEASE)

CLINICAL PICTURE

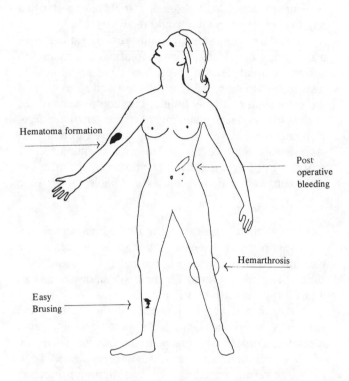

Hematoma formation →

Post operative bleeding ←

Hemarthrosis ←

Easy Brusing →

Pattern of inheritance: Autosomal recessive

PHYSICAL PROPERTIES AND ACTION OF α_2-ANTIPLASMIN

Glycoprotein, molecular weight of 70,000
Regulates fibrinolysis by
   Blocking active site of plasmin
   Blocking lysine-binding sites
   Binding to fibrin in presence of factor XIIIa, making lysis of fibrin more difficult

LABORATORY FINDINGS

A. Screening Procedures

Test	Patient's Result	Normal Range
Prothrombin time	Normal	10–12 seconds
APTT	Normal	<42 seconds
Platelet count	Normal	130,000–400,000/μl
Bleeding time	Normal	1–8 minutes

B. Confirmatory Procedures

Test	Patient's Result	Normal Range
Factor VIII R:Ag	Normal	50% to 150%
Factor VIII R:RCo	Normal	50% to 150%
Clot solubility in 5 molar urea	Normal	Insoluble
Euglobulin clot lysis	Abnormal	>60 minutes
α_2-Antiplasmin (functional)	Abnormal	50% to 150%
α_2-Antiplasmin (immunologic)	Abnormal	5.2–6.9 mg/dl

TREATMENT

Fresh-frozen plasma
ε-Aminocaproic acid (EACA) or tranexamic acid

Table 1
Clinical States with Altered α_2 Antiplasmin Levels

Decreased

  Hereditary

    Homozygous α_2 antiplasmin deficiency

    Heterozygous α_2 antiplasmin deficiency

  Acquired

    DIC

    Severe liver disease

    Septicemia

    Urokinase or streptokinase therapy

    Obstructive peripheral vascular disease

    Primary fibrinolysis (e.g. with neoplastic diseases)

Increased

  Post-operative thrombosis

  Diabetes mellitus

  Post-partum

  Metastatic malignancy

deficiency of factor XIII and deficiency of α_2-antiplasmin.

von Willebrand's disease was ruled out by normal findings for all three components of the factor VIII complex. A qualitative abnormality of platelet function was ruled out by normal results on platelet aggregation studies. A urea clot solubility test was within normal limits, thus eliminating the possibility of deficiency of factor XIII. Assays for factors IX and XI were within normal limits. However, the α_2-antiplasmin assay and the euglobulin clot lysis test were markedly abnormal. α_2-Antiplasmin was quantified by use of S-2251, a synthetic substrate for plasmin. This assay procedure involves the addition of plasmin in excess to a patient's plasma. After incubation, S-2251 is added, and the rate of release of p-nitroaniline is measured photometrically at 405 nm. This reaction may be conducted in a kinetic manner or with an end-point (nonrecording spectrophotometer). The rate of the reaction decreases as the plasma concentration of α_2-antiplasmin increases.

Pathophysiologic Basis. As was discussed in Chapter 2, fibrinolysis is a fibrin-oriented process. Activation of plasminogen on the surface of fibrin results in effective fibrinolysis. After lysis of fibrin, plasminogen activator and plasmin are released and bound to their respective plasma inhibitors. The primary physiologic inhibitor of plasmin is α_2-antiplasmin. In the absence of α_2-antiplasmin, plasmin is free to lyse fibrinogen and other plasmin-sensitive proteins.

The lysine-binding sites on plasmin are important not only in the binding to fibrin but also in the interaction with α_2-antiplasmin. α_2-Antiplasmin forms a complex with plasmin by binding to the lysine-binding sites, thus decreasing the ability of plasmin(ogen) to localize to fibrin clots. α_2-Macroglobulin and other physiologic inhibitors of plasmin do not inhibit binding of plasminogen to fibrin. In patients who lack α_2-antiplasmin, it would be expected that any fibrin formed in vivo would readily lyse.

Results of laboratory screening tests in patients with a hereditary deficiency of α_2-antiplasmin are characteristically normal. However, there is rapid and complete lysis in the whole blood clot lysis test and shortening of the euglobulin clot lysis time. Other components of the fibrinolytic system, including plasminogen, α_2-macroglobulin and fibrin split products, are normal. α_2-Antiplasmin may be quantified with an immunologic procedure or a synthetic substrate procedure by means of a chromogenic or fluorogenic assay (Table 1).

Clinical Picture. Patients with a hereditary deficiency of α_2-antiplasmin have a lifelong history of severe bleeding. In some instances, the pattern of bleeding is suggestive of hemophilia. The first patient described had a history of hemarthrosis (Table 2).

In each patient who has been studied to date, the pattern of inheritance appears to have been autosomal recessive. Persons who are heterozygous for deficiency of α_2-antiplasmin have few bleeding problems. Typically, the results on assays for α_2-antiplasmin function and antigenicity are markedly abnormal. Patients rarely demonstrate spontaneous bleeding. Bleeding usually is associated with trauma and often is delayed. Postoperative bleeding is characteristic. Although persons who are heterozygous for the deficiency have few bleeding problems, they are relatively easily detected by virtue of their decreased level of α_2-antiplasmin.

Treatment. Patients with a deficiency of α_2-antiplasmin may be treated with fresh-frozen plasma alone or in combination with a plasmin inhibitor, such as aminocaproic acid or tranexamic acid.

Bibliography

Aoki N, Saito H, Kamiya T, et al: Congenital deficiency of α_2 antiplasmin inhibitor associated with severe hemorrhagic tendency. *J Clin Invest* 63:877–884, 1979.

Haupt H, Heimburger N: Human serum proteine mit hoher Affinität zu Carboxymethylcellulose. I.

Table 2*

Hereditary α₂ - Antiplasmin Deficiency

			Clinical Findings				Laboratory Results						
Author	Patient	Consanguinity	Clinical Picture	Symptomatic Heterozygotes	Pattern of Inheritance	Treatment	Euglobulin clot lysis	Whole Blood Clot Lysis	FSP**	Clot Solubility in urea	α₂ Antiplasmin antigen	α₂ antiplasmin activity	Misc
Koie et al	25 y.o. male Japan	Yes	Hemothorax Hemarthroses, etc.	No	Autosomal recessive	Tranexamic acid and plasma	65 min (N90-240)	4 hrs (N>24 hrs)	0-5 µg/ml (N 0.5 µg/ml)	—	0 mg/dl (N 6.13 ± 0.88)	3% (N 100%)	Heterozygotes 50% α₂ antiplasm
Kluft et al	17 y.o. male Netherlands	No	Spon. joint, muscle, CNS hemorrhage	Yes	Autosomal recessive	Tranexamic	Normal	Normal	<10 µg/ml (N<10 µg/ml)	—	No detectable antigen	2% of normal	
Miles et al	35 y.o. Female USA	Yes	Bleeding following trauma hemarthroses	Yes	Autosomal recessive	—	150 min (N>120 min)	5 hrs (N>24 hrs)	<10 µg/ml	Yes	<1 µg/ml (N 75.0 µg/ml)	< 10%	Platelet α₂ APT- 20.8 µg (N 68 µg)
(1 family)	Male USA	Yes	Bleeding following trauma	Yes	Autosomal recessive	—	—	—	—	—	<1 µg/ml	12%	
Yoshioka et al (1 family)	5 y.o. female Japan	No	Umbilical bleeding hematomata	No	Autosomal recessive	Tranexamic acid	1.5 hr (N 6-12 hrs)	3 hrs (N >24 hrs)	10 µg/ml (N<10 µg/ml)	—	<1.5% (N 70-150%)	<10% (N70-130%)	
	2 y.o. female Japan	No	Umbilical bleeding hematomata	No	Autosomal recessive	Tranexamic acid	2 hours	3 hrs	5 µg/ml	—	<1.5%	<10%	
	3 mo. old female Japan	No	Umbilical bleeding	No	Autosomal recessive	Tranexamic acid	1.5 hrs	4 hrs	5 µg/ml	—	<1.5%	<10%	
Niewenhuis et al	15 y.o. male Netherlands	No	Posttraumatic bleeding	—	Autosomal recessive	—	Abnormal	—	—	—	83% of normal	4% of normal	Poor binding to plasmin
(1 family)	5 y.o. female Netherlands	No	No symptoms	—	Autosomal recessive	—	Abnormal	—	—	92% of normal	2% of normal	Named α₂ AP-Enschede
Evatt	40 y.o. female USA	?	Post-op bleeding menorrhagia	—	—	—	—	—	—	—	Normal antigen	Very low	

*From Triplett DA: Hereditary α₂ antiplasmin deficiency. *Thrombosis and Hemostasis.* Check Sample TH 84-2, Chicago: ASCP.
**FSP = *Fibrin Split Products*

Isolierung von Lysozym, Clq und bisher unbekannten Globulinen. *Hoppe Seyler's Z Physiol Chem* 353:1125–1132, 1133–1140, 1972.

Kluft C, Vellenga E, Brommer EJP: Homozygous α_2 antiplasmin deficiency. (Letter to the editor) *Lancet* 2:206–210, 1979.

Kluft C, Vellenga E, Brommer EJP, et al: Familial hemorrhagic diathesis in a Dutch family: An inherited deficiency of α_2 antiplasmin. *Blood* 59:1169–1180, 1982.

Koie K, Ogata K, Kamiya T, et al: α_2 Plasmin inhibitor deficiency (Miyasato's disease). *Lancet* 1:1334–1335, 1978.

Miles LA, Plow EF, Donnelly KJ, et al: A bleeding disorder due to deficiency of α_2 antiplasmin. *Blood* 59:1246–1251, 1982.

Yoshioka A, Kamitsuji H, Takase T: Congenital deficiency of α_2 plasmin inhibitor in three sisters. *Haemostasis* 11:176–184, 1982.

CASE
27

PATIENT: 29-year-old woman

CHIEF COMPLAINT: This patient was admitted from the emergency room. She had presented because of pain and tenderness in the right calf.

MEDICAL HISTORY: This hospitalization was the third one for the patient. Eight years earlier, she had been hospitalized because of right-sided pleuritic chest pain and symptoms of thrombophlebitis of the left leg. A presumptive diagnosis of pulmonary embolism was established on the basis of an abnormal ventilation perfusion scan.

After her first admission, the patient was seen approximately 3 years later because of complaints of pain in the right leg and tenderness in the medial aspect of the middle portion of the right thigh. A venogram confirmed the diagnosis of thrombophlebitis. On both previous occasions, the patient had responded to anticoagulant therapy, which consisted of heparinization followed by oral anticoagulation. Her physician had continued the oral anticoagulants for approximately 1 year after each hospitalization.

FAMILY HISTORY: There was a family history of deep-vein thrombosis and pulmonary embolism. The patient's mother had several episodes of thrombophlebitis complicated by pulmonary embolism. Her first episode of thrombophlebitis occurred after childbirth at 22 years of age. The mother died suddenly at 45 years of age, and an autopsy was not performed. However, the medical examiner had signed the death certificate, indicating pulmonary embolism as the cause of death.

The maternal uncle had also died suddenly, at 52 years of age. He had been hospitalized on several occasions because of recurrent pulmonary embolism. The maternal grandfather had also died suddenly, after minor surgery, at 59 years of age.

The patient had one child, 6 years of age, who was asymptomatic.

DRUG HISTORY: At the time of hospitalization, the patient was taking no medication. However, as has been noted above, she had received oral anticoagulants and heparin in the past for management of thrombotic disease.

PHYSICAL EXAMINATION: Swelling of the right calf and Homans' sign were noted. Doppler and impedance plethysmography demonstrated a thrombus in the right proximal popliteal area, extending into the lower portion of the thigh. Venography was not performed.

Laboratory Results

A. Screening Procedures

	Patient	Normal
Prothrombin time	11.5 seconds	10–12 seconds
APTT	37 seconds	<42 seconds
Platelet count	390,000/μl	130,000–400,000/μl
Bleeding time	6 minutes and 30 seconds	1–8 minutes

Questions

1. What additional laboratory procedures are indicated?
2. What abnormalities have been associated with an inherited predisposition to thrombotic disease?
3. What is the treatment of choice?

Laboratory Results

B. Confirmatory Procedures

	Patient	Normal
Fibrinogen (clottable)	300 mg/dl	170–410 mg/dl
Fibrinogen (immunologic)	275 mg/dl	170–410 mg/dl
Prothrombin antigen	85%	60% to 150%
Antithrombin III (activity)	90%	85% to 115%
Antithrombin III (immunologic)	30 mg/dl	23–40 mg/dl
Protein C (immunologic)	40%	68% to 152%
Plasminogen (activity)	5.7 CTA units	3.8–8.4 CTA units
Protein S	85%	61–130%

DIAGNOSIS: Hereditary deficiency of protein C

Discussion

This patient's history and her family history suggest an autosomal dominant predisposition to thromboembolic disease. Thus, the differential diagnosis would include abnormalities of antithrombin III, fibrinogen, plasminogen protein S and protein C. Also, clinical studies have suggested that patients with an abnormality of tissue plasminogen activator may be predisposed to recurrent

HEREDITARY DEFICIENCY OF PROTEIN C

CLINICAL PICTURE

PHYSICAL PROPERTIES OF PROTEIN C

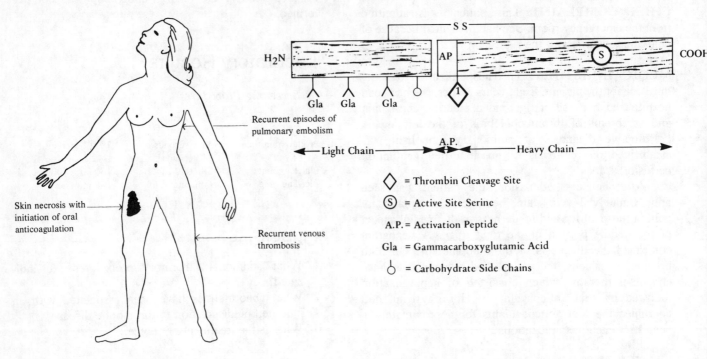

Recurrent episodes of pulmonary embolism

Skin necrosis with initiation of oral anticoagulation

Recurrent venous thrombosis

◇ = Thrombin Cleavage Site

Ⓢ = Active Site Serine

A.P. = Activation Peptide

Gla = Gammacarboxyglutamic Acid

⌀ = Carbohydrate Side Chains

Pattern of inheritance: Autosomal dominant

LABORATORY FINDINGS

A. Screening Procedures

Test	Patient's Result	Normal Range
Prothrombin time	Normal	10–12 seconds
APTT	Normal	<42 seconds
Platelet count	Normal	130,000–400,000/μl
Bleeding time	Normal	1–8 minutes

B. Confirmatory Procedures

Test	Patient's Result	Normal Range
Fibrinogen, clottable	Normal	170–410 mg/dl
Fibrinogen, immunologic	Normal	170–410 mg/dl
Antithrombin III, immunologic	Normal	23–40 mg/dl
Antithrombin III, activity	Normal	85% to 115%
Plasminogen, (activity)	Normal	3.8–8.4 CTA units
Protein C, (immunologic)	Abnormal	68% to 152%
Protein S (immunologic)	Normal	61–130%

TREATMENT

Long-term oral anticoagulants
?Stanazol or other anabolic steroids

thromboembolic disease; however this clinical state remains poorly characterized.

In this case, the antigenic and functional levels of antithrombin III were within normal limits. Also, the values for clottable and antigenic fibrinogen were normal. Protein C antigen was decreased. It was evaluated with an enzyme-linked immunosorbent assay. The functional assay for protein C was not performed.

Biochemical Aspects. Initial work by Walter Seegers in 1960 suggested that a potent anticoagulant activity occurred in preparations of bovine prothrombin that had been digested with purified thrombin. This anticoagulant activity was termed autoprothrombin IIA. Subsequently, in 1970, Marciniak suggested that the anticoagulant was, in fact, a separate protein not derived from prothrombin. Stenflo, in 1976, described a "new" protein that he called protein C. This designation was based on the sequence of elution of vitamin K-dependent proteins during chromatographic separation. Following this report, Seegers showed that protein C was immunologically identical to autoprothrombin IIA.

Stenflo was then able to isolate protein C and to show that it was a serine protease. In addition, it was found to require vitamin K for its synthesis. The structure of bovine protein C has been well characterized. Human protein C has also been purified and found to be similar to the bovine molecule. Protein C is a glycoprotein composed of a heavy chain and a light chain linked by disulfide bonds. The molecular weight of unreduced human protein C has been estimated to be 62,000 on the basis of sodium dodecyl sulfate-polyacrylamide gel electrophoresis. The heavy chain has a molecular weight of approximately 41,000; the light chain has a molecular weight of approximately 21,000. The human protein C molecule appears to be more glycosylated than is bovine protein C and contains approximately 23% carbohydrate. The γ-carboxyglutamic acid residues are located on the light chain, whereas the active serine residue is found on the heavy chain. Recently, a new amino acid, β-hydroxyaspartic acid, has been found in protein C.

In contrast to the other vitamin K-dependent coagulation factors (II, VII, IX and X), activated protein C is a potent anticoagulant. Protein C is thought to be activated in vivo by thrombin after the latter has formed a complex with a cofactor, thrombomodulin, on the surfaces of endothelial cells. In vitro, protein C can be activated by trypsin and by Russell's viper venom. Protein C functions in plasma by inactivating the activated cofactors Va and VIIIa. Activated protein C inactivates the activated forms of these cofactors much more rapidly than it inactivates the native forms (i.e., factors V and VIII).

Inactivation of factor Va has been studied more extensively than has inactivation of factor VIIIa because of the recent purification and isolation of human factor V. Activated protein C inactivates plasma factor Va by means of limited proteolysis. This reaction is dependent on calcium ions and on a negatively charged phospholipid surface. Proteolysis of factor Va involves breakdown of the heavy chain of factor Va (molecular weight, 115,000) to a fragment with a molecular weight of approximately 85,000. Recently, protein S, another vitamin K-dependent protein, has been implicated as a cofactor in accelerating the activity of activated protein C. Presumably, this reaction takes place on the surfaces of activated platelets.

The nature of the degradation of activated factor VIII:C by activated protein C is thought to be analogous to the inactivation of factor Va. Activated factor VIII:C contains a heavy chain of approximately 95,000 daltons that is cleaved by activated protein C.

In addition to its anticoagulant action, activated protein C accelerates fibrinolytic activity. Recent work suggests that activated protein C enhances release of tissue plasminogen activator from the endothelial cells that line the vascular lumina. In addition to stimulation of release of endogenous stores of tissue plasminogen activator, there is experimental evidence that protein C may stimulate synthesis of tissue plasminogen activator by endothelial cells.

In vivo, optimal activation of protein C involves a cofactor found in membranes of endothelial cells. This cofactor has been termed thrombomodulin. Thrombomodulin increases the rate of thrombin-catalyzed activation of protein C by more than 20,000-fold. Purified thrombomodulin has been found to have a molecular weight of approximately 74,000. Thrombin readily forms a complex with thrombomodulin on surfaces of endothelial cells. Once thrombin has formed a complex with thrombomodulin, the substrate specificity of thrombin is greatly altered. It no longer activates factors V and VIII or converts fibrinogen to fibrin. In addition, the thrombin-thrombomodulin complex does not activate platelets. Thus, it would appear that once thrombin has formed a complex with thrombomodulin, it undergoes a structural or conformational change that promotes activation of protein C and at the same time inhibits the other activities that are associated with thrombin.

Down regulation of activated protein C has also been investigated. Initial work suggested that an inhibitor of activated protein C was present. Recently, this inhibitor has been isolated from human plasma and found to have an apparent molecular weight of 57,000. Suzuki and colleagues have estimated that the plasma concentration is approximately 5 μg/ml. The inhibitor of activated protein C appears to form a complex in a 1:1 molar ratio with activated protein C.

Clinical Picture. As mentioned earlier, deficiency of protein C has been associated with an autosomal dominant pattern of inherited predisposition to thrombotic disease. In the affected families who have been studied to date, the level of protein C has been approximately 40% to 50% of the normal level. Thus, hereditary deficiency of protein C is similar to hereditary deficiency of antithrombin III in that both clinical situations are not associated with an absolute deficiency.

At least 24 families have now been identified in whom deficiency of protein C is associated with venous thromboembolic disease. The prevalence of deficiency of protein C has not been well established, although preliminary studies from the Netherlands suggest that there may be as many cases as 1 per 16,000 people.

The clinical picture in patients with a deficiency of protein C is similar to the clinical picture in those with a deficiency of antithrombin III. Thrombophlebitis frequently is the first clinical event. The first episode of thrombophlebitis often occurs after trauma or surgical intervention. Arterial thrombosis is relatively rare. By 30 years of age, more than one-half of patients have presented with various thromboembolic complaints, and by 40 years of age, more than 80% of patients are symptomatic. Another interesting observation in such patients has been the occurrence of skin necrosis at an early stage after institution of oral anticoagulant therapy. Newborn infants with apparent homozygous deficiency of protein C present with purpura fulminans which is usually fatal.

All the initial cases of this deficiency were diagnosed on the basis of a decreased antigenic level of protein C. Recently, several functional assays for protein C have been described. One functional assay makes use of a newer synthetic chromogenic substrate, S-2366. Use of an antigenic assay in combination with a functional assay has enabled the identification of several families with a normal level of protein C antigen but only approximately 50% of the normal functional activity. Thus, there appears to be a distinct heterogeneity in deficiency of protein C that is analogous to the heterogeneity seen in deficiencies of other vitamin K-dependent proteins.

Recent studies have also identified acquired deficiencies of protein C. Liver disease and disseminated intravascular coagulation have been documented in association with an acquired decrease of protein C antigen. In addition, acquired deficiency of protein C has developed after major and minor surgical procedures. Thus, it would appear that acquired deficiency of protein C may be associated with an increased tendency toward thrombosis.

Marlar and Griffin initially proposed that deficiency of the inhibitor of activated protein C would result in abnormal levels of factors V and VIII. They suggested that combined deficiency of factors V and VIII, a rare autosomal recessive disorder, could be explained on the basis of an absence or decrease in activity of the physiologic inhibitor of activated protein C. However, recent work from other laboratories has demonstrated a normal amount of inhibitor of protein C in patients with a hereditary deficiency of factors V and VIII. Thus, the pathophysiologic basis of combined deficiency of factors V and VIII is still a subject of controversy.

The discovery of protein C and its physiologic importance has opened a fertile field of investigation in the characterization of thrombotic disease. Antigenic as well as functional abnormalities of protein C have now been identified, and it would appear that abnormalities of thrombomodulin and protein S might also be associated with a predisposition to thrombosis. Currently, investigators are evaluating the level of protein S antigen in families with an inherited predisposition to thromboembolic disease. Hereditary deficiency of protein S has been associated with recurrent thromboembolic disease.

Treatment. The treatment of choice for patients with a deficiency of protein C is long-term oral anticoagulant therapy. However, clinicians should be aware of the association of skin necrosis with the introduction of oral anticoagulant therapy in such patients. Thus, patients in whom skin necrosis has developed in association with management of thrombotic disease by use of oral anticoagulants should be thoroughly evaluated for an underlying deficiency of protein C.

Another interesting therapy that has been suggested is the use of oral anabolic steroids. Recently, oral anabolic steroids have been used in the treatment of patients with hemophilia A and B, with surprising clinical results. Stanazol increases the level of protein C 1.6 times over baseline. However, clinical experience with Stanazol® has not been well documented; consequently, oral anticoagulants remain the treatment of choice.

In establishing a diagnosis of deficiency of protein C, clinicians should be aware of medical problems that may lead to acquired deficiency of protein C. Thus, liver disease and disseminated intravascular coagulation must be ruled out before a diagnosis of hereditary deficiency of protein C can be made.

Bibliography

History

Kisiel W, Davie EW: Protein C (a review). *Methods Enzymol* 80:320–332, 1981.

Mammen EF, Thomas WR, Seegers WH: Activation of purified prothrombin to autoprothrombin I or autoprothrombin II (platelet cofactor III) or autoprothrombin II-A. *Thromb Diath Haemorrh* 5:218–249, 1960.

Marciniak E: Coagulation inhibitor elicited by thrombin. *Science* 170:452–453, 1970.

Marciniak E: Inhibitor of human blood coagulation elicited by thrombin. *J Lab Clin Med* 79:924–934, 1972.

Seegers WH, Nova E, Henry RL, et al: Relationship of "new" vitamin K dependent protein. A phospholipid-binding zymogen of a serine esterase. *J Biol Chem* 251:3052–3056, 1976.

Stenflo JA: A new vitamin K dependent protein. Purification from bovine plasma and preliminary characterization. *J Biol Chem* 251:355–363, 1976.

Biochemical Aspects

Bern MM, Klumper DI, Wheeler WE, et al: Factor VIII complex in chronic renal failure: Influence of protein C, fibrinolysis and diabetes mellitus. *Thromb Res* 31:177–181, 1983.

Comp PC, Esmon CT: Activated protein C inhibits platelet prothrombin converting activity. *Blood* 54:1272–1281, 1979.

Comp PC, Esmon CT: Generation of fibrinolytic activity by infusion of activated protein C into dogs. *J Clin Invest* 68:1221–1228, 1981.

Fulcher C, Gardiner J, Griffin J, et al: Proteolysis of human factor VIII procoagulant protein with thrombin and activated protein C. *Fed Proc Fed Amer Soc Exp Biol* 42:1176, 1983.

Fulcher CA, Gardiner JE, Griffin JH, et al: Proteolytic inactivation of human factor VIII procoagulant protein by activated protein C and its analogy with factor V. *Blood* 63:486–489, 1984.

Holmberg L, Ljung R, Nilsson IM: The effects of plasmin and protein Ca on factor VIII:C and VIII:CAg. *Thromb Res* 31:41–50, 1983.

Kisiel W: Human plasma protein C: Isolation, characterization and mechanism of activation by α thrombin. *J Clin Invest* 64:761–769, 1979.

Marlar RA, Kleiss AJ, Griffin JH: Human protein C: Inactivation of factors V and VIII in plasma by the activated molecule. *Ann NY Acad Sci* 370:303–310, 1981.

Marlar RA, Kleiss AJ, Griffin JH: Mechanism of action of human activated protein C, a thrombin dependent anticoagulant enzyme. *Blood* 59:1064–1072, 1982.

Stenflo J, Dahlback B, Fernlund P, et al: Protein C, a regulator of prothrombin activation. In Nossel HL, Vogel HJ (eds): *Pathobiology of the Endothelial Cell.* New York: Academic Press, 1982, pp 103–119.

Suzuki K, Stenflo J, Dahlback B, et al: Inactivation of human coagulation factor V by activated protein C. *J Biol Chem* 258:1914–1920, 1983.

Thrombomodulin and Endothelial Cells

Comp PC, Jacocks RM, Ferrell GL, et al: Activation of protein C in vivo. *J Clin Invest* 70:127–134, 1982.

Esmon CT, Esmon NL, Harris KW: Complex formation between thrombin and thrombomodulin: Inhibits both thrombin-catalyzed fibrin formation and factor V activation. *J Biol Chem* 257:7944–7947, 1982.

Esmon CT, Esmon NL, Saugstad J, et al: Activation of protein C by a complex between thrombin and endothelial cell surface protein. In Nossel HL, Vogel HG (eds): *Pathobiology of the Endothelial Cell.* New York: Academic Press, 1982, pp 121–136.

Esmon CT, Owen WG: Identification of an endothelial cell cofactor for thrombin-catalysed activation of protein C. *Proc Natl Acad Sci USA* 78:2249–2252, 1981.

Esmon NL, Carroll RC, Esmon CT: Thrombomodulin inhibition of platelet activation by thrombin. (Abstract) *Thromb Haemostasis* 50:81, 1983.

Esmon NL, Owen WG, Esmon CT: Isolation of membrane-bound cofactor for thrombin-catalysed activation of protein C. *J Biol Chem* 257:859–864, 1982.

Owen WG, Esmon CT: Functional properties of an endothelial cell cofactor for thrombin-catalysed activation of protein C. *J Biol Chem* 256:5532–5535, 1981.

Roles of Protein S and Factor V

DiScipio RG, Davie EW: A characterization of protein S, a γ-carboxyglutamic acid containing protein from bovine and human plasma. *Biochemistry* 18:899–904, 1979.

Salem HH, Broze GJ, Miletich JP, et al: The light chain of factor Va contains the activity of factor Va that accelerates protein C activation by thrombin. *J Biol Chem* 258:8531–8534, 1983.

Salem HH, Broze GJ, Miletich JP, et al: Human coagulation factor Va is a cofactor for the activation of protein C. *Proc Natl Acad Sci USA* 80:1584–1588, 1983.

Walker FJ: Regulation of activated protein C by a new protein—A possible function for bovine protein S. *J Biol Chem* 255:5521–5524, 1980.

Walker FJ: Regulation of activated protein C by protein S—The role of protein C in factor Va inactivation. *J Biol Chem* 256:11128–11131, 1981.

Clinical Picture

Broekmans AW, Bertina RM, Loeliger EA, et al: Protein C and the development of skin necrosis during anticoagulant therapy. (Abstract) *Thromb Haemostasis* 49:244, 1983.

Broekmans AW, van der Linden IK, Veltkamp JJ, et al: Prevalence of isolated protein C deficiency in patients with thrombotic disease and in the population. (Abstract) *Thromb Haemostasis* 50:350, 1983.

Broekmans AW, Veltkamp JJ, Bertina RM: Clinical

manifestations of isolated protein C deficiency. (Abstract) *Thromb Haemostasis* 50:343, 1983.

Broekmans AW, Veltkamp JJ, Bertina RM: Congenital protein C deficiency and venous thromboembolism. *N Engl J Med* 309:340–344, 1983.

Griffin JH, Evatt BL, Zimmerman TS, et al: Deficiency of protein C in congenital thrombotic disease. *J Clin Invest* 68:1370–1373, 1981.

Griffin JH, Mosher DF, Zimmerman TS, et al: Protein C, an antithrombotic protein is reduced in hospitalized patients with intravascular coagulation. *Blood* 60:261–264, 1982.

Hoffmann V, Frick PG: Repeated occurrence of skin necrosis twice following coumarin intake and subsequently during decrease of vitamin K dependent coagulation factors associated with cholestasis. *Thromb Haemostasis* 48:245–246, 1982.

Horellou MH, Samama M, Conard J, et al: Protein C deficiency in three unrelated French patients with venous thrombosis. (Abstract) *Thromb Haemostasis* 50:351, 1983.

Mannucci PM, Vigano S: Deficiencies of protein C, an inhibitor of blood coagulation. *Lancet* 2:463–466, 1982.

Marlar RA, Endres-Brooks J: Recurrent thromboembolic disease due to heterozygous protein C deficiency. (Abstract) *Thromb Haemostasis* 50:351, 1983.

Pabinger-Fasching I, Bertina RM, Lechner K, et al: Hereditary protein C deficiency in two Austrian families. (Abstract) *Thromb Haemostasis* 50:343, 1983.

Seligsohn N, Berger A, Abend M, et al: Homozygous protein C deficiency manifested by massive venous thrombosis in the newborn. *NEJM* 310:559–562, 1984.

Van Amstel WJ, Boekhout-Musrert MJ, Loeliger EA: Successful prevention of coumarin-induced hemorrhagic skin necrosis by timely administration of vitamin K. *Blut* 36:89–93, 1978.

Factor V and VIII Deficiency

Bauer F, Schapira M, Mannucci PM, et al: In vivo inactivation of factor V by a vitamin K dependent factor. Study of an individual with combined V/VIII deficiency. *Thromb Res* 29:453–457, 1983.

Giddings JC, Surgrue A, Bloom AL: Quantitation of coagulant antigens and inhibition of activated protein C in combined V/VIII deficiency. *Brit J Haematol* 52:495–502, 1982.

Kisiel W, Canfield WM: Evidence of normal functional levels of activated protein C inhibitor in combined factor V/VIII deficiency disease. *J Clin Invest* 70:1260–1272, 1982.

Marlar RA, Griffin JH: Deficiency of protein C inhibitor in combined factor V/VIII deficiency. *J Clin Invest* 66:1186–1189, 1980.

Mazzone D, Fichera A, Practico G, et al: Combined congenital deficiency of factor V and factor VIII. *Acta Haematol* 68:337–338, 1982.

Suzuki K, Nishioka J, Hashimoto S: Characterization of protein C inhibitor purified from human plasma. (Abstract) *Thromb Haemostasis* 50:342, 1983.

Suzuki K, Nishioka J, Hashimoto S: Protein C inhibitor: Purification from human plasma and characterization. *J Biol Chem* 258:163–168, 1983.

Vicente V, Alberca I, Lopez Borrasca A: Inhibitor of protein C and combined deficiency of factors V and VIII. (Abstract) *Brit J Haematol* 53:686, 1983.

Functional Assay

Bertina RM, Broekmans AW, van Es-Krommenhoek T, et al: The use of a functional assay for plasma protein C in the diagnosis of protein C deficiency. (Abstract) *Thromb Haemostasis* 50:350, 1983.

Francis RB, Patch MJ: A functional assay for protein C in human plasma. *Thromb Res* 32:605–613, 1983.

Ohno Y, Kato H, Morita T, et al: A new fluorogenic peptide substrate for vitamin K dependent blood coagulation factor, bovine protein C. *J Biochem* 90:1387–1395, 1981.

Sala N, Owen WG, Collen D: Functional assay of protein C in human plasma. (Abstract) *Thromb Haemostasis* 50:353, 1983.

Sala M, Owen WG, Collen D: A functional assay for protein C in human plasma. *Blood* 63:671–675, 1984.

Treatment

Bertina RM, Broekmans AW: Protein C concentrates for therapeutic use. *Lancet* 2:1348, 1982.

Mannucci PM, Vigano S: Protein C concentrates for therapeutic use. (Letter to the editor) *Lancet* 1:875, 1983.

Preston FE, Malia RG, Greaves M, et al: Effect of stanazol on antithrombin III and protein C. *Lancet* 2:517–518, 1983.

Seghatchian MJ: Protein C in clinical factor IX concentrates. *Lancet* 1:1047, 1983.

Protein S Deficiency

Comp PC, Esmon CT: Recurrent venous thromboembolism in patients with a partial deficiency of protein S. *NEJM* 311:1525–1528, 1984.

Schwartz HP, Fischer M, Hopmeier P, et al: Plasma protein S deficiency in familial thrombotic disease. *Blood* 64:1297–1300, 1984.

CASE
28

PATIENT: 56-year-old woman

CHIEF COMPLAINT: This patient presented to the emergency room because of abdominal pain together with nausea and vomiting of 3 to 4 weeks' duration.

MEDICAL HISTORY: The patient had never been hospitalized, with the exception of obstetric admissions. For the year immediately preceding her visit to the emergency room, the patient had noted difficulties with food intolerance and postprandial epigastric discomfort.

FAMILY HISTORY: Noncontributory

DRUG HISTORY: The patient had taken aspirin fairly regularly for the past year for abdominal pain. Other medications included Diabinese (chlorpropamide) for adult-onset diabetes and Dyazide for hypertension.

PHYSICAL EXAMINATION: The patient was a pale woman in obvious pain. There was abdominal distention and absence of bowel sounds on auscultation. Rebound tenderness was noted.

Laboratory Results

A. Screening Procedures

	Patient	Normal
Prothrombin time	19 seconds	10–12 seconds
APTT	48 seconds	<42 seconds
Platelet count	180,000/μl	130,000–400,000/μl
Bleeding time	9 minutes and 30 seconds	1–8 minutes

HOSPITAL COURSE: The patient immediately underwent endoscopic examination. The examination revealed a gastric ulcer, and the patient then underwent partial gastrectomy and vagotomy. Twelve hours after the operation, the patient became hypotensive, and oozing was noted from the surgical site. Before reoperation, further laboratory tests were performed.

Questions

1. Why are the prothrombin time and the activated partial thromboplastin time (APTT) prolonged?
2. What is the most likely explanation for the prolonged bleeding time?
3. What blood components should this patient receive before undergoing surgery?

Laboratory Results

B. Confirmatory Procedures

	Patient	Normal
APTT (50% patient plasma/ 50% pooled normal plasma)	40 seconds	<42 seconds
Prothrombin time (50% patient plasma/50% pooled normal plasma)	13 seconds	10–12 seconds
Factor X assay	25%	50% to 150%
Factor VII assay	10%	50% to 150%
Factor V assay	90%	50% to 150%

DIAGNOSIS: Deficiency of vitamin K; aspirin-induced qualitative abnormality of platelets

Discussion

This case is an excellent example of two acquired hemostatic abnormalities. Deficiency of vitamin K and drug-induced qualitative abnormalities of platelet function are frequently encountered. Patients with a deficiency of vitamin K usually are seen postoperatively or in intensive care units. However, deficiency of vitamin K also is encountered in outpatients who have had gastrointestinal problems, such as diarrhea or nausea and vomiting, and occasionally is seen in patients with peculiar dietary habits. In this patient, who had a history of nausea and vomiting, the most likely explanation for deficiency of vitamin K is inadequate dietary intake.

The acquired qualitative abnormality of platelets is secondary to a history of frequent ingestion of aspirin for abdominal pain. Aspirin acetylates cyclooxygenase, thus inhibiting the platelet prostaglandin pathway. This inhibition of cyclooxygenase is irreversible and persists for the life span of platelets (7 to 10 days). Consequently, patients who frequently ingest aspirin show abnormal

DEFICIENCY OF VITAMIN K; ASPIRIN-INDUCED QUALITATIVE ABNORMALITY OF PLATELETS

CLINICAL PICTURE

PHYSICAL PROPERTIES OF VITAMIN K

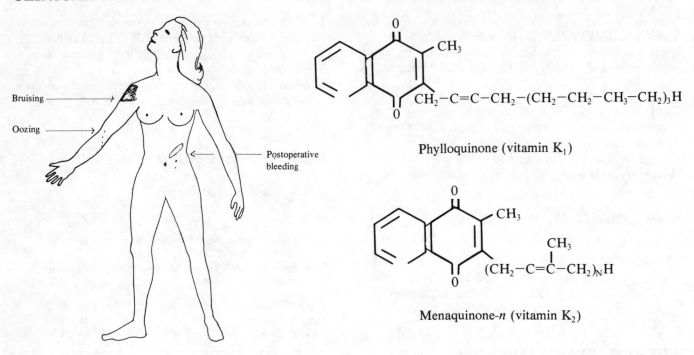

Bruising

Oozing

Postoperative bleeding

Phylloquinone (vitamin K_1)

Menaquinone-n (vitamin K_2)

LABORATORY FINDINGS

A. Screening Procedures

Test	Patient's Result	Normal Range
Prothrombin time	Abnormal	10–12 seconds
APTT	Abnormal	<42 seconds
Platelet count	Normal	130,000–400,000/μl
Bleeding time	Abnormal	1–8 minutes

B. Confirmatory Procedures

Mixing APTT	Normal	<42 seconds
Mixing prothrombin time	Normal	10–12 seconds
Factor V assay	Normal	50% to 150%
Factor X assay	Abnormal	50% to 150%

TREATMENT

Fresh-frozen plasma in acute bleeding

Phytonadione may be given intramuscularly or intravenously. 10 to 20 mg, repeat in 2 to 3 days.

Prothrombin complex concentrates in life threatening situations results on platelet aggregation studies and a prolonged bleeding time.

Before this patient was returned to the operative suite, fresh-frozen plasma and platelet concentrates were administered.

Biochemical Aspects. Vitamin K is a fat-soluble vitamin. Actually, vitamin K is a generic term for a group of fat-soluble vitamins that consist of 2-methyl-1,4-naphthoquinone derivatives. Vitamin K_1 is synthesized by plants; vitamin K_2 refers to a series of vitamins that contain unsaturated side chains that differ in the number of isoprenyl units. Menadione (vitamin K_3) is a provitamin. Menadione is converted to menaquinone-4 in animals and birds. The alkylating enzyme for menadione is present in the liver microsomes of animals and birds.

Vitamin K in the diet is supplied mostly by leafy green vegetables. Absorption of vitamin K requires bile and pancreatic secretions. Patients with malabsorption syndromes lose as much as 90% of an oral dose of vitamin K in their stools.

The role of vitamin K in coagulation is related to a vitamin K-dependent carboxylase system found in microsomes of the liver and other organs. The active form of the vitamin constitutes an electron donor, or a microsomal electron transport system, for which oxygen is the terminal acceptor. This electron transport system is coupled to a carbon dioxide fixation reaction that converts peptide-bound glutamic acid to γ-carboxyglutamic acid. γ-Carboxyglutamic acid is found in all the vitamin K-dependent coagulation proteins (i.e., factors II, VII, IX, X and others). γ-Carboxyglutamic acid is essential in the localization of these proteins to lipid surfaces. In the absence of vitamin K, these coagulation proteins are not effectively bound to the phospholipid surfaces, and the surface-bound localization of coagulation does not occur.

Clinical Picture. A number of vitamin K deficiency states have been described. They include hemorrhagic disease of the newborn, dietary inadequacy, malabsorption syndromes and biliary obstruction; administration of broad-spectrum antibiotics and total parenteral nutrition also may lead to deficiency of vitamin K.

Newborn infants represent a special case of vitamin K nutrition. In healthy infants, levels of the vitamin K-dependent coagulation factors are less than those in adults and may decrease to as low as 30% of adult levels on the second and third days of life. If the prothrombin activity falls below 10%, hemorrhagic disease of the newborn may occur. Typically, such infants may bleed from the umbilicus, skin, nose, mouth and intestines and,

occasionally, they suffer cerebral hemorrhage. Premature infants are more susceptible to deficiency of vitamin K than are term infants.

Infants who are breast-fed are at higher risk for hemorrhage than are formula-fed infants. Human milk contains only 1 to 2 μg of vitamin K per liter, whereas cow's milk contains 15 to 17 μg of vitamin K per liter. The requirement for vitamin K in newborn infants has been estimated to be 5 μg per day. It should also be emphasized that breast milk is sterile and delays colonization of the gut with bacteria, which are another source of vitamin K. It has been recommended that breast-fed babies should receive 1 mg of phytonadione intramuscularly at birth.

Babies born to mothers who are receiving hydantoin anticonvulsants should also receive vitamin K as a prophylactic measure because phenytoin is an antagonist to vitamin K.

Healthy adults may acquire a deficiency of vitamin K as a result of dietary inadequacy or use of antibiotics that sterilize the intestinal tract. Debilitated patients acquire a deficiency of vitamin K much more quickly regardless of antibiotic usage. Patients who receive total parenteral nutrition via a subclavian vein may also suffer hemorrhage due to a deficiency of vitamin K. Fat-soluble vitamins, particularly vitamins D and K, are not metabolized normally when introduced into the central venous circulation. In such patients, it is advisable to give doses of 1 mg of phylloquinone per week to prevent deficiency of vitamin K.

An important source of vitamin K is intestinal bacteria. Vitamin K is not well absorbed from the colon. It appears that the microorganisms that synthesize vitamin K in the gut reside in the ileum. Sulfa drugs, neomycin and other broad-spectrum antibiotics are capable of sterilizing the intestinal tract. Therefore, it is not uncommon for patients who are receiving broad-spectrum antibiotics postoperatively to acquire a deficiency of vitamin K. Such patients should receive vitamin K as a prophylactic measure.

Treatment. Patients with a deficiency of vitamin K may be treated effectively with phytonadione. The usual oral dose of vitamin K_1, is 10–20 mg. Following administration, the abnormal clotting studies should be corrected in 6 to 12 hours. The dose should be repeated every 2 to 3 days until nutrition is improved. If the patient is unable to absorb vitamin K_1, it may be given either intramuscularly or intravenously in daily doses of 10 to 20 mg. Following intravenous administration the clotting defect should be corrected in 3 to 6 hours. If patients have severe vitamin K deficiency and hemorrhage, fresh frozen plasma should be administered.

Bibliography

Biochemical Aspects

Barkhan P, Shearer MJ: Metabolism of vitamin K in man. *Proc R Soc Med* 70:93–96, 1977.

Rodriquez-Erdmann F, Hoff JV, Carmody G: Interaction of antibodies with vitamin K. (Letter to the editor) *J Amer Med Ass* 246:937, 1981.

Clinical States with Vitamin K Deficiency

Bhanchet P, Karshemsant C: A bleeding syndrome in infants: Acquired prothrombin complex deficiency of unknown aetiology. *S Asian J Trop Med Public Health* 6:592–598, 1975.

Fujimara Y, Mimura Y, Kinoshita S, et al: Studies of vitamin K dependent factor deficiency during early childhood with special reference to prothrombin activity and antigen level. *Haemostasis* 11:90–95, 1982.

Goldman HI, Desposito F: Hypoprothrombinemic bleeding in young infants: Association with diarrhea, antibiotics and milk substitutes. *Amer J Dis Chil* 111:430–432, 1966.

Mann KG, Owen CA: Symposium on vitamin K. *Mayo Clin Proc* 49:911–944, 1974.

Nanmacher MA, Willemin M, Hartmann JR, et al: Vitamin K deficiency in infants beyond the neonatal period. *J Pediatr* 76:549–554, 1970.

Shearer MJ, Rahim S, Barkhan P, et al: Plasma vitamin K_1 mothers and their newborn babies. *Lancet* 2:460–463, 1982.

CASE
29

PATIENT: Term male infant

CHIEF COMPLAINT: This patient was the product of an uncomplicated pregnancy. On the day after delivery, circumcision was performed. Subsequently, oozing from the circumcision site was noted, and coagulation studies were ordered.

MEDICAL HISTORY: See above

FAMILY HISTORY: The infant had a sister (3 years of age) and a brother (2 years of age). Neither sibling had hemorrhagic problems, and the remaining family members had no history of bleeding abnormality.

DRUG HISTORY: Noncontributory

PHYSICAL EXAMINATION: Several large ecchymoses were noted over the scalp, and there was active oozing from the circumcision site.

Laboratory Results

A. Screening Procedures

	Patient	Normal
Prothrombin time	24 seconds	13–17 seconds (newborn infant)
APTT	90 seconds	<65 seconds (infant)
Platelet count	350,000/μl	130,000–400,000/μl
Bleeding time	Not performed	1–8 minutes

Questions

1. What additional laboratory procedures are indicated?
2. Is it necessary to have different values for the prothrombin time and the activated partial thromboplastin time (APTT) for newborn infants and children?
3. What is the differential diagnosis?
4. Does the absence of a family history of hemophilia rule out the possibility of deficiency of factor VIII or IX?

Laboratory Results

B. Confirmatory Procedures

	Patient	Normal
Factor VIII:C assay	100%	50% to 150%
Factor IX assay	8%	15% to 42% (term infant)
Factor VII assay	15%	40% to 72% (term infant)
Factor X assay	16%	40% to 72% (term infant)

DIAGNOSIS: Hemorrhagic disease of the newborn (deficiency of vitamin K)

Discussion

This case represents a fairly classical presentation of hemorrhagic disease of the newborn. The laboratory results highlight a major problem that is frequently encountered by laboratory technicians and clinicians who are unfamiliar with perinatal coagulation problems. Acceptable normal ranges for newborn infants and children are essential for making the diagnosis.

Levels of the vitamin K-dependent coagulation factors are uniformly decreased in fetuses and newborn infants. The levels of all four factors are decreased to 30% to 60% of normal adult levels at the time of delivery, and in the absence of vitamin K administration, the levels drop to approximately one-half of their initial levels by days 2 and 3 and then gradually increase over the next few days.

Prothrombin in small, preterm infants has approximately 30% activity, whereas it has approximately 52% activity in term infants. Coagulant activity reaches adult levels by 60 to 120 days. In term infants, factor X has a cord blood activity of approximately 55%; factor VII has an activity of approximately 41%. Results for factor IX activity have been variable, ranging from 14% to 55%. Factor IX activity reaches adult levels by the second to third month of age.

It should be recalled in the differential diagnosis of hemophilia that there is no family history of bleeding abnormality in approximately one-third of patients. Consequently, the medical history of this patient does not rule out the possibility of hemophilia A or B. Factor VIII activity and factor VIII-related antigen in term infants are within the normal adult ranges. Consequently, the finding of normal factor VIII activity in this patient would rule out the possibility of hemophilia A or von

HEMORRHAGIC DISEASE OF THE NEWBORN
(DEFICIENCY OF VITAMIN K)

CLINICAL PICTURE

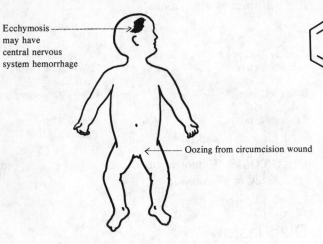

Ecchymosis may have central nervous system hemorrhage

Oozing from circumcision wound

Bleeding usually most evident on days 2 and 3

PHYSICAL PROPERTIES OF VITAMIN K

$$CH_2-C=C-CH_2-(CH_2-CH_2-CH_3-CH_2)_3H$$

Phylloquinone (vitamin K_1)

$$(CH_2-C=C-CH_2)_NH$$

Menaquinone-n (vitamin K_2)

LABORATORY FINDINGS

A. Screening Procedures

Test	Patient's Result	Normal Range
Prothrombin time	Abnormal	10–12 seconds
APTT	Abnormal	<42 seconds
Platelet count	Normal	130,000–400,000/μl
Bleeding time	Normal	1–8 minutes

B. Confirmatory Procedures

Factor VIII:C assay	100%	50 to 150%
Factor IX assay	Abnormal	15 to 42%
Factor VII assay	Abnormal	40 to 72%
Factor X assay	Abnormal	40 to 72%

TREATMENT

Vitamin K_1, 0.5 to 1 mg

Willebrand's disease. The parallel decreases in the levels of factors II, VII, IX and X would rule out hemophilia B as the cause of the clinical bleeding.

Biochemical Aspects. As has been previously discussed, vitamin K is necessary for carboxylation of glutamic acid residues in the vitamin K-dependent proteins: factors II, VII, IX and X. This carboxylation reaction results in the production of γ-carboxyglutamic acid, which is necessary for localization of vitamin K-dependent coagulation proteins to activated phospholipid surfaces, which are provided in vivo by stimulated platelets.

Hemorrhagic disease of the newborn is defined as a bleeding disorder in a newborn infant that is due to severe depression of the coagulant activity of factors II, VII, IX and X secondary to deficiency of vitamin K.

Clinical Picture. Hemorrhagic disease of the newborn is characterized by clinical bleeding in the first week of life. Usually, the second or third day of life is the time of onset of bleeding manifestations.

Breast-fed infants who do not receive vitamin K at birth have lower levels of vitamin K-dependent coagulation factors and a greater incidence of bleeding manifestations than do formula-fed infants and those who have received vitamin K as a prophylactic measure. Human milk contains approximately 1–2 μg of vitamin K per liter, whereas cow's milk contains 15 μg per liter. In addition, it has been found that the intestinal flora of breast-fed infants has a lower content of vitamin K_2-producing bacteria than does that of infants who are fed cow's milk.

All newborn infants should receive 0.5 to 1.0 mg of vitamin K_1 as soon after delivery as is possible. In addition, infants who have a complicating disease, such as chronic diarrhea, cystic fibrosis, biliary atresia or other causes of malabsorption, should receive supplemental vitamin K periodically. Such infants may be at risk for serious bleeding, such as intracranial hemorrhage. Another clinical situation that should be emphasized is use of anticonvulsant medications, such as barbiturates and phenytoin, by pregnant women. Infants whose mothers were taking anticonvulsant medications during pregnancy are at high risk for hemorrhagic disease of the newborn.

Infants whose mothers were taking oral anticoagulants during pregnancy also are vulnerable to neonatal hemorrhage, and death can result from intracranial hemorrhage in such cases. When possible, heparin should be used for anticoagulation during pregnancy. If sodium warfarin or coumarin is used, the drug should be stopped at least 3 to 4 weeks before delivery, and heparin therapy should be initiated. Because breast milk from women who are taking warfarin does not contain appreciable amounts of the drug, breast-feeding can be carried out safely.

Treatment. As has been noted above, all newborn infants should receive 0.5 to 1 mg of vitamin K_1 as soon after delivery as is possible. In patients with hemorrhagic disease of the newborn, the response of the prothrombin time to administration of vitamin K is striking. The prothrombin time often becomes normal in less than 12 hours.

Bibliography

(See Bibliography for Case 28)

CASE
30

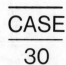

PATIENT: 41-year-old man

CHIEF COMPLAINT: This patient was admitted with a history of chronic alcoholism. At the time of admission, there were mental as well as physical signs of liver failure. Immediately before admission, there had been an episode of massive gastrointestinal bleeding.

MEDICAL HISTORY: The patient had been hospitalized on a number of occasions because of liver disease. He had a 20-year history of ethanol abuse.

FAMILY HISTORY: Noncontributory

DRUG HISTORY: The patient had taken folic acid, Mi-Cebrin (multivitamins with minerals), thiamine hydrochloride, pyridoxine hydrochloride, neomycin, lactulose, nafcillin, emperin, Librium (chlordiazepoxide hydrochloride) and Tylenol (acetaminophen).

PHYSICAL EXAMINATION: The patient was a jaundiced, disoriented man. He was febrile, with a temperature of 105°F. Apparently, the jaundice had begun approximately 3 weeks before admission. There was marked ascites and ankle edema, and numerous ecchymoses were noted over the abdomen and arms. The blood pressure was 100/50 mm Hg, and stools contained blood.

Laboratory Results

A. Screening Procedures

	Patient	Normal
Prothrombin time	19 seconds	10–12 seconds
APTT	52 seconds	<42 seconds
Platelet count	21,000/μl	130,000–400,000/μl
Bleeding time	10 minutes and 30 seconds	1–8 minutes

Questions

1. What laboratory procedures would be helpful in distinguishing liver disease from disseminated intravascular coagulation?
2. Is there more than one possible explanation for the marked thrombocytopenia?
3. Which coagulation factor is not produced in the liver?

Laboratory Results

B. Confirmatory Procedures

	Patient	Normal
Thrombin time	30 seconds	<24 seconds
Factor VIII:C activity	200%	50% to 150%
Fibrinogen (clottable)	150 mg/dl	170–410 mg/dl
Antithrombin III (activity)	33%	85% to 115%
Antithrombin III (immunologic)	8 mg/dl	23–40 mg/dl
Fibrin split products	>40 μg/ml	<10 μg/ml
Protamine sulfate	Positive	Negative

DIAGNOSIS: Alcoholic cirrhosis and liver failure (secondary to ethanol abuse)

Discussion

Abnormalities of hemostasis may arise in persons with liver disease as a result of several pathophysiologic processes, including failure of synthesis, defective hepatic clearance of activated coagulation factors, disseminated intravascular coagulation, abnormal fibrinolysis and qualitative and quantitative abnormalities of platelets.

Biochemical Aspects. The liver is the site of synthesis of all coagulation proteins except von Willebrand factor which is synthesized in megakaryocytes and endothelial cells. The exact site of synthesis of factor VIII:C is currently unknown, although evidence from the porcine model of von Willebrand's disease suggests that the liver is the site of synthesis of this component of the factor VIII complex. In addition, the liver is the site of synthesis of plasminogen and various physiologic inhibitors, such as antithrombin III and α_2-antiplasmin.

In the end stage of chronic liver disease, there often is a low plasma concentration of fibrinogen. By contrast, in uncomplicated cirrhosis, chronic hepatitis, obstructive jaundice, biliary cirrhosis and hepatoma, a high plasma level of fibrinogen is found. Despite its high concentration, fibrinogen may clot poorly. Thus, acquired dysfibrinogenemia is a fairly common complication in patients with liver disease. The abnormality of fibrinogen has been attributed to a high content of sialic acid or, perhaps, a defect of the A alpha chains.

Levels of other coagulation proteins may be variably decreased in liver disease. Members of the vitamin

ALCOHOLIC CIRRHOSIS AND LIVER FAILURE
(SECONDARY TO ETHANOL ABUSE)

CLINICAL PICTURE

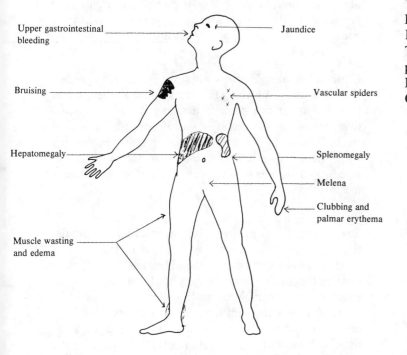

Upper gastrointestinal bleeding

Bruising

Hepatomegaly

Muscle wasting and edema

Jaundice

Vascular spiders

Splenomegaly

Melena

Clubbing and palmar erythema

PATHOPHYSIOLOGIC BASIS OF BLEEDING IN LIVER DISEASE

Decreased production of coagulation proteins
Decreased clearance of activated coagulation factors
Thrombocytopenia due to decreased production of platelets or increased sequestration by the spleen
Increased fibrinolysis
Qualitative abnormalities of platelets

LABORATORY FINDINGS

A. Screening Procedures

Test	Patient's Result	Normal Range
Prothrombin time	Abnormal	10–12 seconds
APTT	Abnormal	<42 seconds
Platelet count	Abnormal	130,000–400,000/μl
Bleeding time	Abnormal	1–8 minutes

B. Confirmatory Procedures

Thrombin time	Abnormal	< 24 seconds
Factor VIII:C activity	Normal	50% to 150%
Fibrin split products	Abnormal	<10 μg/ml

TREATMENT

Supportive care
Fresh-frozen plasma
Vitamin K if deficiency of vitamin K exists concomitantly
Platelet transfusions if indicated

K, or prothrombin, family are synthesized by hepatocytes in the same general way as other plasma glycoproteins are synthesized. The final carboxylation step occurs in microsomes of hepatocytes. In persons with liver failure, complete molecules are synthesized, whereas in those with obstructive jaundice, malabsorption of vitamin K may result in failure of the carboxylation step without abnormality of the synthesis of the precursor protein. In the latter instance, administration of vitamin K corrects the abnormalities of hemostasis. It should be remembered that factor VII has the shortest half-life of any coagulation protein. Therefore, patients with early liver disease may present with a minimally prolonged prothrombin time, and the remainder of the hemostatic evaluation is within normal limits.

It often is difficult to differentiate disseminated intravascular coagulation from liver failure. Patients with severe liver disease may show hypofibrinogenemia, elevated levels of fibrin split products, positive results on tests of paracoagulation and thrombocytopenia. Many clinicians use factor VIII coagulant activity as a means of differentiating primary liver disease from disseminated intravascular coagulation. In most instances, patients with disseminated intravascular coagulation have decreased factor VIII:C activity, whereas those with liver failure have normal or increased activity. However, it should be emphasized that this activity is not an absolute means for differentiating between the two situations. Presumably, a low degree of intravascular coagulation is common in patients with liver disease.

The clearance mechanisms of the liver are important in normal hemostasis. The liver plays a part in clearing fibrin split products and vascular plasminogen activator from the blood. In patients with severe liver disease, the half-life of the plasminogen activator is prolonged.

The fibrinolytic mechanism may also be abnormal in patients with liver disease. Because the liver is the site of synthesis of plasminogen, the level of plasminogen is decreased. The half-life of vascular plasminogen activator is prolonged, leading to accelerated consumption of plasminogen. In addition, α_2-antiplasmin, the primary inhibitor of plasmin, is synthesized in the liver and thus is also found at a decreased level in patients with severe liver disease.

Patients with liver disease often have thrombocytopenia and a prolonged bleeding time. The thrombocytopenia may be due to several mechanisms, including ineffective thrombopoiesis, which is frequently seen in patients who have ingested large quantities of alcohol. Also, in patients with long-standing liver disease and portal hypertension, there may be appreciable sequestration of platelets by an enlarged spleen. Patients with chronic liver disease frequently present with a platelet count of approximately 50,000 to 60,000/μl. Such a low count may be due primarily to sequestration, although decreased production and increased peripheral destruction of platelets cannot be ruled out. Patients who have recently ingested alcohol often show qualitative abnormalities of platelet function. Ultrastructural features include variation in size, disruption of microtubules, abnormal morphologic appearance of granules and vacuolation. Results of platelet aggregation studies are consistent with storage pool disease.

Clinical Picture. Patients with liver failure may present with bleeding from the gastrointestinal tract as well as from the upper respiratory tract. In patients with acute liver failure, the bleeding from the upper gastrointestinal tract is frequently due to superficial erosions. In patients with chronic liver disease, the most common site of bleeding is esophageal varices manifested by hematemesis or melena.

Treatment. In acute liver failure, replacement of deficient coagulation factors by infusion of fresh-frozen plasma may avert catastrophic bleeding. In addition, platelet transfusions may be helpful. It must be emphasized that prothrombin complex concentrates should be avoided in patients with liver failure because they have been reported to precipitate acute episodes of disseminated intravascular coagulation or thrombosis. Other measures, such as balloon tamponade of esophageal varices, may be indicated in a given patient.

Bibliography

Fletcher AP, Biederman O, Moore D, et al: Abnormal plasminogen-plasmin system activity (fibrinolysis) in patients with hepatic cirrhosis: Its causes and consequences. *J Clin Invest* 43:681–695, 1964.

Flute PT: Clotting abnormalities in liver disease. *Prog Liver Dis* 6:301–310, 1979.

Lane DA, Sully MF, Thomas DP, et al: Acquired dysfibrinogenemia in acute and chronic liver disease. *Brit J Haematol* 35:301–308, 1977.

Lechner K, Niessner H, Tholen E: Coagulation abnormalities in liver disease. *Semin Thromb Haemostasis* 4:40–56, 1977.

Ruiz F, Grainger SL, Hall RJC, et al: Relation of simple clotting tests to clotting factor levels in liver disease. *Clin Lab Haematol* 4:247–256, 1982.

Verstraete M, Vermylen J, Collen D: Intravascular coagulation in liver disease. *Annu Rev Med* 25:447–455, 1974.

CASE
31

PATIENT: 35-year-old man

CHIEF COMPLAINT: This patient was brought to the emergency room unconscious. He had been discovered in a boardinghouse where there had been a serious fire.

MEDICAL HISTORY: Not obtainable

FAMILY HISTORY: Not obtainable

DRUG HISTORY: Not obtainable

PHYSICAL EXAMINATION: Approximately 70% of the body surface area was covered by second- and third-degree burns. When blood was drawn, it was noticed that the venipuncture sites bled profusely.

Laboratory Results

A. Screening Procedures

	Patient	Normal
Prothrombin time	18 seconds	10–12 seconds
APTT	49 seconds	<42 seconds
Platelet count	27,000/μl	130,000–400,000/μl
Bleeding time	Not performed	1–8 minutes

Questions

1. What is the most likely diagnosis?
2. What additional laboratory procedures are needed to confirm the clinical impression?

Laboratory Results

B. Confirmatory Procedures

	Patient	Normal
Fibrinogen (clottable)	110 mg/dl	170–410 mg/dl
Antithrombin III (activity)	55%	85% to 115%
Fibrin split products	>40 μg/ml	<10 μg/ml
Protamine sulfate	Positive	Negative

Examination of a peripheral blood smear revealed marked anisocytosis and poikilocytosis of the red cells.

In addition, the platelet count was markedly decreased. The specimen also appeared to be hemolyzed.

DIAGNOSIS: Acute disseminated intravascular coagulation (due to massive burn injury)

Discussion

Disseminated intravascular coagulation is a common acquired coagulopathy that is seen with a number of underlying disease states. It is important to emphasize that disseminated intravascular coagulation is not a disease but, rather, a symptom of an underlying disease (Table 1).

Table 1
Classification of Clinical States Associated with Disseminated Intravascular Coagulation

Obstetric Complications
  Abruptio placentae
  Placenta previa
  Dead fetus
  Amniotic fluid infusion
  Placenta accreta
  Toxemia of pregnancy
  Cesarean section
  Abortion
  Hydatid mole
  Extrauterine pregnancy
  Forceps delivery
  Normal delivery
Tissue Trauma
  Major surgery (especially extracorporeal circulation)
  Severe trauma and burns
  Fat embolism
  Rejection of transplant
  Heatstroke
Hemolytic Processes
  Transfusion of mismatched blood
  Drowning
  Acute hemolysis secondary to infection

ACUTE DISSEMINATED INTRAVASCULAR COAGULATION (DUE TO MASSIVE BURN INJURY)

CLINICAL PICTURE

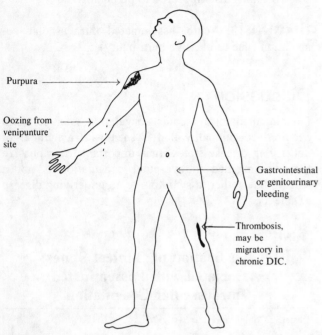

Purpura

Oozing from venipuncture site

Gastrointestinal or genitourinary bleeding

Thrombosis, may be migratory in chronic DIC.

Underlying disease often dominates clinical picture; multiple bleeding sites frequently encountered

PATHOPHYSIOLOGIC BASIS

Generation of thrombin and its consequences
Generation of plasmin and its consequences

LABORATORY FINDINGS

A. Screening Procedures

Test	Patient's Result	Normal Range
Prothrombin time	Abnormal	10–12 seconds
APTT	Abnormal	<42 seconds
Platelet count	Abnormal	130,000–400,000/µl
Bleeding time	Abnormal	1–8 minutes

B. Confirmatory Procedures

Test	Patient's Result	Normal Range
Thrombin time	Abnormal	<24 seconds
Antithrombin III, activity	Abnormal	85% to 115%
Fibrin split products	Abnormal	<10 µg/ml
Protamine sulfate	Present	Absent

TREATMENT

Manage underlying disease
Fresh-frozen plasma or cryoprecipitate
Platelet concentrates
Heparin (promyelocytic leukemia, purpura fulminans)

Table 1 (continued)

Immune mechanisms

Ingestion of acid and other causes

Neoplastic Diseases

Solid Tumor

Leukemia (Promyelocytic M-3, and Monocytic M-5)

Snakebites

Infections (especially acute forms)

Bacterial: gram negative, meningococcal and pneumococcal septicemia

Rickettsial: Rocky Mountain spotted fever

Viral: hemorrhagic smallpox and hemorrhagic fever (Thai, Korean and others)

Mycotic: acute histoplasmosis

Parasitic: malaria (blackwater fever)

Miscellaneous

Cirrhosis of the liver

Glomerulonephritis

Acute pancreatitis

Purpura fulminans

Thrombotic thrombocytopenic purpura

Hemolytic-uremic syndrome

Shock

Severe progressive stroke

Severe heart failure

Giant hemangioma (Kasabach-Merritt)

Large aortic Aneurysm

Disseminated intravascular coagulation occurs when there is generalized or diffuse activation of the coagulation mechanism in vivo, resulting in conversion of fibrinogen to fibrin. In many respects, the pathophysiologic features in vivo mimic the sequence of events that occurs in vitro when plasma is allowed to clot in a glass test tube. On the basis of this simple analogy, the consequences of generation of thrombin in vivo can be readily appreciated. After formation of a fibrin clot, there is also generation of plasmin, which lyses the fibrin clot. Thus, the pathophysiologic features can be understood by knowing the effects of the enzymes thrombin and plasmin on the various components of the coagulation system.

Disseminated intravascular coagulation may be initiated by several mechanisms. The most common mechanisms are escape of tissue substances into circulating blood, endothelial damage with exposure of components of vessel walls and stasis with acidosis and electrolyte imbalances. The findings in most clinical cases reflect generation of thrombin in the systemic circulation. Thrombin converts fibrinogen to fibrin and also promotes consumption of specific procoagulants,

prothrombin and factors V and VIII. In addition, there is an associated thrombocytopenia due to activation and consumption of platelets.

Although disseminated intravascular coagulation results in a consumptive coagulopathy, it should be realized that a consumptive coagulopathy may also occur secondary to a localized event. This phenomenon is best exemplified by the giant hemangioma syndrome (Kasabach-Merritt syndrome) in children and large dissecting aneurysms in adults. In these situations, there is local generation of thrombin, resulting in depletion of coagulation factors and circulating platelets. Also, it should be stressed that disseminated intravascular coagulation may have an abrupt or insidious onset, may be acute or chronic and may be compensated or decompensated, depending on the degree of consumption and utilization of the various procoagulants and platelets. When consumption exceeds synthesis or production of procoagulants and platelets, the plasma levels are reduced, thus leading to decompensated disseminated intravascular coagulation (Figure 1).

In this patient, the disseminated intravascular coagulation was due to massive burns, which resulted in endothelial damage, escape of tissue fluid into the circulation with electrolyte imbalance and shock. Thus, all three major mechanisms involved in the pathogenesis of disseminated intravascular coagulation are present in this patient.

PATHOPHYSIOLOGY OF DISSEMINATED INTRAVASCULAR COAGULATION

ACUTE

Synthesis   Consumption

CHRONIC

Synthesis   Consumption

Net Results:
Low levels of fibrinogen, factors V and VIII and platelets
High levels of fibrin split products

Net Results:
Normal or high levels of fibrinogen and factors V and VIII
Low or normal platelet count
High levels of fibrin split products (diagnostic)

Levels of Procoagulants

1. Related to half-lives and synthesis as well as consumption.
2. In chronic cases, levels may well be increased due to compensatory synthesis.
3. In acute cases, levels usually are decreased—but not always! (i.e., preceding chronic inflammation).
4. Thrombocytopenia is last abnormality to be corrected (may be only finding in chronic cases).
5. Half-lives of fibrin split products are approximately 9 to 12 hours (cleared by reticuloendothelial system).

Figure 1

Biochemical Aspects. Conversion of fibrinogen to fibrin is the final common pathway in all clinical entities that are associated with disseminated intravascular coagulation. Table 1 lists the clinical states that are frequently associated with disseminated intravascular coagulation. As has been noted above, the mechanisms that are involved in the initiation of coagulation in vivo are in many instances speculative. For example, the disseminated intravascular coagulation that is seen in association with gram-negative septicemia has several possible mechanisms of initiation. Endotoxin or the formation of immune complexes may participate in direct activation of the intrinsic system via factor XII or through platelet injury or, alternatively, through endothelial injury with exposure of elements of vessel walls. In most cases, however, it appears that disseminated intravascular coagulation is initiated through the extrinsic system by release of thromboplastic material from injured cells (e.g., monocytes) or tissues.

Thrombin is generated in all cases of disseminated intravascular coagulation. The effects of thrombin on circulating blood are used to diagnose this disorder. Thrombin converts fibrinogen to fibrin, generating two peptides: fibrinopeptides A and B. Specific radioimmunoassays for these two peptides have been described. Also, a commercially available enzyme-linked immunosorbent assay for fibrinopeptide A has recently become available. Although the assays for fibrinopeptides are specific for in vivo generation of thrombin, their technical difficulty has prevented application in routine practice.

Fibrin monomer is also produced as a result of thrombin's action on fibrinogen. Fibrin monomer may polymerize and form an insoluble fibrin clot in the presence of activated factor XIII. Thrombin also activates factor XIII (Table 2). In addition to forming an insoluble fibrin clot, fibrin monomers may form soluble

Table 2
Effects of Thrombin

Coagulation Mechanism

  Degradation of factors V and VIII

  Activation of protein C

  Conversion of fibrinogen to fibrin monomer with generation fibrinopeptides A and B

  Activation of factor XIII

Platelets

  Irreversible aggregation

  Release reaction

Fibrinolysis

  Indirect activation of fibrinolysis

Inhibitors

  Consumption of Antithrombin III with formation of ATIII-Thrombin complexes

DIGESTION OF FIBRINOGEN BY PLASMIN

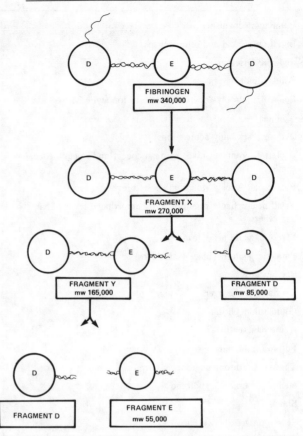

Figure 2. The prerequisite for activation of plasminogen is cleavage of a single arginine-valine bond that links the A and B chains. This cleavage is mediated by urokinase or other plasminogen activators (2 in the figure indicates this site). In addition to this cleavage, the A chain is involved in a second series of reactions; the amino-terminal end is further cleaved at the bonds between Lys-62 and Ser-63 and between Arg-67 and Met-68 and subsequently at the bond between Lys-66 and Lys-77, yielding fragments with a total molecular weight of between 4000 and 7000 (preactivation peptides). The order of bond cleavage is still a matter of controversy. Removal of the preactivation peptides may be mediated by urokinase or through plasmin autodigestion.

complexes with fibrinogen or other fibrin monomers. Such soluble fibrin complexes have been used to detect generation of thrombin in vivo. Fibrin monomers may also form complexes with fibrin split products.

Several techniques have been used for the laboratory detection of fibrin monomer complexes; the techniques include protamine sulfate gelation, ethanol gelation and a ristocetin test. The protamine sulfate test is inexpensive, rapid and technically simple. Protamine sulfate has a specific action on soluble fibrin, causing fibrin monomers to initiate a process of "paracoagulation," with formation of visible fibrin strands. This procedure is relatively simple; however, it is necessary to use a standardized protamine sulfate reagent. More importantly, visualization of strands represents the only acceptable criterion for a positive test result. False-positive results may be due to turbidity, granularity or granular precipitates. Storage of plasma at cold temperature can lead to false results, as can contamination by thrombin, which results from poor venipuncture technique. Unexplained positive test results occur in about 10% of patients with liver disease and occasionally in late pregnancy.

Formation of plasmin is a necessary part of a normal physiologic response to formation of fibrin. Fibrin, fibrinogen or fibrin monomer may then be lysed by plasmin. The fibrin (or fibrinogen) split products are referred to as fragments X, Y, D and E. The sequential degradation of fibrin is illustrated in Figure 2.

The best diagnostic evidence of disseminated intravascular coagulation is the demonstration of high serum levels of fibrin split products. Mild elevations occur in many clinical situations; however, marked elevations are virtually pathognomonic of disseminated intravascular coagulation. The original test used to detect fibrin split products was the tanned red cell hemagglutination inhibition test. More recently, a simpler test, the latex agglutination test, has been introduced. In this test, latex particles coated with antibodies to fragments D and E or antibodies to fibrinogen are exposed to a patient's serum. Agglutination of the latex particles is considered a positive test result. False-positive results may occur in patients with rheumatoid arthritis. Another test that has been used to identify fibrin split products is the staphylococcal clumping test, which is sensitive to early fibrin split products (fragments X and Y).

For many years, measurement of fibrinogen has been a standard procedure in the laboratory evaluation of patients who are suspected of having disseminated intravascular coagulation. The hypofibrinogenemia in such patients results from generation of thrombin with consumption of fibrinogen as well as from generation of plasmin with degradation of fibrinogen. There are certain pitfalls relating to the laboratory measurement of fibrinogen. Results are often affected by improper collection of a blood sample. Poor technique for venipuncture, storage and transportation of blood samples may produce spurious results. For instance, a small degree of contamination by heparin in a blood sample may result in an apparent hypofibrinogenemia when the sample is analyzed for fibrinogen. Heparin inhibits the thrombin-fibrinogen reaction, which is used to quantify fibrinogen. Heparin may contaminate the sample in several ways. Occasionally, coagulation samples are drawn immediately after samples are obtained for blood gas analysis. If a syringe that has been used for administration of heparin is used to make an arterial puncture to obtain samples for blood gas analysis, a small amount of heparin in the hub of the needle may contaminate the coagulation samples. Also, frequently, errors are introduced when blood samples are drawn through indwelling vascular catheters. The unknown presence of heparin in collected blood samples may, in fact, account for more cases of pseudo-disseminated intravascular coagulation (DIC) than true DIC.

In addition to improper sample collection, there are other uncertainties surrounding the quantification of fibrinogen. Although most patients with disseminated intravascular coagulation have a decreased level of fibrinogen, the level may at times fall within the normal range. Fibrinogen is an acute-phase protein; consequently, with certain underlying disease states, such as malignant disease, patients may present with an abnormally high level of fibrinogen as a baseline. Therefore, unless a decline in fibrinogen is "caught," it may be difficult to identify consumption of fibrinogen with accuracy; thus, reliance on the fibrinogen level as the primary diagnostic sign of disseminated intravascular coagulation is not recommended. As has been noted previously, measurement of the levels of fibrin split products is a much more accurate laboratory means of establishing the diagnosis.

Antithrombin III, the major physiologic inhibitor of coagulation, may also be consumed in patients with disseminated intravascular coagulation. Antithrombin III inactivates thrombin and other serine proteases through the formation of a tight stoichiometric complex that possesses neither enzyme nor inhibitor activity. A decrease in the circulating level of antithrombin III may indicate disseminated intravascular coagulation in an early stage of evolution.

In addition, plasma levels of prekallikrein and kallikrein inhibitors and plasminogen and plasmin inhibitors may also be decreased in patients with disseminated intravascular coagulation. Recent studies have demonstrated that the level of fibronectin is appreciably reduced in patients with this disorder. Fibronectin had previously been demonstrated to be associated with circulating soluble fibrin or fibrinogen complexes. It is also incorporated covalently into cross-linked fibrin. Consumption of fibronectin in acute disseminated intravascular coagulation is thought to be dependent on adsorption of fibronectin to circulating particulate matter and removal by the reticuloendothelial system.

Clinical Picture. Patients with disseminated intravascular coagulation usually present with bleeding at more than a single site. Bleeding may take the form of purpura of the skin and mucous membranes, oozing from cutdown and venipuncture sites or bleeding from the genitourinary tract and/or gastrointestinal tract. In many cases, the clinical picture is dominated by the underlying disease. Thus, patients with promyelocytic leukemia may present with severe anemia and infection in addition to evidence of disseminated intravascular coagulation.

Treatment. The only truly effective approach for the management of disseminated intravascular coagulation is elimination of the underlying disease in concert with therapy for associated conditions, such as shock. In some instances, however, management of the underlying disease does not effectively limit the bleeding or thrombosis. In cases in which bleeding is the primary clinical problem, replacement of coagulation factors and/or platelets is indicated. Platelet concentrates, fresh-frozen plasma or cryoprecipitate may be used. Subsequent replacement is determined by the half-life of the factors and platelets.

In some instances, it may be necessary to institute anticoagulant therapy. Heparin is the treatment of choice. Heparin should be given as a continuous intravenous infusion that can be interrupted promptly if bleeding is accentuated. An initial dose of 50 to 100 units per kilogram of body weight with a maintenance dosage of 10 to 15 units per kilogram per hour is usually sufficient. The dosage should be reduced by 25% to 50% in patients with marked thrombocytopenia.

There have been few controlled studies on the use of heparin in disseminated intravascular coagulation. It appears that heparin has been helpful in patients with acute promyelocytic leukemia, giant hemangioma syndrome, purpura fulminans and LaVeen shunts; premature and dysmature infants may also receive some benefit from infusion of heparin. In acute promyelocytic leukemia and purpura fulminans, heparin is strongly recommended. Heparin has not been effective in patients with bacterial septicemia and shock. In addition, it seems to have little effect in patients in whom disseminated intravascular coagulation is complicating liver disease, pregnancy or snakebites. In cases that are associated with snakebites, antivenom is the treatment of choice.

Another effect of transfusion with fresh-frozen plasma or cryoprecipitate may be worthy of mention. It has recently been suggested that fibronectin, an opsonic glycoprotein, might be useful in patients with septicemia, posttraumatic shock or severe burns. Several studies have indicated a positive response in such patients when disseminated intravascular coagulation has been a complicating feature. Theoretically, restoration of the fibronectin level to normal may improve the capacity of phagocytic cells to remove circulating fibrin complexes and platelet aggregates, thereby decreasing the likelihood of microcirculatory thrombosis.

ε-Aminocaproic acid, a fibrinolytic enzyme inhibitor, has little if any role in the management of disseminated intravascular coagulation.

Bibliography

Clinical Picture and Pathophysiologic Basis

Beard MEJ, Hickton CM: Haemostasis in heat stroke. *Brit J Haematol* 52:269–274, 1982.

Cornfield DB, Rossman RE: Diethylstilbestrol-diphosphate induced disseminated intravascular coagulation in prostatic carcinoma. *South Med J* 75:248–249, 1982.

Gralnick HR, Marchesi S, Givelber H: Intravascular coagulation in acute leukemia: Clinical and subclinical abnormalities. *Blood* 40:709–718, 1972.

Miner ME, Graham SH, Gildenberg PL: Disseminated intravascular coagulation fibrinolytic syndrome following head injury in children: Frequency and prognostic implications. *J Pediatr* 100:687–691, 1982.

Muller-Berghaus G: Pathophysiology of generalized intravascular coagulation. *Semin Thromb Hemostasis* 3:209–246, 1977.

Diagnosis

Bick RL, Dukes ML, Wilson WL, et al: Antithrombin III (AT III) as a diagnostic aid in disseminated intravascular coagulation. *Thromb Res* 10:721–729, 1977.

McDuffie FC, Giffin C, Miedringhaus R, et al: Prothrombin, thrombin and prothrombin fragments in plasma of normal individuals and of patients with laboratory evidence of disseminated intravascular coagulation. *Thromb Res* 16:759–773, 1979.

Mertens BF: Fibrinolytic split products (FSP) and ethanol gelation test in preoperative evaluation of patients with prostatic disease. *Mayo Clin Proc* 49:642–649, 1974.

Sandler RM, Liebman HA, Patch MJ, et al: Antithrombin III and anti-activated factor X activity in patients with acute promyelocytic leukemia and disseminated intravascular coagulation treated with heparin. *Cancer* 50:2106–2110, 1982.

Seaman A: The recognition of intravascular clotting. *Arch Intern Med* 125:1016–1021, 1970.

Whitaker AN, Rowe EA, Masci PP, et al: Identification of D-dimer-E complex in disseminated intravascular coagulation. *Thromb Res* 18:453–459, 1980.

Treatment

Feinstein DI: Diagnosis and management of disseminated intravascular coagulation: The role of heparin therapy. *Blood* 60:284–287, 1982.

Heene DL: Disseminated intravascular coagulation: Evaluation of therapeutic approaches. *Semin Thromb Haemostasis* 3:291–317, 1977.

Review Articles

Cash JD: Disseminated intravascular coagulation. In Poller L (ed): *Recent Advances in Blood Coagulation* (2nd edition). Edinburgh: Churchill Livingstone, 1981, pp 293–311.

Colman RW, Robboy SJ, Minna JD: Disseminated intravascular coagulation (DIC), an approach. *Amer J Med* 52:679–689, 1972.

Deykin D: The clinical challenge of disseminated intravascular coagulation. *N Engl J Med* 283:636–644, 1970.

Hamilton PJ, Stalker AJ, Douglas AS: Disseminated intravascular coagulation: A review. *J Clin Pathol* 31:609–613, 1978.

Merskey C, Johnson AJ, Kleiner GJ, et al: The defibrination syndrome, clinical features, and laboratory diagnosis. *Brit J Haematol* 13:528–549, 1967.

CASE
32

PATIENT: 23-year-old woman

CHIEF COMPLAINT: This patient was admitted to the hospital in the ninth month of gestation. The patient's pregnancy had been uneventful, although she had missed several clinic appointments during the last trimester. At the time of admission, she was found to be hypertensive, with a blood pressure of 180/100 mm Hg, and 4+ proteinuria was noted on urinalysis.

MEDICAL HISTORY: This pregnancy was the patient's first.

FAMILY HISTORY: Noncontributory

DRUG HISTORY: The patient had taken Darvon (propoxyphene hydrochloride) and Vistaril (hydroxyzine).

PHYSICAL EXAMINATION: There was a trace of pitting edema of the legs. Fetal heart tones were satisfactory.

Laboratory Results

A. Screening Procedures

	Patient	Normal
Prothrombin time	11 seconds	10–12 seconds
APTT	31.5 seconds	<42 seconds
Platelet count	28,500/μl	130,000–400,000/μl
Bleeding time	8 minutes and 30 seconds	1–8 minutes

Questions

1. What is the primary diagnosis in this case?
2. What is the most likely mechanism for the thrombocytopenia?
3. What additional laboratory procedures are indicated?
4. How should this patient be treated?

Laboratory Results

B. Confirmatory Procedures

	Patient	Normal
Fibrinogen (clottable)	200 mg/dl	170–410 mg/dl
Antithrombin III (activity)	60%	85% to 115%
Fibrin split products	>40 μg/ml	<10 μg/ml
Protamine sulfate	Positive	Negative

Examination of a peripheral blood smear revealed a few microspherocytes, helmet cells and schistocytes. Most of the platelets were large.

DIAGNOSIS: Disseminated intravascular coagulation complicating preeclampsia

Discussion

This case is an example of disseminated intravascular coagulation complicating a clinical picture of preeclampsia. In patients with preeclampsia, a decrease in the platelet count is a common finding, as are elevations in the serum levels of fibrin split products and other laboratory test results that are indicative of disseminated intravascular coagulation. It has been emphasized that a decrease in the platelet count is one of the first findings in patients with preeclampsia. In fact, the platelet count decreases before the serum levels of fibrin split products increase.

The levels of fibrin split products are usually elevated in patients with preeclampsia. In patients who progress to eclampsia, further increases in the levels of fibrin split products usually occur 24 to 48 hours after eclamptic fits.

Other laboratory changes that are typically seen in patients with preeclampsia include an elevation in the level of circulating soluble fibrin-fibrinogen complexes and decreases in the levels of plasminogen, fibrinogen, antithrombin III and α_2-antiplasmin.

The treatment of choice is delivery of the fetus after the blood pressure is controlled if the hypertension is marked. Recently, antithrombin III concentrates have been used in patients with preeclampsia in an attempt to control the intravascular coagulation.

Bibliography

Bonnar J, McNichol GP, Douglas AS: Coagulation and fibrinolytic systems in pre-eclampsia and eclampsia. *Brit Med J* 2:12–18, 1971.

DISSEMINATED INTRAVASCULAR COAGULATION COMPLICATING PREECLAMPSIA

CLINICAL PICTURE

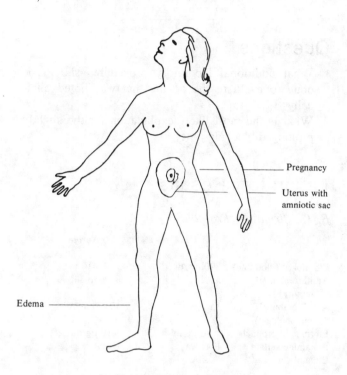

Pregnancy

Uterus with amniotic sac

Edema

Hypertension and proteinuria

PATHOPHYSIOLOGIC BASIS OF DISSEMINATED INTRAVASCULAR COAGULATION

Generation of thrombin and its consequences
Generation of plasmin and its consequences
Underlying disease state and time course of disease

LABORATORY FINDINGS

A. Screening Procedures

Test	Patient's Result	Normal Range
Prothrombin time	Normal	10–12 seconds
APTT	Normal	<42 seconds
Platelet count	Abnormal	130,000–400,000/μl
Bleeding time	Normal	1–8 minutes

B. Confirmatory Procedures

Fibrinogen (clottable)	Normal	170–410 mg/ml
Antithrombin III (activity)	Abnormal	85–115%
Fibrin split products	Abnormal	<10 μg/ml
Protamine sulfate	Abnormal	Negative

TREATMENT

Control hypertension
Deliver fetus
Antithrombin III concentrates have been used in Europe

CASE

33

PATIENT: 62-year-old woman

CHIEF COMPLAINT: This patient was admitted with severe gastrointestinal bleeding of recent onset.

MEDICAL HISTORY: The patient's medical history was complex. She had undergone two breast biopsies for fibrocystic disease with no postoperative complications. In addition, she had undergone a surgical procedure for hemorrhoids, and approximately 2 years before admission, she had undergone aortocoronary artery bypass for coronary artery disease.

FAMILY HISTORY: There was no family history of bleeding problems. There was a history of atherosclerotic heart disease on the maternal and paternal sides of the family.

DRUG HISTORY: The patient had recently taken aspirin on a daily basis for cramping abdominal pain that had preceded the onset of the gastrointestinal bleeding. In addition, she had taken Casyllium for the past 27 years.

PHYSICAL EXAMINATION: The patient was a somewhat obese woman. A number of ecchymotic and purpuric areas were noted over the arms and legs. Auscultation of the heart was unremarkable, and no mass was palpable in the abdomen.

Laboratory Results

A. Screening Procedures

	Patient	Normal
Prothrombin time	11 seconds	10–12 seconds
APTT	28.5 seconds	<42 seconds
Platelet count	90,000/μl	130,000–400,000/μl
Bleeding time	9 minutes and 20 seconds	1–8 minutes

HOSPITAL COURSE: After admission, upper and lower gastrointestinal series were performed. A fungating mass was noted in the rectosigmoid colon; biopsy demonstrated the mass to be a mucin-secreting, well-differentiated adenocarcinoma. An admitting chemistry profile showed elevated levels of alkaline phosphatase and lactate dehydrogenase. Before surgical intervention took place, oozing from venipuncture sites was noted, and additional purpuric areas had appeared over the arms.

Questions

1. What additional laboratory procedures should be done to evaluate the oozing that was noted clinically?
2. What is the most likely explanation for the slightly prolonged bleeding time?

Laboratory Results

B. Confirmatory Procedures

	Patient	Normal
Fibrinogen (clottable)	200 mg/dl	170–410 mg/dl
Antithrombin III (activity)	50%	85% to 115%
Antithrombin III (immunologic)	15 mg/dl	17–30 mg/dl
Fibrin split products	>40 μg/ml	<10 μg/ml
Protamine sulfate	Positive	Negative
Ethanol gel	Positive	Negative

DIAGNOSIS: Chronic disseminated intravascular coagulation (secondary to metastatic adenocarcinoma)

Discussion

At operation, disseminated adenocarcinoma was found in the mesenteric lymph nodes, pericolonic lymph nodes and liver. The laboratory findings and clinical picture are consistent with a diagnosis of chronic disseminated intravascular coagulation. However, the laboratory findings also are consistent with partial compensation of the consumptive coagulopathy. The prothrombin time and activated partial thromboplastin time (APTT) were within normal limits. Also, the fibrinogen level was near the lower limit of the normal range. The most important laboratory evidence in support of a diagnosis of disseminated intravascular coagulation was the finding of elevated levels of fibrin split products. Also, the slightly decreased platelet count was helpful in establishing the diagnosis.

CHRONIC DISSEMINATED INTRAVASCULAR COAGULATION (SECONDARY TO METASTATIC ADENOCARCINOMA)

CLINICAL PICTURE

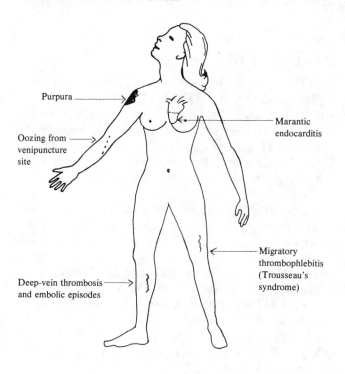

Purpura

Oozing from venipuncture site

Marantic endocarditis

Migratory thrombophlebitis (Trousseau's syndrome)

Deep-vein thrombosis and embolic episodes

PATHOPHYSIOLOGIC BASIS

Activity in mucin that directly activates factor X
Tissue factor activity of malignant cells
Vitamin K-dependent cancer cell procoagulant
Cysteine protease (activates factor X)

LABORATORY FINDINGS

A. Screening Procedures

Test	Patient's Result	Normal Range
Prothrombin time	Normal	10–12 seconds
APTT	Normal	<42 seconds
Platelet count	Variable	130,000–400,000/μl
Bleeding time	Normal	1–8 minutes

B. Confirmatory Procedures

Test	Patient's Result	Normal Range
Fibrinogen (clottable)	Normal or abnormal	170–410 mg/dl
Antithrombin III activity	Abnormal	85% to 115%
Fibrin split products	Abnormal	<10 μg/ml
Protamine sulfate	Abnormal	Negative

TREATMENT

Manage underlying malignant disease
Anticoagulate with heparin, followed by oral anticoagulants if patient has thrombotic complications

Pathophysiologic Basis. Disseminated intravascular coagulation has been reported in association with a number of malignant lesions, including carcinoma of the lungs, breasts, pancreas and colon. Patients with malignant neoplasms are however, unique among patients who have disseminated intravascular coagulation. The hemorrhagic tendency often is mild and associated with laboratory findings of chronic disseminated intravascular coagulation. Concomitant vascular thrombosis frequently is seen in association with the clinical bleeding.

In chronic disseminated intravascular coagulation, the prothrombin time and APTT are often within normal limits and, in fact, the fibrinogen level may also be normal. It should be emphasized that an apparently "normal" level of fibrinogen in the setting of disseminated malignant disease may reflect appreciable consumption of fibrinogen in vivo. Patients with underlying disseminated malignant disease often have a markedly elevated level of fibrinogen as a baseline. Consequently, with the onset of underlying chronic disseminated intravascular coagulation, even thought there is appreciable consumption of fibrinogen, patients may initially present with the clinical picture of chronic disseminated intravascular coagulation and a normal level of fibrinogen; however, a normal level of fibrinogen is *not* a normal finding in such a clinical setting.

Perhaps the most helpful finding in establishing a diagnosis of chronic disseminated intravascular coagulation is elevated levels of fibrin split products. The platelet count often is slightly decreased as well. In this patient, the platelet count was decreased and the bleeding time was slightly prolonged. The slight lengthening of the bleeding time was most likely due to the recent ingestion of aspirin.

Clinical Picture. Patients with chronic disseminated intravascular coagulation often present with a picture of a mild hemorrhagic tendency. In approximately one-fourth of patients, there may also be evidence of thromboembolic disease. Marantic endocarditis may also be evident in such patients.

In some patients with underlying malignant disease, there may be a migratory thrombophlebitis (Trousseau's syndrome). The basis of the underlying thrombosis in such patients is thought to be a factor X-activating substance that has been identified in mucin-secreting adenocarcinomas.

Treatment. Treatment is usually directed toward the underlying malignant disease. In patients with thrombotic complications, heparin therapy, followed by oral anticoagulants, is indicated.

Bibliography

Caprini JA, Sener SF: Altered coagulability in cancer patients. *Ca J Clinic* 32:162–172, 1982.

Delaini F, Colucci M, DeBellis Vitti G, et al: Cancer cell procoagulant: A novel vitamin K dependent activity. *Thromb Res* 24:263–266, 1981.

Donati MB, Davidson JF, Garattini S: *Malignancy and the Hemostatic System*. New York: Review Press, 1981.

Edwards RL, Rickles FR: Abnormalities of blood coagulation in patients with cancer: Mononuclear cell tissue factor generation. *J Lab Clin Med* 98:917–928, 1981.

Garg S, Niemetz J: Tissue factor activity of normal and leukemic cells. *Blood* 42:729–735, 1973.

Gordon SC, Cross BA: A factor X activating cysteine protease from malignant tissue. *J Clin Invest* 67:1665–1671, 1981.

O'Meara RAQ: Coagulative properties of cancer. *Ir J Med Sci* 394:474, 1958.

Owen CA, Oeles HC, Bowie EJW, et al: Chronic intravascular coagulation (ICF) syndrome. (Abstract) *Thromb Diath Haemorrh* 36(Suppl 30):197–213, 1969.

Sack G, Levin J, Bell WR: Trousseau's syndrome and other manifestations of chronic disseminated coagulation in patients with neoplasia: Clinical, pathophysiologic and therapeutic features. *Medicine (Baltimore)* 56:1–9, 1977.

Sakuragawa N, Takahashi K, Hoshiyama M, et al: The extract from the tissue of gastric cancer as procoagulant in disseminated intravascular coagulation syndrome. *Thromb Res* 10:457–462, 1977.

CASE
34

PATIENT: 30-year-old man

CHIEF COMPLAINT: This patient was in good health until 1 day before admission, when pain and swelling developed in his left elbow.

MEDICAL HISTORY: Noncontributory

FAMILY HISTORY: There was a history of diabetes mellitus on the maternal and paternal sides of the family.

DRUG HISTORY: The patient had taken several aspirin tablets during the 24 hours preceding admission.

PHYSICAL EXAMINATION: The patient was a febrile, acutely ill young man. There was no palpable lymphadenopathy or hepatosplenomegaly. Several ecchymotic areas were noted over the arms.

Laboratory Results

	Patient	Normal
Hemoglobin level	12 g/dl	14–18 g/dl
White cell count	39 × 10⁹/liter	4.8–10.8 × 10⁹/liter

A. Screening Procedures

	Patient	Normal
Prothrombin time	14.6 seconds	10–12 seconds
APTT	78.8 seconds	<42 seconds
Platelet count	63,000/μl	130,000–400,000/μl
Bleeding time	10 minutes and 30 seconds	1–8 minutes

Examination of a peripheral blood smear revealed that immature cells accounted for approximately 50% of the white cell population. These cells had nuclear features that wre reniform and cytoplasm that lacked distinct granulation. Special staining tests were performed, including Sudan black B and peroxidase, both of which yielded positive results. Staining with alphanaphthol butyrate gave negative results. A bone marrow aspirate and biopsy sample was subsequently obtained, and the sample showed replacement of normal cells by immature cells similar to those seen in the peripheral smear.

Questions

1. On the basis of the cytochemical findings, what type of leukemia does the patient most likely have?
2. Do the coagulation values influence or contribute to the diagnosis and classification of the leukemia?
3. What additional laboratory procedures should be done to further evaluate the coagulation defect?

Laboratory Results

B. Confirmatory Procedures

	Patient	Normal
Antithrombin III (activity)	50%	85% to 115%
Antithrombin III (immunologic)	18 mg/dl	23–40 mg/dl
Fibrin split products	>40 μg/ml	<10 μg/ml
Protamine sulfate	Positive	Negative

DIAGNOSIS: Disseminated intravascular coagulation complicating acute promyelocytic leukemia (M-3, hypogranular variant)

Discussion

Examination of the peripheral blood smear and bone marrow sample suggested the possibility of hypogranular, acute nonlymphocytic leukemia (M-3) or monocytic leukemia (M-5). The nuclear features of these two types of leukemia cells may be confusing; consequently, it is necessary to perform special staining studies to establish the diagnosis. In this case, special staining techniques were performed; positive results were obtained with Sudan black B and peroxidase, and negative results were obtained with alphanaphthol butyrate. The strongly positive peroxidase and Sudan black B test results are suggestive of granulocytic leukemia. Auer bodies were identified when peroxidase stain was used.

Chromosomal studies revealed a translocation of a fragment of chromosome 17 to chromosome 15. (15q+, 17q−) This specific chromosomal abnormality is seen in approximately 69% of patients with acute promyelocytic leukemia.

Disseminated intravascular coagulation complicates promyelocytic leukemia more frequently than it complicates other forms of acute myelogenous leukemia. Patients with acute promyelocytic leukemia tend to be

DISSEMINATED INTRAVASCULAR COAGULATION COMPLICATING ACUTE PROMYELOCYTIC LEUKEMIA (M-3, HYPOGRANULAR VARIANT)

CLINICAL PICTURE

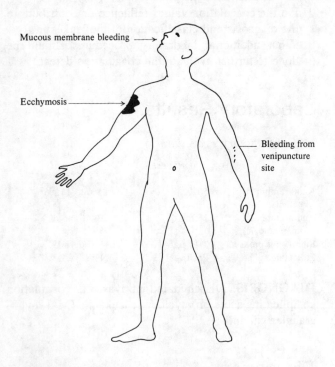

Mucous membrane bleeding

Ecchymosis

Bleeding from venipuncture site

PATHOPHYSIOLOGIC BASIS

Granules in promyelocytes contain a thromboplastin substance

LABORATORY FINDINGS

A. Screening Procedures

Test	Patient's Result	Normal Range
Prothrombin time	Abnormal	10–12 seconds
APTT	Abnormal	<42 seconds
Platelet count	Abnormal	130,000–400,000/μl
Bleeding time	Abnormal	1–8 minutes

B. Confirmatory Procedures

Antithrombin III, activity	Abnormal	85% to 115%
Fibrin split products	Abnormal	<10 μg/ml
Protamine sulfate	Abnormal	Negative

TREATMENT

Institute heparin therapy before starting chemotherapy
Chemotherapy for leukemia
Supportive care (i.e., platelet transfusions)

younger and have a lower white cell count and platelet count and less organ infiltration than do patients with other forms of acute myelogenous leukemia.

The patient was hydrated and placed on Zyloprim (allopurinol) and also given heparin before chemotherapy was instituted. Chemotherapy consisted of Adriamycin (doxorubicin hydrochloride) and cytarabine. During the patient's hospital course, bleeding developed from the oral cavity and gastrointestinal tract, and complete remission was not attained. The patient died after several weeks of hospitalization.

An important aspect of this case was the recognition that the morphologic features of the cells were consistent with a hypogranular promyelocytic leukemia. In contrast to typical M-3 leukemia, the hypogranular forms usually present with a slightly higher white cell count. It is important in treating any patient with the promyelocytic variant of acute myelogenous leukemia to make the correct diagnosis and to institute heparin therapy before starting chemotherapy.

The pathophysiologic basis of the disseminated intravascular coagulation that is seen in association with acute promyelogenous leukemia is thought to be release of a thromboplastin-like substance from granules in the cytoplasm of the promyelocytes.

The other acute myelogenous leukemia that is frequently associated with disseminated intravascular coagulation is M-5, or acute monocytic, leukemia. The pathophysiologic basis of the disseminated intravascular coagulation that complicates M-5 leukemia may be related to two recent observations. It appears that monocytes can express tissue factor activity, which may be a property of their membranes, and, in addition, recent evidence has suggested that monocytes possess factor VII activity.

Bibliography

Gralnick HR, Abrell E: Studies of the procoagulant and fibrinolytic activity of promyelocytes in acute promyelocytic leukemia. *Brit J Haematol* 24:89–99, 1973.

CASE
35

PATIENT: 55-year-old woman

CHIEF COMPLAINT: This patient was admitted because of intractable chest pain. The pain had often been associated with the anxiety that the patient experienced during renal dialysis.

MEDICAL HISTORY: The patient had experienced progressive renal failure over the preceding 3 years. The exact nature of the renal disease had not been established. She had been on renal dialysis for approximately 2 years and had arteriovenous fistulas in both arms.

FAMILY HISTORY: There was a history of diabetes mellitus on the paternal and maternal sides of the family.

DRUG HISTORY: The patient had taken Lanoxin (digoxin), Capoten (Captopril), digoxin, Natabec (multivitamins with minerals), Colace (docusate sodium), Valium (diazepam), cimetidine and nitroglycerin.

PHYSICAL EXAMINATION: The patient appeared slightly cachectic. There was a suggestion of hyperpigmentation, and numerous ecchymotic areas were noted over the arms and trunk. There was no palpable organomegaly.

Laboratory Results

A. Screening Procedures

	Patient	Normal
Prothrombin time	10.7 seconds	10–12 seconds
APTT	21 seconds	<42 seconds
Platelet count	159,000/μl	130,000–400,000/μl
Bleeding time*	>15 minutes	1–8 minutes

°The bleeding time was performed on the right leg because there were arteriovenous, fistulas in both arms.

Hemoglobin level	8 g/dl	12–16 g/dl
Blood urea nitrogen	60 mg/dl	7–18 mg/dl
Creatinine	6.0 mg/dl	0.5–1.1 mg/dl
Hematocrit	25%	36% to 46%

HOSPITAL COURSE: The above tests were obtained prior to undergoing a coronary artery bypass procedure.

Questions

1. Is the prolonged bleeding time related to the underlying renal disease?
2. Is hemorrhage a significant potential complication in this patient?
3. What forms of therapy should this patient receive?

Laboratory Results

B. Confirmatory Procedures

	Patient	Normal
Platelet Aggregation Studies		
ADP	Weak primary wave, no evidence of secondary wave	Biphasic aggregation
Collagen	Minimal response	Full-range monophasic aggregation
Epinephrine	Minimal response	Biphasic aggregation
Ristocetin	Weak agglutination (30% optical density change)	Full-range monophasic agglutination or biphasic agglutination
Platelet retention (glass-bead column)	35%	40% to 90%

DIAGNOSIS: Qualitative abnormality of platelets (secondary to chronic renal insufficiency)

Discussion

Uremia is commonly associated with an abnormal bleeding tendency. A number of hemostatic disorders have been described; they include a prolonged bleeding time, defective platelet aggregation (adenosine diphosphate, collagen and epinephrine), decreased platelet retention in glass-bead columns and decreased availability of platelet factor 3. In addition, it has been noted that patients often have increases in factor VIII:C activity, factor VIII R:RCo and factor R:Ag. Of the various laboratory findings, the prolonged bleeding time correlates best with the clinical picture.

This patient presented with a markedly prolonged bleeding time, greater than 15 minutes. This value should not, however, be accepted without question. As has been noted, because of the presence of arteriovenous fistulas

QUALITATIVE ABNORMALITY OF PLATELETS
(SECONDARY TO CHRONIC RENAL INSUFFICIENCY)

CLINICAL PICTURE

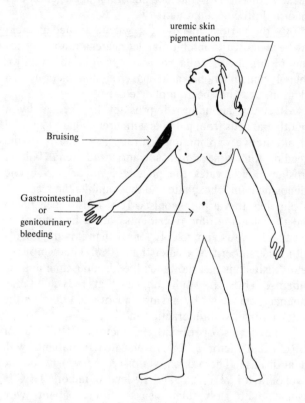

uremic skin pigmentation

Bruising

Gastrointestinal or genitourinary bleeding

PATHOPHYSIOLOGIC BASIS OF UREMIC BLEEDING

Retained metabolites (guanidinosuccinic acid or phenolic acid) affect platelet function
Increased prostacyclin-like activity
Low hematocrit (<30%)

LABORATORY FINDINGS

A. Screening Procedures

Test	Patient's Result	Normal Range
Prothrombin time	Normal	10–12 seconds
APTT	Normal	<42 seconds
Platelet count	Normal	130,000–400,000/μl
Bleeding time	Abnormal	1–8 minutes

B. Confirmatory Procedures

| Platelet aggregation | Abnormal | See tracings |
| Platelet retention | Abnormal | 40% to 90% |

TREATMENT

Dialysis
Cryoprecipitate
1-Desamino-8-D-arginine vasopressin (DDAVP)
Packed red cells if there is severe anemia

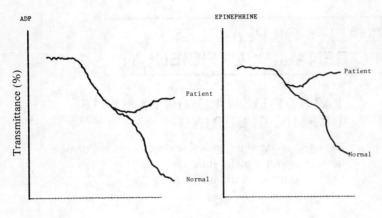

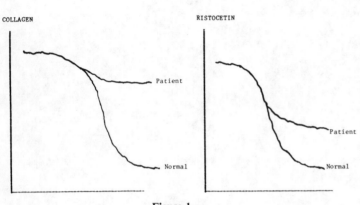

Figure 1

in both arms, it was necessary to perform the bleeding time on a leg. Thus, no normal range is available for comparison of this bleeding time.

Other findings included elevation of the blood urea nitrogen and creatinine secondary to the chronic renal failure. The patient had frequently been on dialysis but was evaluated 2 days after the most recent dialysis procedure. Another interesting observation was the relatively short activated partial thromboplastin time (APTT). A shortened APTT may be seen in a number of different clinical situations, including acute disseminated intravascular coagulation, liver disease and, occasionally, severe anemia. In this case, the hematocrit was 25%, which may account for the shortened APTT.

The results of platelet aggregation studies were typical of chronic renal disease. There were abnormalities in the responses to adenosine diphosphate, collagen and epinephrine. In addition, the ristocetin agglutination response was slightly blunted.

Biochemical Aspects. In acute and chronic renal disease, there is a bleeding tendency that is often multifactorial. Various abnormalities have been described; they include qualitative defects of platelets, deficiencies of coagulation factors, disseminated intravascular coagulation and abnormal fibrinolysis.

A qualitative abnormality of platelet function is perhaps the most common finding. This defect is extrinsic and appears to parallel the levels of retained metabolites in the blood. Unless the metabolites are removed, the function of transfused platelets will also be impaired. As noted above, a number of laboratory abnormalities have been described; they include decreased adhesion of platelets, abnormal aggregation and abnormal procoagulant activity.

Of the various metabolites, guanidinosuccinic acid has been shown to inhibit platelet aggregation to adenosine diphosphate, collagen and epinephrine in vitro. Phenol and phenolic acid have similar actions. In addition, urea has been implicated.

Recently, an increase in prostacyclin-like activity in endothelial cells from patients with uremia has suggested an alternative explanation for the pathogenesis of the bleeding that is seen in association with renal failure. Prostacyclin elevates the platelet level of 3',5'-cyclic adenosine monophosphate and thus inhibits the response of platelets to various agonists. It has also been noted that the bleeding time of patients with a hemotacrit of less than 30% is appreciably longer than it is in patients with a hematocrit of greater than 30%. The use of red cell transfusions has shortened the bleeding time in such patients. Thus, it would appear that red cells may enhance hemostasis by having a favorable effect on the platelet-vessel wall interaction in vivo.

The levels of fibrinogen, factor VIII:C, factor R:RCo and factor R:Ag are elevated in patients with renal disease. There often is a discrepancy between the level of factor VIII R:Ag and the level of factor VIII:C in patients with glomerular disease. Some patients with nephrotic syndrome have decreased levels of antithrombin III as well as loss of factor IX in the urine.

Clinical Picture. The clinical picture often is characteristic of a primary hemostatic abnormality, with epistaxis and ecchymosis being predominant. Also, occasionally, bleeding occurs from the gastrointestinal and genitourinary tracts.

Treatment. Uremic bleeding rarely occurs in patients who are on regular dialysis. If such patients bleed, the differential diagnosis would include inadequate heparin neutralization and/or disseminated intravascular coagulation in association with another underlying clinical condition, such as septicemia. In patients who are not on dialysis, hemorrhage may be difficult to manage unless metabolic defects are first corrected by dialysis. As has been noted, unless the metabolites are removed by proper dialysis, transfused platelets will acquire the uremic defect.

Cryoprecipitate shortens the bleeding time and reduces the complications of bleeding in patients with severe uremia. Typically, the bleeding time becomes shortened within 1 hour after infusion of cryoprecipitate, although the maximal effect is not manifest for several hours. The mechanism of action of cryoprecipitate is not clear. Patients with uremia typically have increased quantities of the various components of the factor VIII complex as well as fibronectin.

A synthetic analog of vasopressin (1-desamino-8-D-arginine vasopressin, DDAVP) has also been found to be effective in treating patients with uremia. DDAVP induces the release of components of the factor VIII molecule from the endothelium. Again, the mechanism whereby DDAVP shortens the bleeding time is not fully understood. It should be stressed that this form of therapy is often a "one-shot" treatment. After repeated doses, patients become relatively refractory to further treatment.

Bibliography

Carvalho ACA: Bleeding in uremia—A clinical challenge. *N Engl J Med* 308:38–39, 1983.

Eknoyan G, Wacksman SJ, Glueck HI, et al: Platelet function in renal failure. *N Engl J Med* 280:677–681, 1969.

Janson PA, Jubelirer SJ, Weinstein MJ, et al: Treatment of the bleeding tendency in uremia with cryoprecipitate. *N Engl J Med* 303:1318–1322, 1980.

Larsson SO, Hedner U, Nilsson IM: On coagulation and fibrinolysis in conservatively treated chronic uraemia. *Acta Med Scand* 189:433–441, 1971.

Livio M, Gotti E, Marchesi D, et al: Uraemic bleeding: Role of anaemia and beneficial effect of red cell transfusions. *Lancet* 2:1013–1015, 1982.

Mannucci PM, Remuzzi G, Pusineri F, et al: Deamino-8-D-arginine vasopressin shortens the bleeding time in uremia. *N Engl J Med* 308:8–12, 1983.

Rabiner SF: Uremic bleeding. *Prog Hemostasis Thromb* 1:233–250, 1972.

Remuzzi G, Cavenaghi AE, Mecca G, et al: Prosta-cyclin-like activity and bleeding in renal failure. *Lancet* 2:1195–1197, 1977.

Stein IM, Cohen BD, Kornhauser RS: Guanidino-succinic acid in renal failure, experimental azotemia and inborn errors of urea cycle. *N Engl J Med* 280:926–930, 1969.

Stewart JH, Castaldi PA: Uraemic bleeding: A reversible platelet defect corrected by dialysis. *Q J Med* 36:409–423, 1967.

CASE
36

PATIENT: 18-year-old man

CHIEF COMPLAINT: This patient was admitted with a diagnosis of nephrotic syndrome complicating membranous glomerulonephritis.

After admission, pain developed in the patient's left leg and was localized primarily to the ilial femoral area.

MEDICAL HISTORY: When 16 years of age, the patient had been diagnosed as having membranous glomerulonephritis. There was no known clinical condition that would have predisposed to the membranous glomerulonephritis. At the time of his original presentation, the patient had asymptomatic proteinuria.

A renal biopsy was performed. The glomeruli exhibited varying degrees of capillary wall thickening. The changes were uniform throughout the biopsy specimen. Methenamine silver stain demonstrated that the basement membranes of the peripheral capillary loops possessed subepithelial spikes, or clubs. Immunofluorescence studies revealed localization of IgG in a diffuse, generalized, granular pattern outlining the entire glomerular capillary bed.

FAMILY HISTORY: Noncontributory

DRUG HISTORY: The patient was taking prednisone and thiazide diuretics.

PHYSICAL EXAMINATION: There was anasarca and pain localized to the left ilial femoral area.

Laboratory Results

A. Screening Procedures

	Patient	Normal
Prothrombin time	12 seconds	10–12 seconds
APTT	42 seconds	<42 seconds
Platelet count	250,000/μl	130,000–400,000/μl
Bleeding time	6 minutes	1–8 minutes

Questions

1. Does the patient's underlying nephrotic syndrome have any relationship to the deep-vein thrombosis?

2. What is a possible explanation for the borderline value for the activated partial thromboplastin time (APTT)?

Laboratory Results

B. Confirmatory Procedures

	Patient	Normal
Antithrombin III (activity)	30%	85% to 115%
Antithrombin III (immunologic)	16.5 mg/dl	23–40 mg/dl

DIAGNOSIS: Acquired deficiency of antithrombin III (secondary to nephrotic syndrome)

Discussion

This case is an example of acquired deficiency of antithrombin III. Nephrotic syndrome has been documented in many instances to be associated with thrombotic complications, such as renal vein thrombosis and deep-vein thrombosis. It has only recently been appreciated that a primary underlying pathophysiologic mechanism is urinary loss of antithrombin III secondary to massive proteinuria.

In addition to loss of antithrombin III, acquired deficiency of factor XII has been described in association with nephrotic syndrome. This deficiency may account for the borderline value for the APTT that was noted in this patient. However, the level of factor XII was not measured.

Bibliography

Lau SO, Tkachuck JY, Hasegawa DK, et al: Plasminogen and antithrombin III deficiencies in the childhood nephrotic syndrome associated with plasminogenuria and antithrombinuria. *J Pediatr* 96:390–392, 1980.

Sullivan MJ, Hough DR, Agodoa LCY: Peripheral arterial thrombosis due to nephrotic syndrome: The clinical spectrum. *South Med J* 76:1011–1016, 1983.

ACQUIRED DEFICIENCY OF ANTITHROMBIN III
(SECONDARY TO NEPHROTIC SYNDROME)

CLINICAL PICTURE

PATHOPHYSIOLOGIC BASIS OF DEFICIENCY OF ANTITHROMBIN III

Loss of antithrombin III in urine due to proteinuria

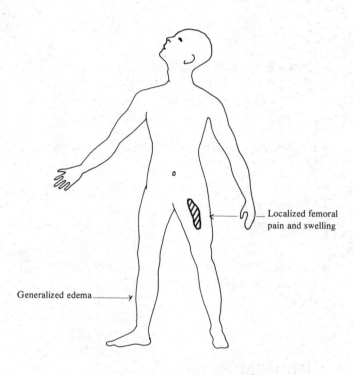

Localized femoral pain and swelling

Generalized edema

Massive proteinuria and hyperlipidemia

LABORATORY FINDINGS

A. Screening Procedures

Test	Patient's Result	Normal Range
Prothrombin time	Normal	10–12 seconds
APTT	Normal	<42 seconds
Platelet count	Normal	130,000–400,000/μl
Bleeding time	Normal	1–8 minutes

B. Confirmatory Procedure

Antithrombin III, activity	Abnormal	85% to 115%

TREATMENT

Anticoagulants
Fresh-frozen plasma as source of antithrombin III or antithrombin III concentrates

CASE
37

PATIENT: 43-year-old man.

CHIEF COMPLAINT: This patient was hospitalized in November 1980 because of nephrotic syndrome. The urinary level of protein at the time of admission was 1290 mg/dl (total urine volume, 920 ml). The amount of protein in the urine in a 24-hour period was calculated to be 11.9 g. The serum level of cholesterol was 276 mg/dl (normal, 140–310 mg/dl), and the level of triglycerides was 1096 mg/dl (normal, 56–298 mg/dl). The total amount of protein in the serum was 4.2 g, with an albumin of 1.9 g.

MEDICAL HISTORY: The patient had previously been diagnosed as having mild hypertension, which had been responsive to thiazide diuretics. In addition, he had been diagnosed as having hypothyroidism and was being treated with Synthroid (levothyroxine sodium). There was no history of surgical intervention or bleeding problems.

FAMILY HISTORY: Noncontributory

DRUG HISTORY: Thiazides and Synthroid

PHYSICAL EXAMINATION: Pitting edema was noted over the anterior tibial surfaces.

Laboratory Results

A. Screening Procedures

	Patient	Normal
Prothrombin time	11.6 seconds	10–12 seconds
APTT	50 seconds	<40 seconds
Platelet count	285,000/μl	130,000–400,000/μl
Bleeding time	7 minutes and 30 seconds	1–8 minutes

HOSPITAL COURSE: The patient was scheduled for a renal biopsy to determine the cause of the nephrotic syndrome. Before the biopsy was performed, the above coagulation screening profile was obtained.

Questions

1. What additional laboratory procedures are indicated?
2. What coagulation abnormalities have been associated with nephrotic syndrome?

Laboratory Results

B. Confirmatory Procedures

	Patient	Normal
APTT (50% patient plasma/ 50% pooled normal plasma)	35 seconds	<42 seconds
Factor VIII:C assay	194%	50% to 150%
Factor IX:C assay	131%	50% to 150%
Factor XI assay	124%	50% to 150%
Factor XII assay	20%	30% to 150%
Antithrombin III (activity)	82%	85% to 115%

DIAGNOSIS: Acquired deficiency of factor XII (secondary to nephrotic syndrome)

Discussion

This patient was placed on prednisone and responded well. One month after admission, the amount of protein in the urine had decreased to 2.3 g/24 hours and the clinical status had improved markedly.

A variety of coagulation abnormalities, including elevated plasma levels of fibrinogen, factor V and factor VIII:C, have been described in association with nephrotic syndrome. Acquired deficiencies of coagulation factors have been less frequently reported. Deficiency of Christmas factor (factor IX) due to urinary loss of factor IX has been recognized, as have deficiencies of Hageman factor (factor XII) and Fletcher factor (prekallikrein).

The pathophysiologic basis of acquired deficiency of Hageman factor in persons with nephrotic syndrome has not been established. Urine from persons with severe nephrotic syndrome contains appreciable amounts of Hageman factor, as detected by immunologic assay.

DEFICIENCY OF FACTOR XII (SECONDARY TO NEPHROTIC SYNDROME)

CLINICAL PICTURE

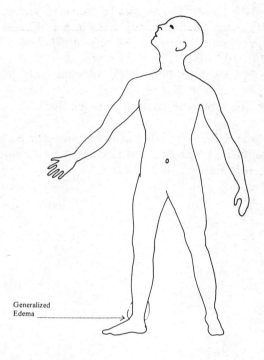

Generalized
Edema

Proteinuria and hyperlipidemia

PATHOPHYSIOLOGIC BASIS OF ACQUIRED DEFICIENCY OF FACTOR XII

?Loss of factor XII in urine
Factor XII:Ag factor XII:C ratio >1 in plasma
No inhibitor demonstrated

LABORATORY FINDINGS

A. Screening Procedures

Test	Patient's Result	Normal Range
Prothrombin time	Normal	10–12 seconds
APTT	Abnormal	<42 seconds
Platelet count	Normal	130,000–400,000/μl
Bleeding time	Normal	1–8 minutes

B. Confirmatory Procedures

Mixing APTT	Normal	<42 seconds
Factor XII assay	Abnormal	30% to 150%

TREATMENT

Manage nephrotic syndrome

Because the molecular weight of Hageman factor is approximately 80,000, it is not surprising that this plasma protein is excreted in the urine. However, urinary loss of Hageman factor alone may not account for the reduced plasma activity of Hageman factor because there is no relationship between plasma and urinary levels of this factor. In several series, the plasma level of Hageman factor has been decreased; however, the level of Hageman factor antigen, as measured by radio-immunoassay, has been within the normal range. Thus, the ratio of the level of Hageman factor antigen to its activity in the plasma of persons with nephrotic syndrome has been greater than one. No circulating antibody to Hageman factor has been detected; consequently, it appears that a nonfunctional Hageman factor exists in the plasma of such persons. These findings have been reported in children and adults.

Currently, there are insufficient data to determine whether deficiency of Factor XII in persons with nephrotic syndrome is associated with thrombosis. Also, no correlation between acquired deficiency of factor XII and the histologic type of nephrotic syndrome has been established.

Bibliography

Hurby MA, Honig GR, Shapira E: Immunoquantitation of Hageman factor in urine and plasma of children with nephrotic syndrome. *J Lab Clin Med* 96:501–510, 1980.

Royen EA, van de Boer JEG, Wilmink JM, et al: Acquired factor XII deficiency in a patient with nephrotic syndrome. *Acta Med Scand* 205:535–539, 1979.

Thompson AR: Factor XII and other hemostatic protein abnormalities in nephrotic syndrome patients. *Thromb Haemostasis* 48:27–32, 1982.

CASE
38

PATIENT: 59-year-old woman

CHIEF COMPLAINT: This patient noted the onset of her illness approximately 1 year before her initial visit. At that time, she had noticed bruising of a spontaneous nature. In addition to a number of minor bruises, there was a large bruise over the ventral aspect of the left forearm. After the appearance of this ecchymosis, large ecchymoses were also noted over the legs.

Immediately before the onset of bruising, the patient had an episode of otitis media and was placed on Cleocin (clindamycin). After several days of therapy with Cleocin, an allergic reaction developed; it was characterized by urticaria and marked facial edema. The Cleocin was discontinued.

Following the onset of the ecchymosis, the patient again consulted her family physician, who ordered a number of laboratory tests and placed the patient on vitamin K together with vitamin C. She did not respond to the vitamin therapy and was subsequently admitted to a hospital, where a bone marrow aspirate and biopsy was performed; the specimen was interpreted as being within normal limits. During the patient's hospitalization, she was found to have a factor VIII:C activity of 2% together with a prolonged activated partial thromboplastin time (APTT). The provisional diagnosis was von Willebrand's disease despite a medical history of no bleeding complications after tonsillectomy at 18 years of age and hysterectomy at 47 years of age. Additional laboratory test results included a prothrombin time of 12 seconds (normal, 10–12 seconds), Ivy bleeding time of 8 minutes (normal, 2–10 minutes) and a platelet count of 265,000/μl (normal, 150,000–400,000/μl). The APTT was 56.8 seconds (normal, less than 35 seconds).

MEDICAL HISTORY: There was no history of bruising or bleeding problems. The patient had been diagnosed as having gout.

FAMILY HISTORY: There was no family history of bleeding problems. The patient had three sons (26, 33 and 35 years of age) all of whom were living and well.

DRUG HISTORY: At the time of evaluation, the patient was taking Benemid (probenecid) and an antihistamine. The patient reported allergies to Cleocin and penicillin.

PHYSICAL EXAMINATION: A number of ecchymoses were noted over the arms and legs. In addition, the patient reported shoulder pain and swelling of the right knee. Although the knee was swollen, there was no evidence of effusion, and it was not tender to palpation.

Laboratory Results

A. Screening Procedures

	Patient	Normal
Prothrombin time	11 seconds	10–12 seconds
APTT	79 seconds	<42 seconds
Platelet count	235,000/μl	200,000–450,000/μl
Bleeding time	7 minutes	1–8 minutes

Questions

1. Is this patient's history compatible with a diagnosis of von Willebrand's disease?
2. Does the history of allergy to Cleocin help explain the abnormal APTT?
3. What additional laboratory procedures are indicated?

Laboratory Results

B. Confirmatory Procedures

	Patient	Normal
APTT (50% patient plasma/50% pooled normal plasma)		
Immediate	45 seconds	<42 seconds
2-hour incubation	75 seconds	<42 seconds
Factor VIII:C activity	<1%	50% to 150%
Factor VIII R:Ag	79%	50% to 150%
Factor VIII R:RCo	110%	50% to 150%
Factor VIII inhibitor titer	>200 Bethesda units	0 Bethesda units

Additional laboratory tests that were performed included antinuclear antibody to rule out the possibility of systemic lupus erythematosus. This test was negative. Immunoglobulins were also quantified, with the following results: IgG, 530 mg/dl (normal, 800–1800 mg/dl); IgA, 100 mg/dl (normal, 90–450 mg/dl); IgM, 460 mg/

ACQUIRED INHIBITOR OF FACTOR VIII
(POSSIBLY DRUG [CLEOCIN] RELATED)

CLINICAL PICTURE

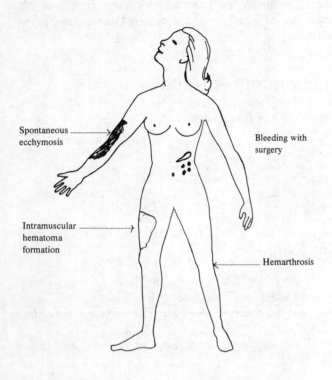

Spontaneous ecchymosis

Bleeding with surgery

Intramuscular hematoma formation

Hemarthrosis

PATHOPHYSIOLOGIC BASIS

Possible drug (Cleocin) allergy

LABORATORY FINDINGS

A. Screening Procedures

Test	Patient's Result	Normal Range
Prothrombin time	Normal	10–12 seconds
APTT	Abnormal	<42 seconds
Platelet count	Normal	130,000–400,000/μl
Bleeding time	Normal	1–8 minutes

B. Confirmatory Procedures

Mixing APTT	Abnormal†	<42 seconds
Factor VIII:C activity	<1%	50% to 150%
Factor VIII inhibitor	Abnormal	0 Bethesda units

†*Accenuated with 2-hour incubation.*

TREATMENT

Immunosuppressive therapy
Factor VIII concentrates for active bleeding

dl (normal, 70–280 mg/dl). Findings on immunoelectrophoresis were unremarkable; there was no evidence of a monoclonal protein.

DIAGNOSIS: Acquired inhibitor of factor VIII, (possibly drug [Cleocin] related)

Discussion

This case is an example of an acquired high titer inhibitor of factor VIII:C. Spontaneous inhibitors of factor VIII:C arise in a number of different clinical situations, including collagen vascular disease (i.e., systemic lupus), pregnancy and the immediate postpartum period, certain dermatologic diseases and after drug reactions (penicillin, sulfa drugs and gold) and occasionally are found in patients with no obvious underlying disease. In this patient, the onset of the illness was related to an allergic reaction to Cleocin. Consequently, it would appear that this patient would be best diagnosed as having a drug-related inhibitor of factor VIII:C.

The patient was extensively evaluated for underlying collagen vascular disease. No autoantibody was demonstrated. The patient was seen 1 year after the onset of the inhibitor, and it was found that the inhibitor persisted, although at a diminished titer (90 Bethesda units). During the interval between the initial and follow-up clinic visits, the patient had received no medication other than that used to manage the underlying gout.*

Biochemical Aspects. Most spontaneous inhibitors of factor VIII:C have been characterized as IgG antibodies. However, there have been three instances of IgM antibodies and one of an IgA antibody to factor VIII:C. Light-chain typing of spontaneous inhibitors has demonstrated heterogeneity (i.e., lambda and kappa light chains).

The kinetics of the neutralization reaction of spontaneous inhibitors is more complex than that of hemophilic inhibitors. There is an initial rapid destruction of factor VIII:C activity, which is followed by a phase of equilibrium in which factor VIII:C activity may still be measured regardless of the antibody titer. It has been suggested that the inhibitor-factor VIII:C complex may continue to express factor VIII:C activity.

The etiologic basis of antibodies to factor VIII:C in persons without hemophilia is unknown. The antibodies are not related to previous exposure to blood or blood products. Typically, such patients do not demonstrate an anamnestic response on exposure to factor VIII.

This patient returned again with a large intrarectus hematoma and spontaneous retroperitoneal bleeding diagnosed by CAT scan.

Clinical Picture. Patients with spontaneous inhibitors of factor VIII:C often have a severe bleeding diathesis, characterized by hematoma formation, hematuria and intramuscular, retroperitoneal and cerebral hemorrhages. Hemarthrosis may also occur but is less common than in severe hemophilia A. Spontaneous remission is commonly seen in women in whom an inhibitor develops during the postpartum period and in patients with an inhibitor associated with allergy to penicillin.

Treatment. Management of an acute bleeding episode in a patient with a spontaneous inhibitor is similar to that of a hemophiliac with an inhibitor. However, replacement by use of factor VIII concentrates may be effective in such patients, whereas such therapy is ineffective in hemophiliacs. Immunosuppressive therapy with azathioprine or cyclophosphamide has also been effective. Prothrombin complex concentrates may be required in patients with extremely high titers of inhibitors of factor VIII.

Bibliography

Clinical Picture

Allain JP, Gaillandre A, Frommel D: Acquired haemophilia: Functional study of antibodies to factor VIII. *Thromb Haemostasis* 45:285–289, 1981.

Coller BS, Hultin MB, Hoyer LW, et al: Normal pregnancy in a patient with a prior postpartum factor VIII inhibitor with observations on pathogenesis and prognosis. *Blood* 58:619–624, 1981.

Green D: Spontaneous inhibitors of factor VIII. *Brit J Haematol* 15:57–75, 1968.

Nakashima K, Miyahara T, Fujii S, et al: Spontaneously acquired factor VIII inhibitor in a 7 year old girl. *Acta Haematol* 68:58–62, 1982.

Nilsson IM, Lamme S: On acquired hemophilia A. *Acta Med Scand* 208:5–12, 1980.

Treatment

Herbst KD, Rapaport SI, Kenoyer DG, et al: Syndrome of an acquired inhibitor of factor VIII responsive to cyclophosphamide and prednisone. *Ann Intern Med* 95:575–578, 1981.

Sultan Y, Maisonneuve P, Bismuth A, et al: Successful management of a patient with an acquired factor VIII inhibitor. *Transfusion* Philadelphia 23:62–64, 1983.

Review Articles

Bidwell E: Acquired inhibitors of coagulants. *Annu Rev Med* 20:63–74, 1969.

Feinstein DI, Rapaport SI: Acquired inhibitors of blood

coagulation. In Spaet T (ed): *Progress in Hemostasis and Thrombosis*. New York: Grune & Stratton, 1972, vol I, pp 75–95.

Green D: Circulating anticoagulants. *Med Clin North Amer* 56:145–151, 1972.

Green D, Lechner K: A study of 215 non-hemophilic patients with inhibitors to factor VIII. *Thromb Haemostasis* 45:200–203, 1981.

Lechner K: Acquired inhibitors in nonhemophilic patients. *Haemostasis* 3:65–93, 1974.

Margolius A, Jackson DP, Ratnoff OD: Circulating anticoagulants: A study of 40 cases and a review of the literature. *Medicine (Baltimore)* 40:145–202, 1961.

Palascak JE: Autoantibodies against clotting factors. In Lusher JM, Barnhardt MI (eds): *Abnormalities of Hemostasis*. New York: Masson Publishing, 1981, vol 3, pp 99–113.

Shapiro SS, Hultin M: Acquired inhibitors to blood coagulation factors. *Semin Thromb Hemostasis* 1:336–385, 1975.

CASE

39

PATIENT: 73-year-old woman

CHIEF COMPLAINT: This patient was admitted with a diagnosis of acute rectal bleeding.

MEDICAL HISTORY: The patient had undergone open heart surgery in 1976 with insertion of a prosthetic mitral valve for mitral stenosis. There was no untoward bleeding associated with this surgical procedure. In 1982, she again underwent major surgery for a possible ovarian tumor. The lesion was found to be a serous cystadenoma and was successfully removed. This operation also was performed without complications.

FAMILY HISTORY: Noncontributory

DRUG HISTORY: The patient had taken Tagamet (cimetidine), Aldactazide (spironolactone with hydrochlorothiazide), Coumadin (sodium warfarin) and Lanoxin (digoxin).

PHYSICAL EXAMINATION: The patient was a pale and slightly obese woman. Surgical scars were noted over the abdomen and chest. Pelvic and rectal examinations were unremarkable.

Laboratory Results

A. Screening Procedures

	Patient	Normal
Prothrombin time	13.5 seconds	10–12 seconds
APTT	60 seconds	<42 seconds
Platelet count	280,000/μl	130,000–400,000/μl
Bleeding time	7 minutes	1–8 minutes

HOSPITAL COURSE: At the time of admission, the patient's hemoglobin level was 7.5 g/dl; consequently, she immediately received 3 units of packed red cells. Barium enema revealed a polypoid mass in the splenic flexure of the colon consistent with an adenomatous polyp. There was also an area in the sigmoid colon consistent with a polyp.

Colonoscopic examination was performed to obtain biopsy specimens from the polypoid masses. A specimen from the larger polyp, the mass in the splenic flexure, was consistent with adenocarcinoma. Therefore, the patient was prepared for exploratory laparotomy. Before coagulation studies were performed, she received vitamin K, 20 mg intramuscularly, for 2 consecutive days.

Questions

1. Can the prolonged prothrombin time and activated partial thromboplastin time (APTT) be explained by the previous administration of Coumadin?
2. What additional laboratory procedures are indicated?

Laboratory Results

B. Confirmatory Procedures

APTT (patient plasma/pooled normal plasma)	Immediate	30-Minute Incubation	60-Minute Incubation
1:9	43 seconds	45 seconds	45 seconds
5:5	51 seconds	53 seconds	57 seconds
9:1	59 seconds	60 seconds	61 seconds

The results of the mixing studies were interpreted as being indicative of a circulating anticoagulant. Appropriate controls were performed in parallel. To rule out the possibility of a nonspecific, or lupus type of, anticoagulant, a tissue thromboplastin inhibition procedure was performed, with the following results:

		Patient
1:100 dilution of thromboplastin	2.9	Normal <1.1
		Borderline 1.1–1.3
1:1000 dilution of thromboplastin	3.3	Abnormal >1.3

To further confirm the impression of a lupus type of inhibitor, a platelet neutralization procedure was performed, and the results were positive.

DIAGNOSIS: Lupus anticoagulant

Discussion

This case illustrates a number of interesting points. Patients with occult lesions of the gastrointestinal tract who are taking oral anticoagulants often present with rectal bleeding. Thus, it is necessary to evaluate thoroughly any patient taking oral anticoagulants who presents with rectal bleeding. It is erroneous to assume that the bleeding is due solely to excess anticoagulation.

After this patient had received intramuscular vitamin K, the prothrombin time and APTT were prolonged. The finding of a prolonged prothrombin time and APTT would raise the possibility of an abnormality in the final common pathway of coagulation. The other

LUPUS ANTICOAGULANT

CLINICAL PICTURE

No bleeding symptoms
Occasionally thrombotic symptoms

Female patient may have recurrent abortions

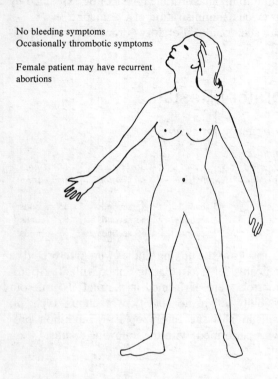

PATHOPHYSIOLOGIC BASIS

IgG or IgM antibody
Directed against phospholipids

LABORATORY FINDINGS

A. Screening Procedures

Test	Patient's Result	Normal Range
Prothrombin time	Normal or abnormal	10–12 seconds
APTT	Abnormal	<42 seconds
Platelet count	Normal	130,000–400,000/μl
Bleeding time	Normal	1–8 minutes

B. Confirmatory Procedures

Test	Patient's Result	Normal Range
Mixing APTT	Abnormal	<42 seconds
Tissue thromboplastin inhibition, 1:100	>1.3	<1.1
Platelet neutralization procedure	Positive	—

TREATMENT

Once a firm diagnosis of a lupus anticoagulant has been established, further treatment is *not* indicated.
Be aware of high frequency of thrombotic complications.

possibility would be a circulating anticoagulant. Mixing studies indicated that there was an anticoagulant. The anticoagulant was subsequently identified as being nonspecific, or of the lupus type.

Biochemical Aspects. Lupus anticoagulants have been identified as being immunoglobulins of the IgG or IgM class. Most inhibitors belong to the IgG class. These immunoglobulins interfere with various phospholipid-dependent coagulation test results without inhibiting the activity of coagulation factors. Most investigators have suggested that lupus inhibitors interfere with the phospholipid component of the complex that is involved in the conversion of prothrombin to thrombin. Such antibodies have been found to have precipitant activity against anionic phospholipids. In addition, they react with cardiolipin, the phospholipid antigen that is used in serologic tests for syphilis. The mechanism of production of antibodies to various lipid components of cell membranes is currently unknown.

Clinical Picture. The term lupus anticoagulants is a misnomer. Perhaps a more appropriate term would be nonspecific inhibitors of the APTT. These inhibitors may be seen in patients with systemic lupus erythematosus. However, they are more commonly seen in patients with other clinical disorders and occasionally in patients with no obvious underlying disease. Approximately 10% of patients with systemic lupus erythematosus may have lupus anticoagulants.

In the absence of any other predisposition to hemorrhage, such patients do not bleed spontaneously or intraoperatively. It is important to appreciate that such patients may have other clinical conditions that predispose to hemorrhage. For instance, patients who have systemic lupus erythematosus may have an isolated deficiency of prothrombin, concomitant thrombocytopenia, acquired von Willebrand's disease or associated specific inhibitors (i.e., inhibitor of factor VIII).

Laboratory evaluation of patients with the nonspecific, or lupus type of, anticoagulant typically demonstrates prolongation of all phospholipid-dependent coagulant test results. These tests include the prothrombin time, APTT and Russell's viper venom time. The APTT is considerably more sensitive than is the prothrombin time to lupus anticoagulants. The sensitivity of the prothrombin time and APTT may depend on the reagents used. Certain reagents appear to be much more sensitive, although the reason for this increased sensitivity is not readily apparent. For instance, the choice of an activator in the APTT does not appear to correlate with sensitivity to lupus anticoagulants.

Some patients with lupus anticoagulants have a false-positive VDRL. Other patients with lupus inhibitors have had recurrent abortions and thromboembolic phenomena. Indeed, it would appear that patients with lupus anticoagulants are at an increased risk for the development of thrombotic complications. Several recent studies have suggested that there is a relationship between recurrent thrombosis and inhibition of synthesis of prostacyclin by endothelial cells.

Treatment. The most important clinical aspects of the lupus anticoagulants is their recognition and correct identification. Because patients with these inhibitors do not have a predisposition to hemorrhage, prophylactic transfusions, vitamin K and other measures are not indicated. However, appropriate vigilance for possible thromboembolic phenomena is necessary.

Bibliography

Laboratory Diagnosis

Clyne LP, Dainiak N, Hoffman R, et al: In vitro correction of anticoagulant activity and specific clotting factor assays in SLE. *Thromb Res* 18:643–655, 1980.

Exner T, Rickard KA, Kronenberg H: A sensitive test demonstrating lupus anticoagulant and its behavioural patterns. *Brit J Haematol* 40:143–151, 1978.

Mannucci PM, Canciani MT, Mari D, et al: The varied sensitivity of partial thromboplastin and prothrombin time reagents in the demonstration of the lupus like anticoagulant. *Scand J Haematol* 22:423–432, 1979.

Thiagarajan P, Shapiro S, DeMarco L: Monoclonal immunoglobulin M coagulation inhibitor with phospholipid specificity. *J Clin Invest* 66:397–405, 1980.

Triplett DA, Brandt JT, Kaczor D, et al: Laboratory diagnosis of lupus inhibitors: A comparison of the tissue thromboplastin inhibition procedure with a new platelet neutralization procedure. *Amer J Clin Pathol* 79:678–682, 1983.

Venous Thrombosis

Carreras LO, Vermylen JG: "Lupus" anticoagulant and thrombosis—Possible role of inhibition of prostacyclin formation. *Thromb Haemostasis* 48:38–40, 1982.

Manoharan A, Gibson L, Rush B, et al: Recurrent venous thrombosis with a 'lupus' coagulation inhibitor in the absence of systemic lupus. *Aust NZ J Med* 7:422–426, 1977.

Mavchin SJ, McVerry BA, Parry H, et al: Inhibition of prostacyclin activity in systemic lupus erythematosus. *Ann Rheum Dis* 39:524–525, 1980.

Mueh JR, Herbst KD, Rapaport SI: Thrombosis in patients with the lupus anticoagulant. *Ann Intern Med* 92:156–159, 1980.

Peck B, Hoffman GS, Franck WA: Thrombophlebitis in systemic lupus erythematosus. *J Amer Med Ass* 240:1728–1730, 1978.

Williams H, Laurent R, Gibson T: The lupus coagulation inhibitor and venous thrombosis: A report of four cases. *Clin Lab Haematol* 2:139–144, 1980.

Other Hemostatic Findings in Systemic Lupus Erythematosus

Castro O, Farber LR, Clyne LP: Circulating anticoagulants against factor IX and XI in systemic lupus erythematosus. *Ann Intern Med* 77:543–548, 1972.

Leone G, Accorra F, Boni P: Circulating anticoagulant against factor XI and thrombocytopenia with platelet aggregation inhibition in systemic lupus erythematosus. *Acta Haematol* 58:240–245, 1977.

Natelson EA, Cyprus GS, Hettig RA: Absent factor II in systemic lupus erythematosus. *Arthritis Rheum* 19:79–82, 1976.

Rapaport SI, Ames SB, Duvall BJ: A plasma coagulation defect in systemic lupus erythematosus arising from hypoprothrombinemia combined with antiprothrombinase activity. *Blood* 15:212–227, 1960.

Sanfelippo MJ, Drayna CJ: Prekallikrein inhibition associated with the lupus anticoagulant. *Amer J Clin Pathol* 77:275–279, 1982.

Vercellotti CM, Mosher DF: Acquired factor XI deficiency in systemic lupus erythematosus. *Thromb Haemostasis* 48:250–252, 1982.

Review Articles

Lee SL, Miotti AB: Disorders of hemostatic function in patients with systemic lupus erythematosus. *Semin Arthritis Rheum* 4:241–252, 1975.

Shapiro SS, Thiagarajan P: Lupus anticoagulants. In Spaet TH (ed): *Progress in Hemostasis and Thrombosis*. New York: Grune & Stratton, 1982, vol 6, pp 263–285.

CASE
40

PATIENT: 62-year-old man

CHIEF COMPLAINT: This patient was admitted because of right upper quadrant pain of some duration. After evaluation, it was thought that he had chronic cholecystitis because cholelithiasis had been demonstrated by ultrasound and cholecystograms.

MEDICAL HISTORY: The patient had no history of bleeding problems. However, he had a history of illnesses, including diabetes, which had been difficult to control with dietary modification in combination with oral hypoglycemic agents. Also, he had a history of coronary artery disease, having an old anterior myocardial infarction.

FAMILY HISTORY: The family history showed a marked prevalence of coronary artery disease and diabetes. There was a history of diabetes on the maternal and paternal sides of the family.

DRUG HISTORY: The patient had taken digitalis, thiazide diuretics and insulin.

PHYSICAL EXAMINATION: There was tenderness in the right upper quadrant, and a trace of pitting edema was noted over the legs.

Laboratory Results

A. Screening Procedures

	Patient	Normal
Prothrombin time	13 seconds	10–12 seconds
APTT	52 seconds	<42 seconds
Platelet count	220,000/μl	130,000–400,000/μl
Bleeding time	2 minutes and 49 seconds	1–8 minutes

Questions

1. What additional laboratory procedures are indicated?
2. Could deficiency of vitamin K account for the above findings?

Laboratory Results

B. Confirmatory Procedures

	Patient	Normal
APTT (50% patient plasma/50% pooled normal plasma)	52 seconds	<42 seconds
Thrombin time	23 seconds	20–24 seconds

Because the above results indicated that there was a circulating inhibitor, an incubation procedure for circulating anticoagulants was performed, with the following results:

APTT (patient plasma/pooled normal plasma)	5-Minute Incubation	15-Minute Incubation	30-Minute Incubation	60-Minute Incubation
1:9	43 seconds	44 seconds	45 seconds	47 seconds
5:5	52 seconds	53 seconds	49 seconds	55 seconds
9:1	53 seconds	53 seconds	52 seconds	46 seconds

APTT (buffer/ pooled normal plasma)				
5:5	34 seconds	22 seconds	21 seconds	21 seconds

To further evaluate the nature of the inhibitor, a tissue thromboplastin inhibition procedure was performed, with the following results:

Thromboplastin dilution	Control	Patient	Ratio	Normal
1:100	35	65	1.9	<1.1
1:1000	81	162	2	<1.1

A platelet neutralization procedure (PNP) was also positive.

DIAGNOSIS: Lupus anticoagulant

Discussion

This case is a classical example of the lupus type of anticoagulant. The prothrombin time and activated partial thromboplastin time (APTT) were prolonged, indicating the effect of the inhibitor in the final common pathway of coagulation. Subsequent mixing studies revealed an inhibitor, which was further characterized with the tissue thromboplastin inhibition procedure. It

LUPUS ANTICOAGULANT

CLINICAL PICTURE

No bleeding symptoms
Occasionally thrombotic symptoms

Female patients may have recurrent abortions

PATHOPHYSIOLOGIC BASIS

IgG or IgM antibodies
Directed against phospholipids

LABORATORY FINDINGS

A. Screening Procedures

Test	Patient's Result	Normal Range
Prothrombin time	Normal or abnormal	10–12 seconds
APTT	Abnormal	<42 seconds
Platelet count	Normal	130,000–400,000/μl
Bleeding time	Normal	1–8 minutes

B. Confirmatory Procedures

Mixing APTT	Abnormal	<42 seconds
Tissue thromboplastin inhibition, 1:100	>1.3	<1.1
Platelet neutralization procedure	Positive	

TREATMENT

Once a firm diagnosis of a lupus anticoagulant has been established, further treatment is *not* indicated.

should be emphasized, however, that the tissue thromboplastin inhibition procedure is not a specific test for the lupus inhibitor. The results of this test may be abnormal in patients who are taking heparin or who have inhibitors to coagulation factors in the final common pathway or inhibitors to factor IX or VIII. The recently described platelet neutralization procedure is more specific and sensitive in detecting and characterizing lupus anticoagulants.

Subsequent studies performed with the platelet neutralization procedure yielded positive results. After a lupus type of anticoagulant had been identified, the patient underwent an uneventful cholecystectomy. There was no bleeding intraoperatively or postoperatively.

Bibliography

(See Bibliography for Case 39)

CASE
41

PATIENT: 50-year-old man

CHIEF COMPLAINT: This patient presented with persistent epistaxis. He had suffered intermittent mild epistaxis for 3 years before admission. One and one-half years before this admission, he had consulted his local physician. A routine workup revealed a monoclonal spike on serum protein electrophoresis. A bone marrow biopsy was obtained, and a diagnosis of multiple myeloma was established. For the past year, the patient had continued to consult his physician for intermittent chemotherapy.

MEDICAL HISTORY: Noncontributory

FAMILY HISTORY: Noncontributory

DRUG HISTORY: The patient had taken melphalan and prednisone. He had been instructed to avoid aspirin and aspirin-containing medications.

PHYSICAL EXAMINATION: There was no palpable lymphadenopathy or organomegaly.

Laboratory Results

A. Screening Procedures

	Patient	Normal
Prothrombin time	16 seconds	10–12 seconds
APTT	44 seconds	<42 seconds
Platelet count	70,000/μl	130,000–400,000/μl
Bleeding time	9 minutes	1–8 minutes

Questions

1. What are the possible explanations for the bleeding episodes?
2. What additional laboratory procedures are indicated?
3. What laboratory results correlate with clinical bleeding in patients with multiple myeloma and Waldenström's macroglobulinemia?

Laboratory Results

B. Confirmatory Procedures

	Patient	Normal
Thrombin time	38 seconds	20–24 seconds

Circulating Anticoagulant Screen
  Thrombin time: pooled normal plasma, 21 seconds
  Thrombin time: patient plasma, 38 seconds
  Thrombin time: patient plasma plus pooled normal plasma (50:50), 29 seconds

Additional laboratory evaluation was undertaken for multiple myeloma. Serum protein electrophoresis showed a fast gamma monoclonal spike of 3.9 g. This spike was subsequently characterized as representing IgG kappa myeloma (subclass IgG_1). Urinary electrophoresis did not demonstrate Bence Jones protein. Bone marrow examination showed that plasma cells accounted for approximately 30% of the marrow cellularity. The marrow was interpreted as being somewhat hypocellular (35%). Serum viscosity was increased to 11 (normal, 1.2–1.9).

DIAGNOSIS: Multiple myeloma (IgG kappa) with hyperviscosity syndrome

Discussion

This patient was treated with a 10-unit plasmapheresis over a 36-hour period. This treatment had a dramatic effect on the epistaxis, and the patient was discharged with instructions to undergo a 1-unit plasmapheresis on a weekly basis and to continue his therapeutic drug regimen.

Biochemial Aspects. There are a number of possible explanations for bleeding in this patient. The prothrombin time, activated partial thromboplastin time (APTT) and thrombin time were prolonged, indicating the nonspecific inhibitory effect of the circulating monoclonal protein. In addition, the platelet count was decreased to 70,000/μl. The thrombocytopenia was probably multifactorial, being secondary to the chemotherapy as well as to marrow replacement by the malignant plasma cells. Perhaps the most readily explainable cause of the epistaxis is the patient's increased serum viscosity. It is well known that patients with hyperviscosity syndrome

MULTIPLE MYELOMA (IgG) WITH HYPERVISCOSITY SYNDROME

CLINICAL PICTURE

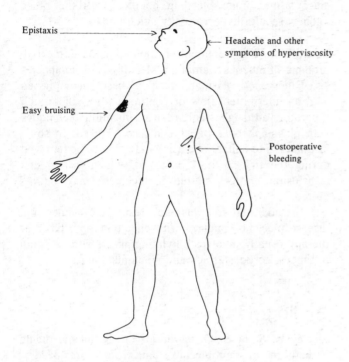

Epistaxis

Headache and other symptoms of hyperviscosity

Easy bruising

Postoperative bleeding

LABORATORY FINDINGS

A. Screening Procedures

Test	Patient's Result	Normal Range
Prothrombin time	Abnormal	10–12 seconds
APTT	Abnormal	<42 seconds
Platelet count	Normal or abnormal	130,000–400,000/μl
Bleeding time	Abnormal	1–8 minutes

B. Confirmatory Procedures

Thrombin time	Abnormal	<24 seconds
Mixing thrombin time	Abnormal	<24 seconds

PATHOPHYSIOLOGY OF BLEEDING IN IMMUNOPROLIFERATIVE DISORDERS

Hyperviscosity syndrome
Qualitative and quantitative abnormalities of platelets
Inhibitors (specific and nonspecific)
Disseminated intravascular coagulation
Isolated deficiency of factor X in amyloidosis

TREATMENT

Plasmapheresis for immediate relief of bleeding
Manage underlying malignant process with chemotherapy and appropriate supportive therapy

frequently present with mucous membrane bleeding in addition to other complaints, such as severe headache. The treatment of choice for patients with hyperviscosity syndrome is plasmapheresis.

Hemorrhagic abnormalities associated with lymphoproliferative disorders are frequently multifactorial in origin. The most frequent causes are thrombocytopenia and acquired qualitative abnormalities of platelets. In addition, circulating inhibitors are frequently seen as in the hyperviscosity syndrome and rarely acquired factor deficiency such as isolated factor X deficiency in primary systemic amyloidosis.

Hemorrhagic manifestations are relatively common, having been reported in 15% of patients with IgG myeloma and in 38% of those with IgA myeloma or Waldenström's macroglobulinemia. Platelet abnormalities are the most common cause of bleeding, accounting for hemorrhagic manifestations in 25% to 60% of patients. Qualitative problems of platelet function are relatively common and have been attributed to coating of the mucopolysaccharide surfaces of platelets with abnormal protein. Of the various screening tests of platelet function, the bleeding time and platelet retention procedure correlate most closely with clinically serious bleeding.

This patient had an inhibitor in his plasma. Of the various inhibitors encountered in lymphoproliferative disorders, the most common is the nonspecific inhibitor of fibrin monomer polymerization. In the older literature, this inhibitor was frequently referred to as antithrombin V. The thrombin time is prolonged due to interference with fibrin monomer polymerization. Also, the reptilase time is abnormal. Fibrin monomer inhibitor is seen in 14% to 71% of patients with IgG myeloma. However, this inhibitor is not correlated with clinical hemorrhage.

In addition to the nonspecific inhibitor, specific inhibitors of factor VIII have been described in Waldenström's macroglobulinemia and IgA myeloma. Patients with these diseases have bleeding problems directly related to the inhibitor.

Disseminated intravascular coagulation has also been described in patients with immunoproliferative disorders. Fifty percent of patients with myeloma have elevated levels of fibrin split products; thus, chronic disseminated intravascular coagulation is another mechanism that would account for decreased levels of coagulation factors in such patients.

Hyperviscosity syndrome frequently is manifest by bleeding from mucous membranes and oozing after minor surgical procedures. The pathophysiologic basis of the hemorrhagic problems in such patients is not known, although expansion of the plasma volume, disruption of small vessels and local hypoxia have been suggested as possible mechanisms. In addition, many such patients have qualitative abnormalities of platelet function.

Clinical Picture. As has been discussed above, such patients present with a clinical picture much like that of abnormalities of primary hemostasis. There is frequently mucous membrane bleeding coupled with the other findings seen in hyperviscosity syndrome.

Treatment. The treatment of choice for the immediate problem of mucous membrane bleeding is plasmapheresis. Emergency plasmapheresis is best accomplished with an intermittent-flow or continuous-flow blood cell separator, although standard centrifugation techniques with plasmapheresis packs can also be used. In some instances, 6 to 8 liters of plasma may have to be removed during the first 2 to 4 days; consequently, red cell transfusion and/or volume replacement may be required.

In addition to plasmapheresis, the underlying disease must be managed with chemotherapy. Chemotherapy usually involves alkylating agents and, in some instances, corticosteroids and vinca alkaloids.

Bibliography

Hurley R, Shaw S: Observations on the haemorrhagic diathesis in multiple myelomas. *Postgrad Med J* 39:480–483, 1963.

Lackner H: Hemostatic abnormalities associated with dysproteinemias. *Semin Hematol* 10:125–133, 1973.

McPherson RA, Onstad JW, Ugoretz RJ, et al: Coagulopathy in amyloidosis: Combined deficiency of factors IX and X. *Amer J Hematol* 3:225–235, 1977.

Pechet L, Kastrul JJ: Amyloidosis associated with factor X (Stuart) deficiency. *Ann Intern Med* 61:316–321, 1964.

Perkins HA, Mackenzie MR, Fudenberg HH: Hemostatic defects in dysproteinemias. *Blood* 35:695–698, 1970.

Stone WJ, Latos DI, Lankford PG, et al: Chronic peritoneal dialysis in a patient with primary amyloidosis, renal failure, and factor X deficiency. *South Med J* 71:764–767, 1978.

Triplett DA, Harms CS, Bang NU, et al: Mechanism of acquired factor X deficiency in primary amyloidosis. (Abstract) *Blood* (Suppl) 50:285, 1977.

CASE
42

PATIENT: 68-year-old woman

CHIEF COMPLAINT: This patient had bloody diarrhea and had suffered from abdominal cramps and bloating 3 days before admission. She had also noticed that dark ecchymoses appeared spontaneously over the arms and legs. In addition, the patient had noted a gradual onset of weakness and "easy bruising" over the preceding 6 months.

MEDICAL HISTORY: A diagnosis of osteoarthritis had been made 10 years before the patient's present illness.

FAMILY HISTORY: No history of hemostatic abnormalities

DRUG HISTORY: The patient had taken Indocin (indomethacin).

PHYSICAL EXAMINATION: There were several large ecchymoses over the arms and legs. Heart rate, pulse and blood pressure were within normal limits. The liver was palpable approximately 4 cm below the right costal margin, but the spleen was not palpable.

Laboratory Results

A. Screening Procedures

	Patient	Normal
Prothrombin time	19 seconds	10–12 seconds
APTT	83 seconds	<42 seconds
Platelet count	157,000/μl	130,000–400,000/μl
Bleeding time	5 minutes	1–8 minutes

Additional admitting laboratory results included

	Patient	Normal
Hemoglobin level	10.7 g/dl	12–16 g/dl
White cell count	8×10^9/liter	$4.8–10.8 \times 10^9$/liter
Platelet count	157×10^9/liter	$200–450 \times 10^9$/liter
Hematocrit	31.8%	37% to 47%
Alkaline phosphatase	220 units/ml	30–85 units/ml
Lactate dehydrogenase	190 units/ml	60–100 units/ml
Serum glutamic-oxaloacetic transaminase	40 units/ml	10–110 units/ml

HOSPITAL COURSE: After admission, the patient continued to have gastrointestinal bleeding. She was given vitamin K; however, the prothrombin time and the activated partial thromboplastin time (APTT) remained prolonged. The patient underwent sigmoidoscopy, and a rectal biopsy specimen was obtained.

Questions

1. Why was a rectal biopsy performed?
2. Would use of special staining techniques on the rectal biopsy specimen be indicated?
3. Why was there no response of the APTT or the prothrombin time to administration of vitamin K?
4. What additional coagulation studies are indicated?

Laboratory Results

B. Confirmatory Procedures

	Patient	Normal
APTT (50% patient plasma/ 50% pooled normal plasma)	40 seconds	<42 seconds
Prothrombin time (50% patient plasma/50% pooled normal plasma)	12 seconds	10–12 seconds
Stypven time	24 seconds	6–10 seconds
Factor X activity	5%	50% to 150%

The rectal biopsy specimen was found to contain amyloid after it had been stained with Congo red.

DIAGNOSIS: Acquired deficiency of factor X in association with primary systemic amyloidosis

Discussion

Isolated deficiency of factor X is not necessarily a congenital abnormality. Acquired deficiency of factor X has been described in a number of cases of primary systemic amyloidosis. Patients with an acquired deficiency may have hemorrhagic complications superimposed on the clinical manifestations of amyloidosis. Recently, acquired deficiency of factors X and IX has been reported in systemic amyloidosis.

Patients with an acquired deficiency of factor X do not have circulating inhibitors of coagulation factors. All such patients are refractory to treatment with vitamin K

ACQUIRED DEFICIENCY OF FACTOR X IN ASSOCIATION WITH PRIMARY SYSTEMIC AMYLOIDOSIS

CLINICAL PICTURE

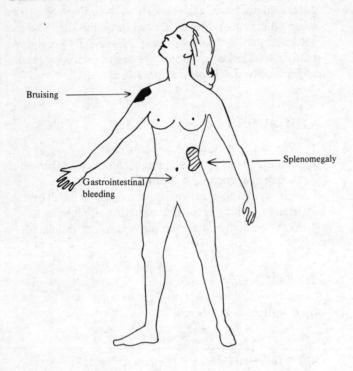

Bruising

Gastrointestinal bleeding

Splenomegaly

PATHOPHYSIOLOGIC BASIS OF ACQUIRED FACTOR X DEFICIENCY

Selective adsorption of circulating factor X to amyloid fibrils

LABORATORY FINDINGS

A. Screening Procedures

Test	Patient's Result	Normal Range
Prothrombin time	Abnormal	10–12 seconds
APTT	Abnormal	<42 seconds
Platelet count	Normal	130,000–400,000/μl
Bleeding time	Normal	1–8 minutes

B. Confirmatory Procedures

Mixing APTT	Normal	<42 seconds
Mixing prothrombin time	Normal	10–12 seconds
Stypven time	Abnormal	6–10 seconds
Factor X activity	Abnormal	50% to 150%
Biopsy	Positive for amyloid	

TREATMENT

Will *not* respond to fresh-frozen plasma or prothrombin complex concentrates
Splenectomy
?Corticosteroids

or fresh-frozen plasma. Treatment with prothrombin complex concentrates (factors II, VII, IX and X) has also been ineffective.

Isolated deficiency of factor X in patients with amyloidosis is apparently due to specific adsorption of factor X to amyloid fibrils. Thus, it would appear that amyloid deposits in some patients may be exposed to circulating blood in the microvasculature or in the open circulation of the spleen; this mechanism would account for the rapid removal of factor X from plasma and immobilization on amyloid deposits. Recently, an immunoperoxidase technique has been used to demonstrate factor X directly in formalin-fixed and paraffin-embedded tissue. Removal of an enlarged spleen infiltrated with amyloid improved the deficiency of factor X in a single patient.

Acquired deficiency of factor X has also been reported in association with renal adenocarcinoma, fungicide exposure and mycoplasmal pneumonia.

Bibliography

Andre MMR, Duhamel G, Vergoz D, et al: Syndrome hemorragique par deficit acquis en facteur Stuart-Prower, amylose. Maladie de Waldenstrome. *Soc Med Hop Paris* 117:41–48, 1966.

Bayer WL, Curiel DC, Szeto JLF, et al: Acquired factor X deficiency in a negro boy. *Pediatrics* 44:1007–1009, 1969.

Bernhardt B, Valletta M, Brook J, et al: Case report, amyloidosis with factor X deficiency. *Amer J Med Sci* 264:411–414, 1972.

Cordonnier D, Puglishi JC, Shaerer R, et al: Syndrome nephrotique et deficit acquis en facteur Stuart revelateurs de l'association amylose-myelome. *J Urol Nephrol* 78:760–764, 1972.

Door GJH, Ottolander EM, Perret LJ: Verworven hemorragische diathese ten gevolge van geisoleerde factor-X-devicientie. *Ned Tijdschr Geneeskd* 109:852–854, 1965.

Furie B, Greene E, Furie BC: Syndrome of acquired factor X deficiency and systemic amyloidosis: In vivo studies of the metabolic fate of factor X. *N Engl J Med* 297:81–85, 1977.

Galbraith PA, Sharma N, Parker WL, et al: Acquired factor X deficiency; altered plasma antithrombin activity and association with amyloidosis. *J Amer Med Ass* 230:1658–1660, 1974.

Greipp PR, Kyle RA, Bowie EJW: Factor X deficiency in primary amyloidosis. *N Engl J Med* 301:1050–1051, 1979.

Howell M: Acquired factor X deficiency associated with systematized amyloidosis. A report of a case. *Blood* 21:739–744, 1963.

Jacobson RJ, Sandler SG: Systemic amyloidosis associated with microangiopathic haemolytic anaemia and factor X (Stuart factor) deficiency. *S Afr Med J* 46:1634–1637, 1972.

Josso PF, Boussen M, Prou-Wartelle O, et al: Anomalies complexes de la coagulation dans deux cas de maladie de Kahler avec syndrome hemorragique. Signification du deficit en facteur Stuart au cours du myelome. *Nouv Rev Fr Hematol* 6:741–744, 1966.

Korsan-Bengsten K, Hijort P, Ygge J: Acquired factor X deficiency in a patient with amyloidosis. *Thromb Diath Haemorrh* 7:558–566, 1962.

Krause JR: Acquired factor X deficiency and amyloidosis. *Amer J Clin Pathol* 67:170–173, 1977.

McPherson RA, Onstad JW, Ugoretz RJ, et al: Coagulopathy in amyloidosis: combined deficiency of factors IX and X. *Amer J Hematol* 3:225–235, 1977.

Pechet L, Kastrull JJ: Amyloidosis associated with factor X (Stuart) deficiency. Case report. *Ann Intern Med* 61:315–318, 1964.

Peuscher FW, van Aken WG, van Mourik JA, et al: Acquired transient factor X (Stuart factor) deficiency in a patient with mycoplasma pneumonial infection. *Scand J Haematol* 23:257–264, 1979.

Stefanini N, Wiggishof CC: Stuart factor (factor X) deficiency associated with renal and adrenal insufficiency. *Ann Intern Med* 64:1285–1291, 1966.

Triplett DA, Bang NU, Harms CS, et al: Mechanism of acquired factor X deficiency in primary amyloidosis. (Abstract) *Blood* 50:285, 1977.

Wolf PL, Fujihara S: Immunoperoxidase identification of factor-X in systemic amyloid tissues formalin-fixed and paraffin-embedded. (Abstract) *Lab Invest* 44:77, 1981.

CASE
43

PATIENT: 65-year-old man

CHIEF COMPLAINT: This patient was admitted because of recurrent headache together with nonspecific feelings of fatigue and a "heavy feeling in the left upper quadrant."

MEDICAL HISTORY: The patient had been hospitalized for appendectomy at 23 years of age.

FAMILY HISTORY: There was a family history of adult-onset diabetes. Also, on the paternal side of the family, there was a history of early death from vascular disease.

DRUG HISTORY: The patient had been taking large doses of aspirin for the headaches. In addition, he admitted to a smoking habit of approximately 1½ packs per day.

PHYSICAL EXAMINATION: The patient appeared plethoric. There was congestion of the vessels of the conjunctiva. The spleen was palpable approximately four fingerbreadths below the left costal margin. There was also a trace of pitting edema over the legs.

Laboratory Results

A. Screening Procedures

	Patient	Normal
Prothrombin time	33 seconds	10–12 seconds
APTT	114 seconds	<42 seconds
Platelet count	550,000/μl	130,000–400,000/μl
Bleeding time	9 minutes and 30 seconds	1–8 minutes

Questions

1. Does this patient have an abnormality of the final common pathway of coagulation?
2. What additional laboratory procedures are indicated?
3. Are the abnormal prothrombin time and activated partial thromboplastin time (APTT) spurious results?

Laboratory Results

B. Confirmatory Procedures

The complete blood count included the following findings:

	Patient	Normal
Hemoglobin level	26.6 g/dl	14–18 g/dl
Red cell count	9.3×10^{12}/Liter	4.7–6.1×10^{12}/Liter
White cell count	12.4×10^{9}/Liter	4.8–10.8×10^{9}/Liter
Hematocrit	80.4%	42% to 52%

Oxygen saturation of hemoglobin was normal.

Examination of a peripheral blood smear revealed a few nucleated red cells and progranulocytes. A differential count showed 7% eosinophils. A bone marrow aspirate and biopsy specimen demonstrated 100% cellularity, with hyperplasia of the myeloid, erythroid and megakaryocytic series. No iron stores were seen in the bone marrow.

DIAGNOSIS: Polycythemia vera

Discussion

The abnormal prothrombin time and APTT in this patient were spurious results. A repeat sample was obtained with a correction of the volume of citrate in the blood collection system (Figure 1). When the volume of

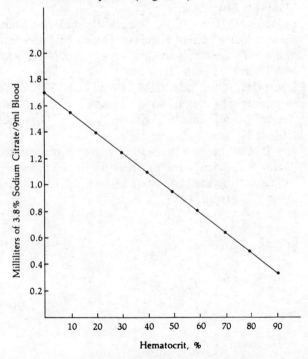

Figure 1

POLYCYTHEMIA VERA

CLINICAL PICTURE

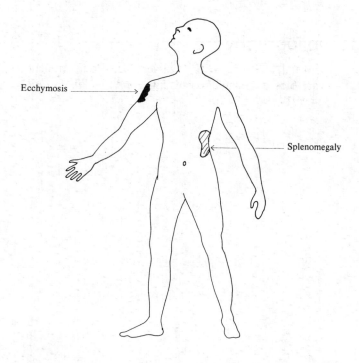

Ecchymosis

Splenomegaly

EXPLANATION OF ABNORMAL RESULTS ON HEMOSTATIC TESTS

Too much citrate for volume of plasma

LABORATORY FINDINGS

A. Screening Procedures

Test	Patient's Result	Normal Range
Prothrombin time	Abnormal*	10–12 seconds
APTT	Abnormal*	<42 seconds
Platelet count	Abnormal	130,000–400,000/μl
Bleeding time	Abnormal	1–8 minutes

B. Confirmatory Procedures

Prothrombin time and APTT corrected when citrate volume is reduced

*With standard collection tubes.

TREATMENT

Manage underlying polycythemia vera

citrate was adjusted to the elevated hematocrit, the repeat prothrombin time and APTT were found to be 12 and 35 seconds, respectively.

This case illustrates the need to be aware of spurious results, which may be due to improper handling of a sample before laboratory tests are done. Perhaps the most common problem is illustrated by this case. In patients with a markedly elevated hematocrit, the volume of citrate must be appropriately reduced to prevent spurious prolongation of the prothrombin time and APTT. It is helpful to keep in mind that such spurious results are also a problem with children, particularly newborn infants, in whom the hematocrit is typically elevated.

Patients with polycythemia vera may have clinical bleeding. The bleeding is usually from mucous membranes and is thought to be due to platelet function abnormalities or hyperviscosity.

Bibliography

Koepke JA, Rodgers JL, Olivier MJ: Preinstrument variables in coagulation testing. *Amer J Clin Pathol* 64:591–596, 1975.

CASE
44

PATIENT: 45-year-old man

CHIEF COMPLAINT: This patient presented with marked exertional angina. The angina had first appeared approximately 3 years earlier and had become progressively more frequent and severe. A number of medications had been tried; however, the patient continued to have exertional angina.

MEDICAL HISTORY: With the exception of angina, the patient had been free of physical illness. As a youngster, the patient had undergone tonsillectomy with adenoidectomy as well as left inguinal herniorrhaphy. No bleeding was associated with either surgical procedure.

FAMILY HISTORY: There was a history of diabetes mellitus on the maternal side of the family. On the paternal side, there was a history of coronary artery disease. A number of male relatives had died at young ages of myocardial infarction.

DRUG HISTORY: The patient had been taking nitroglycerin since the onset of the angina. In addition, he had taken propranolol (beta-adrenergic blocking agent). More recently, the calcium antagonist nifedipine had been added to his regimen. As noted above, none of these medications had been effective in controlling the clinical symptoms.

PHYSICAL EXAMINATION: Unremarkable

Laboratory Results

A. Screening Procedures (Preoperative)

	Patients	*Normal*
Prothrombin time	12 seconds	10–12 seconds
APTT	35 seconds	<42 seconds
Platelet count	300,000/μl	130,000–400,000/μl
Bleeding time	7 minutes	1–8 minutes

HOSPITAL COURSE: After hospitalization, the patient underwent coronary arteriography. Significant narrowing of the left anterior descending coronary artery was noted, with greater than 80% of the lumen being occluded. There was also significant narrowing of the circumflex branch of the left coronary artery. It was thought that the patient would benefit from a bypass

procedure. Before the operation was done, a panel of screening tests was performed.

A two-vessel coronary artery bypass procedure was performed with saphenous vein grafts. After the operation, there was oozing from the surgical site. Consequently, coagulation laboratory personnel were consulted.

Questions

1. What additional laboratory procedures are indicated?
2. What is the differential diagnosis in patients who bleed after cardiopulmonary bypass?

Laboratory Results

B. Confirmatory Procedures (Postoperative)

	Patient	*Normal*
Thrombin time	50 seconds	20–24 seconds
Thrombin time (protamine sulfate corrected)	42 seconds	20–24 seconds
Fibrin split products	>80 μg/ml	<10 μg/ml
Platelet count	100,000/μl	130,000–400,000/μl

DIAGNOSIS: Hyperfibrinolysis following cardiopulmonary bypass

Discussion

When bleeding occurs during or after an operation, a number of possibilities must be considered. In postoperative bleeding, it is important to make a distinction between inadequate surgical hemostasis and a hemostatic defect. The appearance of oozing from venipuncture sites together with hematuria, petechiae or some other systemic hemostatic defect suggests a primary hemostatic problem rather than local surgical bleeding.

A number of laboratory tests are helpful in establishing a diagnosis. Such tests include the thrombin time, levels of fibrin split products, protamine sulfate-corrected thrombin time, platelet count, prothrombin time and activated partial thromboplastin time (APTT). Comparison of the thrombin time and the protamine sulfate-corrected thrombin time will provide information about heparin effect, protamine excess, elevated fibrin

HYPERFIBRINOLYSIS FOLLOWING CORONARY ARTERY BYPASS

CLINICAL PICTURE

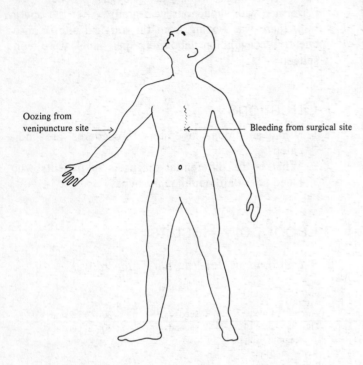

Oozing from venipuncture site →

← Bleeding from surgical site

PATHOPHYSIOLOGIC BASIS OF BLEEDING AFTER CARDIOPULMONARY BYPASS

Heparin excess
Qualitative abnormality of platelets
Thrombocytopenia
Primary fibrinolysis
Disseminated intravascular coagulation

LABORATORY FINDINGS

A. Screening Procedures (Preoperative)

Test	Patient's Result	Normal Range
Prothrombin time	Normal	10–12 seconds
APTT	Normal	<42 seconds
Platelet count	Normal	130,000–400,000/μl
Bleeding time	Normal	1–8 minutes

B. Confirmatory Procedures (Postoperative)

Test	Patient's Result	Normal Range
Thrombin time	Abnormal	<24 seconds
Thrombin time, protamine	Abnormal	<24 seconds
Fibrin split products	Abnormal	<10 mg/ml
Platelet count	100,000/μl	130,000–400,000/μl

TREATMENT

ε-Aminocaproic acid (EACA)
Monitor renal output, blood pressure and electrolyte levels

degradation products and hyperfibrinolysis. If appreciable hyperfibrinolysis occurs, the thrombin time, protamine sulfate-corrected thrombin time and levels of fibrin split products will be abnormal. Also, accelerated lysis of the clot will be observed. If excess heparin is the problem, the protamine sulfate-corrected thrombin time will be normal or nearly normal and appreciable clot lysis will not be noted.

Pathophysiologic Basis

The pathophysiologic basis of bleeding in patients who undergo cardiopulmonary bypass has been extensively debated in the literature. A number of possibilities have been documented; they include heparin excess, qualitative abnormalities of platelets associated with thrombocytopenia and primary fibrinolysis as well as disseminated intravascular coagulation.

Accelerated fibrinolysis occurs in most patients who undergo bypass operations. The fibrinolytic system may be activated via the oxygenation mechanism. The pathogenesis of the fibrinolytic activity that occurs during cardiopulmonary bypass procedures remains unclear.

Clinical Picture. Localized bleeding often is the initial clinical manifestation. However, oozing from a venipuncture site may be the first sign of a bleeding problem. Excessive bleeding tends to occur within the first 3 hours after surgical intervention. Excess bleeding may be defined as chest tube drainage that exceeds 600 ml in an adult within the first 8 hours after open-heart surgery.

Treatment. In patients in whom bleeding appears to be related to excessive fibrinolysis, as would seem to be the case in this patient, administration of ε-aminocaproic acid is indicated. The usual dose is 5 to 10 g given intravenously, followed by a dosage of 1 to 2 g per hour until the bleeding ceases or slows. It should be emphasized that the use of ε-aminocaproic acid may be associated with ventricular arrhythmia, hypotension and hypokalemia. Consequently, during intravenous administration of ε-aminocaproic acid, renal output, blood pressure and electrolyte levels should be monitored.

Bibliography

Bachmann F, McKenna R, Cole ER, et al: The hemostatic mechanism after open heart surgery: I. Studies on plasma coagulation factors and fibrinolysis in 512 patients after extra-corporeal circulation. *J Thorac Cardiovasc Surg* 70:76–81, 1975.

Bachmann F, McKenna R, Whittaker B, et al: The hemostatic mechanism after open heart surgery: II. Frequency of abnormal platelet functions during and after extra-corporeal circulation. *J Thorac Cardiovasc Surg* 70:298–302, 1975.

Bick RL: Alterations of hemostasis associated with cardiopulmonary bypass: Pathophysiology, prevention, diagnosis, and management. *Semin Thromb Hemostasis* 3:59–82, 1976. (Review article)

Fekete LF, Bick RL: Laboratory modalities for assessing hemostasis during cardiopulmonary bypass. *Semin Thromb Hemostasis* 3:83–87, 1976.

Milam JD, Austin SF, Martin RF, et al: Alteration of coagulation and selected clinical chemistry parameters in patients undergoing open heart surgery without transfusions. *Amer J Clin Pathol* 76:155–162, 1981.

Soloway HB, et al: Differentiation of bleeding diatheses which occur following protamine correction of heparin anticoagulation. *Amer J Clin Pathol* 59:188–192, 1973.

CASE
45

PATIENT: 48-year-old man

CHIEF COMPLAINT: This patient presented to the emergency room with severe right-sided chest pain together with pain and tenderness of the calf and lower portion of the thigh of the left leg.

MEDICAL HISTORY: The patient had been hospitalized at 8 years of age because of acute appendicitis and at 22 years of age because of viral hepatitis.

FAMILY HISTORY: Noncontributory

DRUG HISTORY: The patient had taken aspirin for several days before hospitalization in an attempt to alleviate the pain in the left leg.

PHYSICAL EXAMINATION: The left calf was obviously swollen and tender, and Homans' sign was present. In addition, the diameter of the lower portion of the left thigh was appreciably larger than the diameter of the corresponding portion of the right thigh. There also were physical findings suggestive of a pulmonary embolus.

Laboratory Results

A. Screening Procedures

	Patient	Normal
Prothrombin time	12 seconds	10–12 seconds
APTT	36 seconds	<42 seconds
Platelet count	450,000/μl	130,000–400,000/μl
Bleeding time	9 minutes	1–8 minutes

HOSPITAL COURSE: A pulmonary angiogram revealed a large embolus occluding the right pulmonary artery.

SUBSEQUENT HOSPITAL COURSE: Because the x-ray studies and angiographic studies indicated a massive pulmonary embolus, streptokinase therapy was begun. A loading dose of 250,000 units of streptokinase was given over 30 minutes, which was followed by 100,000 units per hour. The intention was to continue this therapy for 48 to 72 hours. However, approximately 36 hours after this therapy had been started, a large hematoma was noted over the right inguinal area. Consequently, streptokinase was stopped, and anticoagulation with heparin was instituted.

Questions

1. What is the most likely explanation for the hematoma in the right inguinal area?
2. What laboratory tests should be obtained?
3. What are the contraindications to streptokinase therapy?

Laboratory Results

B. Confirmatory Procedures

Coagulation studies obtained at the time of discontinuing streptokinase:

	Patient	Normal
Prothrombin time	21 seconds	10–12 seconds
APTT	90 seconds	<42 seconds
Thrombin time	100 seconds	<24 seconds
Fibrinogen (clottable)	30 mg/dl	170–410 mg/dl
Fibrin split products	>40 μg/ml	<10 μg/ml

DIAGNOSIS: Hematoma formation in association with streptokinase therapy

Discussion

Administration of fibrinolytic agents has been associated with hemorrhagic complications; consequently, many clinicians hesitate to use this form of therapy, particularly if they have no experience with it. This case illustrates a relatively common problem in patients who are receiving streptokinase. The hematoma resulted from bleeding at the site of an arterial puncture for blood gas analysis. Appropriate orders for applying pressure to the arterial puncture site were not followed; consequently, there was serious bleeding at the puncture site with formation of a large hematoma. Special care must be exercised for patients receiving streptokinase therapy to present such side effects. Sampling for blood gas analysis should be minimized; if sampling is necessary, pressure should be applied for an appropriate period after the arterial puncture is done.

Streptokinase has been approved by the Food and Drug Administration for use in patients with massive pulmonary emboli and in those with extensive deep-vein thrombosis and occlusion of arteriovenous cannulas. The standard dose is similar to the dose that was used in this patient. A number of laboratory procedures have been used to monitor streptokinase therapy; the most widely

HEMATOMA FORMATION IN ASSOCIATION WITH STREPTOKINASE THERAPY

CLINICAL PICTURE

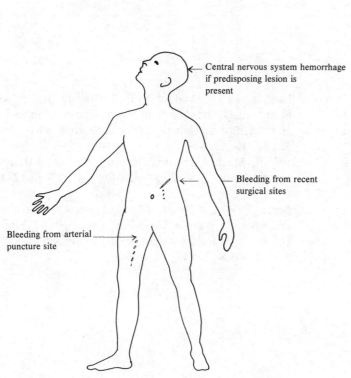

Central nervous system hemorrhage if predisposing lesion is present

Bleeding from recent surgical sites

Bleeding from arterial puncture site

MECHANISM OF ACTION OF STREPTOKINASE

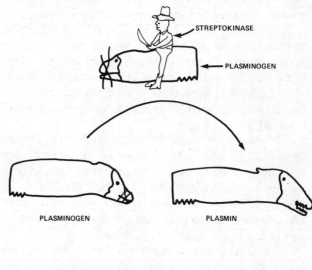

STREPTOKINASE

PLASMINOGEN

PLASMINOGEN   PLASMIN

LABORATORY FINDINGS

A. Screening Procedures

Test	Patient's Result	Normal Range
Prothrombin time	Normal	10–12 seconds
APTT	Normal	<42 seconds
Platelet count	Normal	130,000–400,000/μl
Bleeding time	Abnormal	1–8 minutes

B. Confirmatory Procedures

Test	Result	Normal Range
Thrombin time	Abnormal	<24 seconds
Fibrinogen	Abnormal	170–410 mg/dl
Fibrin split products	Abnormal	<10 μg/ml

TREATMENT

Discontinue streptokinase
Administer fresh-frozen plasma if necessary
ε-Aminocaproic acid (EACA) may be required in some cases

used test is the thrombin time. Typically, the thrombin time is prolonged twofold to sixfold over the baseline value. Thus, this patient's thrombin time was appropriate for adequate thrombolytic therapy; the complication arose because of unfamiliarity with precautions needed in patients receiving streptokinase.

In patients receiving fibrinolytic therapy, there is a significant risk for bleeding, particularly if a patient is subjected to invasive procedures or trauma. Absolute contraindications to thrombolytic therapy include surgical intervention in the preceding 2 weeks, cardiopulmonary resuscitation, percutaneous biopsy, central nervous system lesions, recent stroke and recent delivery. Relative contraindications include mitral valve disease with atrial fibrillation, hypertension, subacute bacterial endocarditis, mucous membrane lesions and recent bleeding from any site.

It should be stressed that thrombolytic therapy should not be administered when any other antithrombotic agent is being used. This patient had been taking aspirin immediately before hospitalization, and his baseline bleeding time was slightly prolonged. Thus, impairment of platelet function may have contributed in part to the hemorrhagic complications.

An area of growing interest in thrombolytic therapy is direct infusion of such agents in the coronary arteries of patients with acute myocardial infarction. In this situation, a lower dose of streptokinase is used (2000 to 8000 units per minute). Typically, an occluded vessel may be reperfused within 30 to 60 minutes in approximately 80% of patients. Vascular patency is reestablished within 3 to 6 hours of the onset of symptoms, and there is increasing evidence that ischemic myocardium may be preserved. Because low doses of streptokinase are used, there is little risk for systemic hemorrhage in such patients.

Bibliography

Albrechtsson U, Anderson J, Einarsson E, et al: Streptokinase treatment of deep venous thrombosis and the post-thrombotic syndrome. *Arch Surg* 116: 33–38, 1981.

Bell WR, Meek AG: Guidelines for the use of thrombolytic agents. *N Engl J Med* 301:1266–1271, 1979.

Sharma GVRK, Burleson VA, Sasahara AA: Effect of thrombolytic therapy on pulmonary-capillary blood volume in patients with pulmonary embolism. *N Engl J Med* 303:842–847, 1980.

CASE
46

PATIENT: 23-year-old man

CHIEF COMPLAINT: This patient was seen in the office of an orthopedic surgeon. He had injured his left knee while playing basketball. The injury had resulted in severe swelling and discoloration of the knee; consequently, the patient sought medical attention. The knee was aspirated, and a large amount of bloody synovial fluid was evacuated. Because of the massive swelling, a complete physical examination was difficult to perform. The orthopedic surgeon believed that there may have been internal derangement of the knee; therefore, the patient was admitted for arthroscopic examination under anesthesia. Before this procedure was performed, a hemostatic evaluation was requested.

MEDICAL HISTORY: At birth, the patient was covered with petechiae; however, a platelet count performed at that time was within normal limits. As a child, the patient had frequent problems with epistaxis, which often lasted as long as 2 to 3 days, and spontaneous bruising. The patient's mother had noted that petechiae appeared spontaneously over his legs and, occasionally, over his trunk and arms. When 5 years of age, the patient had fallen and injured his abdomen, and the injury had necessitated hospitalization. He had been diagnosed as having "internal bleeding" and had been transferred to a hospital in Chicago. During that hospitalization, a number of studies had been performed, and the patient had been diagnosed as being a "bleeder."

As he grew older, the patient had noticed that the epistaxis and spontaneous petechiae were occurring less frequently. He engaged in strenuous activity, including basketball and softball. When playing basketball, he would notice swelling of the knees; consequently, he would wrap them with Ace bandages. This treatment was helpful, although the patient had continued to notice swelling and many petechiae immediately adjacent to the Ace bandages. While the patient was playing softball, his right elbow frequently became swollen and discolored. He had also noticed oozing of blood in the gingival area after tooth brushing. There had also been prolonged bleeding from superficial cuts.

In 1973, the patient had undergone appendectomy with minimal bleeding problems.

FAMILY HISTORY: The patient had one brother and three sisters, all of whom were living and well and had no history of bleeding problems. A maternal grandfather had difficulties with epistaxis, and a maternal female cousin had also been diagnosed as being a "bleeder."

DRUG HISTORY: The patient was taking vitamin K regularly and had been cautioned to avoid aspirin.

PHYSICAL EXAMINATION: Several petechiae were noted over the arms, and gingival bleeding was seen in the area of the right lower molars.

Laboratory Results

A. Screening Procedures

	Patient	Normal
Prothrombin time	11 seconds	10–12 seconds
APTT	35 seconds	<42 seconds
Platelet count	200,000/μl	130,000–400,000/μl
Bleeding time	>15 minutes	1–8 minutes

Questions

1. Does this patient have an abnormality of primary hemostasis or an abnormality of secondary hemostasis?
2. What additional laboratory procedures are indicated?
3. Is the family history helpful in establishing the diagnosis?

Laboratory Results

B. Confirmatory Procedures

	Patient	Normal
Factor VIII:C	100%	50% to 150%
Factor R:Ag	120%	50% to 150%
Factor R:RCo	100%	50% to 150%

Platelet Aggregation Studies (see platelet aggregation tracings)

	Patient	Normal
ADP	No response (high and low concentrations)	Biphasic aggregation
Collagen	Minimal response	Full-range monophasic aggregation
Epinephrine	No response	Biphasic aggregation
Ristocetin	Variable response with prolonged stirring	Full-range monophasic agglutination or biphasic agglutination
Platelet retention (glass-bead column)	0	40% to 90%
Clot retraction	Absent	Present

GLANZMANN'S THROMBASTHENIA

CLINICAL PICTURE

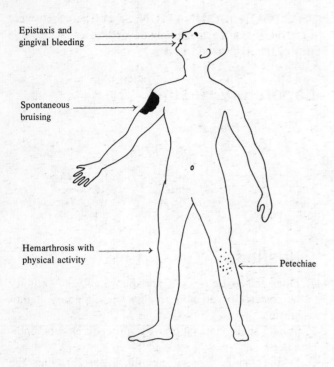

Epistaxis and gingival bleeding

Spontaneous bruising

Hemarthrosis with physical activity

Petechiae

Pattern of inheritance: Autosomal recessive

PATHOPHYSIOLOGIC BASIS

Decreased levels of membrane glycoproteins IIb and IIIa
Stimulated platelets do not bind fibrinogen

LABORATORY FINDINGS

A. Screening Procedures

Test	Patient's Result	Normal Range
Prothrombin time	Normal	10–12 seconds
APTT	Normal	<42 seconds
Platelet count	Normal	130,000–400,000/μl
Bleeding time	Abnormal	1–8 minutes

B. Confirmatory Procedures

Factor VIII:C	Normal	50% to 150%
Factor VIII R:Ag	Normal	50% to 150%
Factor VIII R:RCo	Normal	50% to 150%
Platelet aggregation	See tracings	
Clot retraction	Abnormal	Present
Platelet retention	0	40% to 90%

TREATMENT

Judicious use of platelet concentrates
Avoidance of aspirin containing compounds

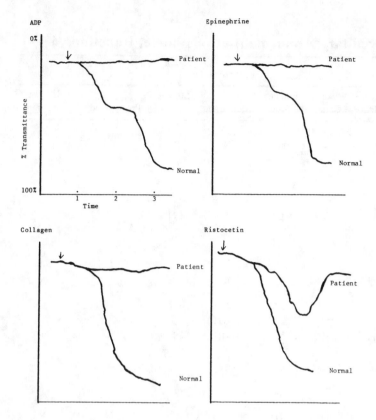

DIAGNOSIS: Glanzmann's thrombasthenia

Discussion

This case is a classical example of an abnormality of primary hemostasis. The patient had a lifelong history of hemostatic difficulty, characterized by easy bruising, spontaneous formation of petechiae and mucous membrane bleeding.

In a patient with such a history, it is necessary to evaluate the factor VIII molecule and platelet function. In this case, all values for factor VIII were within normal limits, thus ruling out the possiblity of von Willebrand's disease. However, results of platelet aggregation studies were strikingly abnormal, with no response to adenosine diphosphate, epinephrine or collagen. These findings, in addition to an absence of clot retraction and essentially no platelet retention in a glass-bead column, are virtually pathognomonic of Glanzmann's thrombasthenia.

The family history in this case is not helpful, although it is suggestive of an autosomal recessive pattern of inheritance.

Biochemical Aspects. Platelets from patients with Glanzmann's thrombasthenia have decreased amounts of the membrane glycoproteins IIb and IIIa. It has also been demonstrated that the level of the platelet-specific alloantigen PL[Al] is decreased in patients with Glanzmann's thrombasthenia. The PL[Al] antigenic marker is associated with membrane glycoprotein IIIa.

The relationship between membrane glycoproteins and functional abnormalities of aggregation and clot retraction is currently unknown. Platelets from patients with Glanzmann's thrombasthenia bind thrombin and adenosine diphosphate normally. In addition, the shape change that is induced by thrombin and adenosine diphosphate is normal. However, platelets from such patients do not bind fibrinogen when they are stimulated with adenosine diphosphate or epinephrine.

Clinical Picture. Glanzmann's thrombasthenia is inherited in an autosomal recessive manner. The hemorrhagic symptoms vary from mild bruising to severe bleeding beginning in infancy. Heterozygous carriers appear to be completely asymptomatic, although selected techniques may demonstrate partial deficiency of membrane glycoproteins.

Major symptoms include bruising, epistaxis, mucous membrane bleeding and, occasionally, petechiae. Recurrent hemarthrosis is uncommon, distinguishing this abnormality of primary hemostasis from abnormalities of secondary hemostasis, such as hemophilia A.

Symptoms become less severe as affected persons grow older; some individuals become virtually asymptomatic during puberty of shortly thereafter.

The differential diagnosis includes disorders of platelet function and von Willebrand's disease (Table 1). A lack of clot retraction in the presence of a normal platelet count is virtually pathognomonic of Glanzmann's thrombasthenia. Other diagnostic possibilities that must be ruled out include gray platelet syndrome and storage pool disease. In a few instances, congenital afibrinogenemia may be a possibility in the differential diagnosis at the time of the initial evaluation.

Treatment. In female patients, menorrhagia may be controlled with oral contraceptives. Platelet transfusions are necessary for managing serious bleeding episodes; however, platelets must be administered judiciously because antibodies to normal platelets often develop, making patients refractory to further transfusions.

Table 1
Clinical and Laboratory Features of Hereditary Abnormalities of Platelet Function*,†

	Platelet Tests						
	Hereditary	Platelet Count	Platelet Size	Membrane	Storage Pool	Prostaglandin	Release Reaction
Abnormalities of Adhesion							
von Willebrand's disease	AD	N	N	N	N	N	N
Bernard-Soulier syndrome	AR	D	L	D-GP I	N	N	N
Ehlers-Danlos syndrome	AD	N	L	N	N	?	D
Abnormalities of Primary Aggregation							
Glanzmann's thromboasthenia	AR	N	N	(D–GP) II–III	N	N	N
Essential athrombia	AR	N	N	?	N	N	N
Abnormalities of Secondary Aggregation							
Storage pool disease	AD–V	N	N	N	D	N	D
Wiskott-Aldrich syndrome	SL	D	Sm	N	D	?	N
Hermansky-Pudlak syndrome	AR	N	N	N	D	N	N

		Platelet Function Tests								
Bleeding Time	Platelet Retention	ADP Aggregation	Epinephrine Aggregation	Collagen Aggregation	Ristocetin Agglutination	Platelet Factor 3	Clot Retraction	Baumgartner Adhesion	Baumgartner Aggregation	Remarks
P	D	N	N	N	D	N	N	D	N	Factor VIII/VWF decreased, characteristic transfusion response
P	D	N	N	N	D	N	N	D	N	Membrane glycoprotein I decreased, sialic acid decreased
P	N	D 2nd	D 2nd	D	N	D	N	?	?	"Cigarette paper" scars, abnormal elastic tissue
P	D	A	A	A	D–N	D	A	N	A	Membrane glycoproteins IIb and III$_a$ decreased, sialic acid and fibrinogen decreased
P	D	A	A	A	N	D	D	N	A	Detectable clot retraction
P	D	D 2nd	D 2nd	D	V	D	N	N	D	Absence of dense bodies on electron microscopy
P	D	D 2nd	D 2nd	D	N	D	N	N	D	Eczema, decreased IgM, infection
P	D	D 2nd	D 2nd	D	N	V	N	N	D	Albinism, ceroid storage cells in bone marrow

(continued)

Table 1 *(continued)*
Clinical and Laboratory Features of Hereditary Abnormalities of Platelet Function*,†

				Platelet Tests			
	Hereditary	Platelet Count	Platelet Size	Membrane	Storage Pool	Prostaglandin	Release Reaction
Thrombocytopenia-absent radius syndrome	AR	D	N	N	D	N	N
Chédiak-Higashi syndrome	AR	N	N	N	D	N	N
"Aspirin-like" defect Deficiency of cyclooxygenase	?	N	N	N	N	D	D
Deficiency of thromboxane synthesis	?	N	N	N	N	D	D
Other "release" abnormalities May-Hegglin anomaly	AD	D–N	L	?	N–D	?	N
Glycogen storage disease, type I	AR	N	N	?	?	?	N
Other connective tissue disorders	AR	N	L	N	N	?	D
Deficiency of platelet factor 3	AR	N	N	N	N	N	N
Afibrinogenemia	AR	N	N	N	N	N	D*
Deficiency of factor VIII, release abnormality	V	N–D	N	?	D	?	?
Macrothrombocytopenia, nephritis, deafness	AD	D	L	D–S	?	?	?
Gray platelet syndrome	?	D	L	N	N	N	N

Bibliography

Caen JP: Glanzmann's thrombasthenia. *Clin Haematol* 1:383–392, 1972.

Caen JP, Castaldi PA, Leclere JC, et al: Congenital bleeding disorders with long bleeding time and normal platelet count. I. Glanzmann's thrombasthenia (report of 15 patients). *Amer J Med* 41:4–26, 1966.

Gerrard JM, Schollmeyer JV, Phillips DR, et al: Alpha actinin deficiency in thrombasthenia: Possible identity of alpha-actinin and glycoprotein III. *Amer J Pathol* 94:509–528, 1979.

Hagen I, Solum NO: Further studies on the protein composition and surface structure of normal platelets from patients with Glanzmann's thrombasthenia and Bernard-Soulier syndrome. *Thromb Res* 13(5):845–855, 1978.

Hardisty RM: Hereditary disorders of platelet function. *Clin Haematol* 12:153–173, 1983.

Hardisty RM, Dormandy KM, Hutton RA: Thrombasthenia: Studies on three cases. *Brit J Haematol* 10:371–387, 1964.

Nurden AT, Caen JP: An abnormal glycoprotein in three cases of Glanzmann's thrombasthenia. *Brit J Haematol* 28:253–260, 1974.

		Platelet Function Tests								
Bleeding Time	Platelet Retention	ADP Aggregation	Epinephrine Aggregation	Collagen Aggregation	Ristocetin Agglutination	Platelet Factor 3	Clot Retraction	Baumgartner Adhesion	Baumgartner Aggregation	Remarks
P	D	D 2nd	D 2nd	D	N	V	N	N	D	Multiple congenital abnormalities
N–P	D	D 2nd	D 2nd	D	N	V	N	N	D	Albinism, giant granules in leukocytes
N–P	D	D 2nd	D 2nd	D	N	V	N	N	D	Mimics "aspirin-like" defect
N–P	D	D 2nd	D 2nd	D	N	V	N	N	D	
P	?	N	?	D	N	N	N	?	?	Döhle's bodies in granulocytes
P	D	D 2nd	D 2nd	D	N	N	N	?	?	Defect corrected by management of metabolic disorder
P	N	D 2nd	D 2nd	D	N	?	N	?	?	Marfan's syndrome, pseudoxanthoma, osteogenesis imperfecta, etc.
N–P	N	N	N	N	N	D	N	N	N	Rare abnormality
P	D	D*	D*	D*	N	D*	N	D*	D*	Corrected by fibrinogen*
P	D	D 2nd	D 2nd	D	N	D	N	N	D	May mimic von Willebrand's disease
P	D	D	D	D	N	D	N	?	?	Foam cells in renal interstitial tissue
P	N	N	N	N	N	?	N	?	?	

*Abbreviations: AD, autosomal dominant; AR, autosomal recessive; SL, sex-linked recessive; V, variable; N, normal; D, decreased; P, prolonged, L, large; GP, glycoprotein; S, sialic acid; A, absent, ?, not known; Sm, small.

†From Triplett DA: Thrombosis and hemostasis check sample program Am Soc Clin Path Chicago, Ill.

CASE
47

PATIENT: 21-year-old man

CHIEF COMPLAINT: This patient was admitted for evaluation of a hemostatic abnormality. He had a lifelong history of easy bruising and abnormal bleeding after dental extractions.

MEDICAL HISTORY: The patient had not been circumcised at birth.

FAMILY HISTORY: There was a possibility of consanguinity.

DRUG HISTORY: No medication

PHYSICAL EXAMINATION: Several large ecchymoses were noted, over the arms and legs.

Laboratory Results

A. Screening Procedures

	Patient	Normal
Prothrombin time	12 seconds	10–12 seconds
APTT	35 seconds	<42 seconds
Platelet count	90,000/μl	130,000–400,000/μl
Bleeding time	>15 minutes	1–8 minutes

Questions

1. What additional laboratory procedures are indicated?
2. Is the family history of possible consanguinity helpful in establishing a diagnosis?

Laboratory Results

B. Confirmatory Procedures

	Patient	Normal
Factor VIII:C	95%	50% to 150%
Factor VIII R:Ag	100%	50% to 150%
Factor VIII R:RCo	95%	50% to 150%

Platelet Aggregation Studies (see platelet aggregation tracings, Figure 1)

	Patient	Normal
Adenosine diphosphate	Biphasic response	Biphasic aggregation
Collagen	Full-range monophasic response	Full-range monophasic aggregation
Epinephrine	Biphasic response	Biphasic aggregation
Ristocetin	Absent	Full-range monophasic agglutination or biphasic agglutination
Platelet retention (glass-bead column)	20%	40% to 90%

A peripheral blood smear was found to contain large platelets.

DIAGNOSIS: Bernard-Soulier syndrome

Discussion

The thrombocytopenia and prolonged bleeding time in this patient raised a number of possibilities, including chronic autoimmune thrombocytopenia and Bernard-Soulier syndrome. Results of platelet aggregation studies

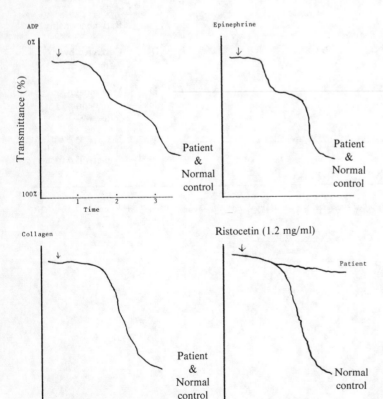

Figure 1

BERNARD-SOULIER SYNDROME

CLINICAL PICTURE

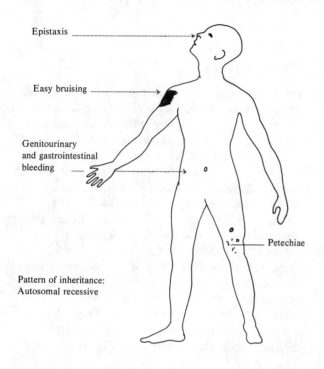

Epistaxis

Easy bruising

Genitourinary
and gastrointestinal
bleeding

Petechiae

Pattern of inheritance:
Autosomal recessive

PATHOPHYSIOLOGIC BASIS

Thrombocytopenia due to shortened life span of platelets
in the circulation
Decreased thrombin binding
Decreased adhesion to subendothelium
Failure to bind and activate factor XI
Decreased levels of glycoproteins Is and Ib
Decreased platelet binding of von Willebrand factor

LABORATORY FINDINGS

A. Screening Procedures

Test	Patient's Result	Normal Range
Prothrombin time	Normal	10–12 seconds
APTT	Normal	<42 seconds
Platelet count	Abnormal	130,000–400,000/μl
Bleeding time	Abnormal	1–8 minutes

B. Confirmatory Procedures

Factor VIII:C	Normal	50% to 150%
Factor VIII R:Ag	Normal	50% to 150%
Factor VIII R:RCo	Normal	50% to 150%
Platelet aggregation	See tracings	
Platelet retention	Abnormal	40% to 90%

TREATMENT

Platelet concentrates
Avoidance of aspirin containing compounds

confirmed the initial impression of Bernard-Soulier syndrome. There was no response to ristocetin but normal aggregation responses to adenosine diphosphate, epinephrine and collagen. A peripheral blood smear contained many large platelets.

Bernard-Soulier syndrome is a disorder that is inherited in an autosomal recessive manner. Consequently, the family history of consanguinity was helpful in establishing the diagnosis.

Biochemical Aspects. Patients with Bernard-Soulier syndrome present with a prolonged bleeding time and a decreased platelet count. Peripheral blood smears from such patients show large platelets. The platelet count ranges from 50,000/μl to nearly normal levels. Platelets often are as large as 20 μm in diameter, with coarse granularity and vacuolation. Transmission electron microscopy demonstrates no specific structural abnormality. The thrombocytopenia is presumably related to the shortened life span of circulating platelets.

Platelets from patients with Bernard-Soulier syndrome appear to exhibit a decreased response to thrombin, as demonstrated by decreased thrombin binding and decreased aggregation with low concentrations of thrombin. Typically, the platelets do not respond to ristocetin and also show diminished adhesion to aortic subendothelium in the platelet adhesion model of Baumgartner.

The level of membrane glycoproteins I_s and I_b are reduced. It appears that glycoprotein I is the membrane receptor for von Willebrand factor and that this glycoprotein therefore participates in the critical platelet-subendothelium interaction that is involved in adhesion. Apparently, glycoprotein I also contains the antigenic site for the drug-dependent antibodies that are related to sensitization to quinidine, quinine and Sedormid.

Clinical Picture. The pattern of bleeding in patients with Bernard-Soulier syndrome is similar to that in patients with other abnormalities of primary hemostasis. Clinical manifestations include purpura, epistaxis, gingival bleeding, gastrointestinal hemorrhage, hematuria, menorrhagia and easy bruising. Hemarthrosis has not been reported.

There is wide variability of clinical bleeding within a given family. No specific correlation has been found between any laboratory parameter of platelet function and bleeding symptoms.

Treatment. Management of hemorrhagic episodes involves transfusion of platelet concentrates. However, such concentrates should be used judiciously because of the possibility of platelet alloimmunization as well as the development of antibody to glycoprotein I.

Bibliography

Caen JP, Nurden AT, Jeanneau C, et al: Bernard-Soulier syndrome—A new platelet glycoprotein abnormality. Its relationship with platelet adhesion to subendothelium and with the factor VIII von Willebrand protein. *J Lab Clin Med* 87:586–596, 1976.

George JN, Reimann TA, Moake JL, et al: Bernard-Soulier disease: A study of four patients and their parents. *Brit J Haematol* 48:459–467, 1981.

Jamieson GA, Okumura T: Reduced thrombin binding and aggregation in Bernard-Soulier platelets. *J Clin Invest* 60:861–864, 1978.

Kissane JM, Cryer PE: Fever, pharyngitis and lymphadenopathy in a patient with Bernard-Soulier syndrome. *Amer J Med* 70:852–857, 1981.

Kunicki TJ, Johnson MM, Aster RH: Absence of the platelet receptor for drug-dependent antibodies in the Bernard-Soulier syndrome. *J Clin Invest* 62:716–721, 1978.

Lusher JM, Barnhardt MI: Congenital disorders affecting platelets. *Semin Thromb Hemostasis* 4:123–186, 1977.

Nurden AT, Caen JP: Specific roles for platelet surface glycoproteins in platelet function. *Nature (London)* 255:720–722, 1975.

Nurden AT, Caen JP: Further studies on glycoprotein composition of normal human, Bernard-Soulier and thrombasthenia platelets. *Thromb Haemostasis* 38:200–208, 1977.

Weiss HJ, Tschopp TB, Baumgartner HR, et al: Decreased adhesion of giant (Bernard-Soulier) platelets to subendothelium. Further implications on the role of the von Willebrand factor in hemostasis. *Amer J Med* 57:920–924, 1974.

CASE
48

PATIENT: 7-year-old boy

CHIEF COMPLAINT: This patient presented for an evaluation of easy bruising.

MEDICAL HISTORY: When the patient was 6 years of age, his mother had noticed the onset of ecchymosis, particularly over the legs. In addition, the patient had had bouts of epistaxis since 2 years of age.

   The patient had undergone tonsillectomy and circumcision without bleeding complications.

FAMILY HISTORY: No history of bleeding

DRUG HISTORY: No medication

PHYSICAL EXAMINATION: Large ecchymotic areas were noted over the legs and the trunk. There was no evidence of telangiectasia or other vascular malformation.

Laboratory Results

A. Screening Procedures

	Patient	Normal
Prothrombin time	11.2 seconds	10–12 seconds
APTT	25 seconds	<42 seconds
Platelet count	190,000/μl	130,000–400,000/μl
Bleeding time	10 minutes and 30 seconds	1–8 minutes

Questions

1. What additional laboratory procedures are indicated?
2. Do the history and physical examination suggest an abnormality of primary hemostasis or an abnormality of secondary hemostasis?

Laboratory Results

B. Confirmatory Procedures

	Patient	Normal
Factor VIII:C	>200%	50% to 150%
Factor VIII R:Ag	>200%	50% to 150%
Factor VIII R:RCo	190%	50% to 150%

Platelet Aggregation Studies (see platelet aggregation tracings, Figure 1)

	Patient	Normal
Adenosine diphosphate	Primary wave with disaggregation	Biphasic aggregation
Collagen	Prolonged lag phase with weak aggregation	Full-range monophasic aggregation
Epinephrine	Primary wave with disaggregation	Biphasic aggregation
Ristocetin	Normal response	Full-range monophasic agglutination or biphasic agglutination

   Because of the prolonged bleeding time and the abnormal results on platelet aggregation studies, lumi aggregation studies were performed. The platelet content of adenosine triphosphate was markedly decreased. Subsequently, transmission electron microscopy was undertaken, and the platelets were found to be deficient in dense bodies.

DIAGNOSIS: Hereditary storage pool disease

Discussion

This case is an example of a qualitative abnormality of platelet function. The abnormal results on platelet aggregation studies indicated an absence of the release reaction. Abnormal platelet release may be due to a deficiency of granules within platelets or an abnormality of prostaglandin synthesis. When deficiency of granules is the cause, the condition is referred to as storage pool disease; if abnormal prostaglandin synthesis is the cause, the condition is called "aspirin-like" defect.

Biochemical Aspects. In the platelet response, platelets undergo a shape change and then adhere to collagen or other components of vessel walls. After adhesion has taken place, platelets synthesize prostaglandin endoperoxides (prostaglandins G_2 and H_2) and thromboxane A_2. They then secrete the contents of several types of granule (dense bodies, alpha granules and lysosomes). It is thought that endoperoxides and thromboxane A_2 as well as secreted adenosine diphosphate have major roles in mediating the platelet response to various stimuli. The final pathway for platelet release is probably regulated by movement of calcium ions from intracellular storage sites (dense tubular system).

HEREDITARY STORAGE POOL DISEASE

CLINICAL PICTURE

Epistaxis

Easy bruising

Postoperative
bleeding

Pattern of inheritance: Varies according to case

PATHOPHYSIOLOGIC BASIS

Absence of dense bodies and storage pool of adenosine
diphosphate and triphosphate
Alpha granules may or may not be absent
Abnormal phospholipase A_2

LABORATORY FINDINGS

A. Screening Procedures

Test	Patient's Result	Normal Range
Prothrombin time	Normal	10–12 seconds
APTT	Normal	<42 seconds
Platelet count	Normal	130,000–400,000/μl
Bleeding time	Abnormal	1–8 minutes

B. Confirmatory Procedures

Factor VIII:C	Normal	50% to 150%
Factor VIII R:Ag	Normal	50% to 150%
Factor VIII R:RCo	Normal	50% to 150%
Platelet aggregation	See tracings	
Platelet granular ATP	Abnormal	Normal

TREATMENT

Platelet concentrates
Cryoprecipitate (?)
Avoid any medications that contain aspirin

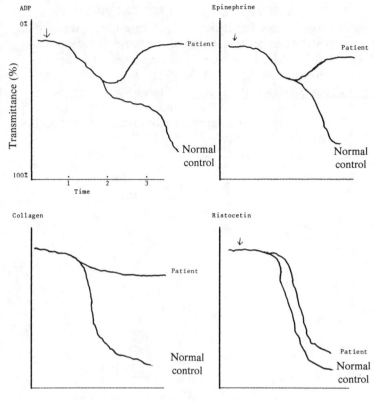

Figure 1

In addition to abnormalities of dense granules, patients with storage pool disease may have abnormal synthesis of prostaglandins and thromboxanes. It has been postulated that phospholipase A_2 is abnormal in patients with storage pool disease. Recently, evidence for a phospholipase A_2 defect has been reported in a patient with Hermansky-Pudlak syndrome.

Clinical Picture. Patients with storage pool disease present with a clinical history typical of a deficiency of primary hemostasis. Chief complaints include easy bruising, bleeding from mucous membranes and prolonged bleeding after minor cuts or surgical intervention. In female patients, abnormally heavy menstrual periods may be the most common complaint.

Treatment. Platelet transfusions usually are effective in controlling bleeding in such patients. However, transfusions should be given judiciously because of the risk for platelet alloimmunization or transmission of viral hepatitis. In one report, administration of cryoprecipitate was described as being effective in controlling bleeding in a patient with storage pool disease and albinism.

Of course, all drugs that inhibit platelet aggregation (e.g., aspirin and antihistamines) should *not* be administered to patients with storage pool disease.

Patients with storage pool disease lack or have diminished amounts of the substances stored in dense granules. They also may have deficiencies of substances stored in alpha granules and lysosomes. Typical platelet aggregation findings include an absence of the second phase of aggregation to adenosine diphosphate and epinephrine and a decreased response to collagen. The initial agglutination response to ristocetin is usually normal, but maximal agglutination (probably due to secretion of adenosine diphosphate) may be decreased.

Storage pool disease has been described in association with a number of clinical conditions, including Hermansky-Pudlak syndrome. In patients with Hermansky-Pudlak syndrome, there is oculocutaneous albinism (tyrosinase positive) and deposition of a ceroid-like pigment in the bone marrow and reticuloendothelial system.

In addition, patients with Chédiak-Higashi syndrome with storage pool disease have been reported. Other congenital disorders in which storage pool disease has been described include Wiskott-Aldrich syndrome and thrombocytopenia-absent radius (TAR) syndrome.

The diminished platelet content of adenosine diphosphate and triphosphate is due to deficiencies of granule-bound nucleotides (storage pool). The platelet content of serotonin, calcium and pyrophosphate are also decreased in patients with storage pool disease.

Bibliography

Gerritsen SM, Akkerman JW, Nijmeijer B, et al: The Hermansky-Pudlak syndrome. Evidence for a lowered 5-hydroxytryptamine content in platelets of heterozygotes. *Scand J Haematol* 18:249–256, 1977.

Gerritsen SM, Akkerman JWN, Sixma JJ: Correction of bleeding time in patients with storage pool deficiency by infusion of cryoprecipitate. *Brit J Haematol* 40:153–160, 1978.

Hermansky F, Pudlak P: Albinism associated with hemorrhagic diathesis and unusual pigmented reticular cells in the bone marrow: Report of two cases with histochemical studies. *Blood* 14:162–169, 1959.

Logan LJ, Rapaport SI, Maher I: Albinism and abnormal platelet function. *N Engl J Med* 284:1340–1345, 1971.

Lorez HP, DaPrada M, Launay JM: Fluorescence microscopy of 5-HT organelles in normal and storage pool deficient blood platelets. *Experientia* 33:823–824, 1977.

Pareti FI, Mannucci PM, Capitanio A, et al: Heterogeneity of storage pool deficiency. *Thromb Haemostasis* 38:3, 1977.

Weiss HG, Witte LD, Kaplan KL, et al: Heterogeneity in storage pool deficiency studies on granule-bound substances in 18 patients including variants deficient in α granules, platelet factor 4, β-thromboglobulin, and platelet derived growth factor. *Blood* 54:1296–1319, 1979.

White JG: Ultrastructural studies of the gray platelet syndrome. *Amer J Pathol* 95:445–462, 1979.

White JG, Gerrard JM, Rao GH, et al: Differences in platelet storage pool deficiency (SPD) of Hermansky-Pudlak syndrome (HPS) and non-albinos (NA).

Thromb Diath Haemorrh 34:360–361, 1975.

Zahavi J, Gale R, Kakkar VV: Storage pool disease of platelets in an infant with thrombocytopenic absent radii (TAR) syndrome simulating Fanconi's anemia. *Haemostasis* 10:121–133, 1981.

Zahavi J, Gale R, Sacks Z: Storage pool disease of platelets in an infant with thrombocytopenia absent radii syndrome simulating Fanconi anemia. (Abstract) *Thromb Haemostasis* 38:283, 1977.

CASE
49

PATIENT: 55-year-old man

CHIEF COMPLAINT: This patient was admitted with a diagnosis of pilonidal cyst.

MEDICAL HISTORY: The patient's medical history was suggestive of a bleeding abnormality. The patient had bled profusely after several dental extractions. However, in each instance, transfusion had not been necessary. At the time of circumcision, there had been no evidence of bleeding.

The patient also stated that he tended to bruise easily and bleed profusely after minor cuts. With the exception of dental surgery and circumcision, no surgical procedure had been performed.

FAMILY HISTORY: Several male members of the family on the maternal side had bleeding problems. In all instances, the bleeding had been associated with surgical intervention or trauma. No coagulation studies had been performed.

The patient had two sisters. One sister had a history of abnormally heavy menstrual periods.

DRUG HISTORY: No medication

PHYSICAL EXAMINATION: An oozing pilonidal cyst was noted.

HOSPITAL COURSE: The patient underwent a surgical procedure. At the time of surgical intervention, profuse bleeding was noted, and the bleeding did not respond to transfusion of 6 units of fresh-frozen plasma. After the operation had been completed, the patient continued to bleed. The following laboratory results were obtained:

Laboratory Results

A. Screening Procedures

	Patient	Normal
Prothrombin time	12 seconds	10–12 seconds
APTT	48 seconds	<42 seconds
Platelet count	160,000/μl	130,000–400,000/μl
Bleeding time	13 minutes and 30 seconds	1–8 minutes

Questions

1. What is the differential diagnosis?
2. What additional laboratory procedures are indicated?

Laboratory Results

B. Confirmatory Procedures

	Patient	Normal
Factor VIII:C	20%	50% to 150%
Factor VIII R:Ag	200%	50% to 150%
Factor VIII R:RCo	150%	50% to 150%

Platelet Aggregation Studies (see platelet aggregation tracings, Figure 1)

	Patient	Normal
Adenosine diphosphate	Primary wave with disaggregation	Biphasic aggregation
Collagen	Blunted single wave of aggregation	Full-range monophasic aggregation
Epinephrine	Primary wave with disaggregation	Biphasic aggregation
Risotocetin	Normal response	Full-range monophasic agglutination or biphasic agglutination
Platelet retention	32%	40% to 90%

Because of the prolonged bleeding time and the abnormal results on platelet aggregation studies, lumi aggregation studies were performed. The platelet content of adenosine triphosphate was within normal limits. Aspirin-treated normal platelets mixed with the patient's platelets did not correct the abnormal results on the previous platelet aggregation studies, suggesting an abnormality of prostaglandin metabolism.

DIAGNOSIS: Qualitative abnormality of platelets ("aspirin-like" defect); deficiency of factor VIII (hemophilia A), mild

Discussion

This case illustrates an interesting combination of findings. The clinical history together with the results on screening tests suggested the possibility of von Willebrand's disease. However, on further evaluation, the patient was found to have a decrease in factor VIII:C

QUALITATIVE ABNORMALITY OF PLATELETS ("ASPIRIN-LIKE" DEFECT) AND HEMOPHILIA A

CLINICAL PICTURE

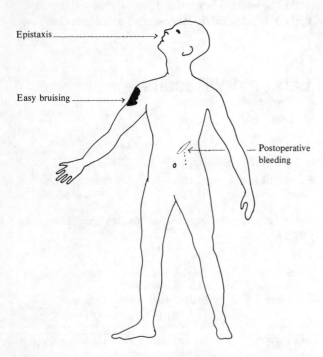

Epistaxis

Easy bruising

Postoperative bleeding

Pattern of inheritance: Hemophilia, sex linked; platelet defect, autosomal recessive

PATHOPHYSIOLOGIC BASIS

Deficiency of factor VIII:C
"Aspirin-like" defect

LABORATORY FINDINGS

A. Screening Procedures

Test	Patient's Result	Normal Range
Prothrombin time	Normal	10–12 seconds
APTT	Abnormal	<42 seconds
Platelet count	Normal	130,000–400,000/μl
Bleeding time	Abnormal	1–8 minutes

B. Confirmatory Procedures

Factor VIII C	Abnormal	50% to 150%
Factor VIII R:Ag	Normal	50% to 150%
Factor VIII R:RCo	Normal	50% to 150%
Platelet aggregation	See tracings	
Platelet ATP	Normal	Normal

TREATMENT

Cryoprecipitate
Platelet concentrates
Avoidance of aspirin containing compounds

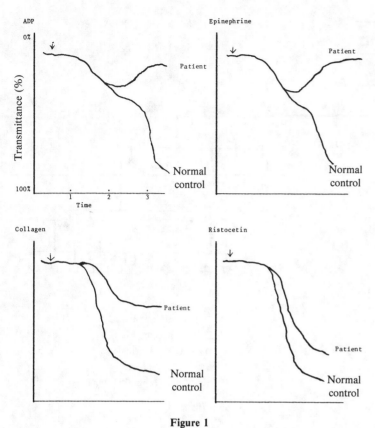

Figure 1

activity but normal levels of factor VIII R:Ag and factor VIII R:RCo. These findings were obtained after the surgical procedure, during which the patient had received fresh-frozen plasma. The patient was reevaluated later, and a similar set of values was obtained for the factor

VIII complex. Thus, the patient appeared to have mild hemophilia A. Family members on the maternal side were evaluated, and the diagnosis of mild hemophilia A was substantiated.

In addition to mild hemophilia A, there was a distinct abnormality of platelet function. The platelet aggregation response was typical of a release defect. Lumi aggregation studies demonstrated a normal platelet content of adenosine triphosphate. Mixing studies performed with aspirin-treated normal platelets and the patient's platelets demonstrated that the defect was an abnormality of prostaglandin metabolism. The various enzymes of the prostaglandin pathway were not fully evaluated in this patient.

After the evaluation had been completed, the patient was treated with cryoprecipitate and platelet concentrates, which controlled the bleeding. Thus, adequate management of this patient's medical problems required the use of cryoprecipitate and platelet concentrates.

Bibliography

Chesney C, Colman RW, Pechet L: A syndrome of platelet release abnormality in mild hemophilia. *Blood* 43:821–827, 1974.

Crowell ED Jr, Eisner EV: Familial association of thrombopathia and anti-hemophiliac deficiency. *Blood* 40:227–231, 1972.

Weiss HG: Abnormalities of factor VIII and platelet aggregation: Use of ristocetin in diagnosing the von Willebrand's syndrome. *Blood* 45:403–409, 1975.

CASE
50

PATIENT: 15-year-old girl

CHIEF COMPLAINT: This patient was admitted with swelling and pain involving the knees and ankles. The swelling and pain had been present for several weeks. In addition, the patient reported a lifelong history of "easy bruising." She also described ill-defined pain in the right lower quadrant.

MEDICAL HISTORY: The patient had been seen on several occasions by her pediatrician because of abdominal pain, which had originally been attributed to the onset of menarche.

FAMILY HISTORY: The paternal grandmother had been evaluated for thrombocytopenia in 1963. At that time, she was found to have a platelet count of 25,000/μl together with a normal hemoglobin and hematocrit. Examination of a bone marrow aspirate and biopsy specimen revealed an increased number of megakaryocytes; consequently, a diagnosis of idiopathic thrombocytopenic purpura was made. She was placed on corticosteroids and discharged; however, she failed to respond and subsequently underwent splenectomy. Her platelet count increased to 487,000/μl 14 days after the surgical procedure had been done. She has been re-evaluated by her family physician on a number of occasions and has consistently been found to have a normal platelet count, in the range of 250,000 to 300,000/μl.

Other family members, including the patient's father, a paternal aunt and four living siblings, had a history of "easy bruising" (see family tree, Figure 1). In addition, the father bled profusely after right inguinal herniorrhaphy in 1968. In 1974, he was admitted with hematochezia.

A 13-year-old sister had been admitted on a number of occasions for easy bruising. In 1976, this sister underwent exploratory laparotomy because of unexplained abdominal pain. At the time of laparotomy, a ruptured corpus luteum cyst was found together with a large amount of blood in the pelvis. She was seen again in 1977 for evaluation of rectal bleeding and abdominal pain.

A 20-year-old brother had severe bleeding into the right knee as a result of trauma associated with sports activities.

DRUG HISTORY: No medication

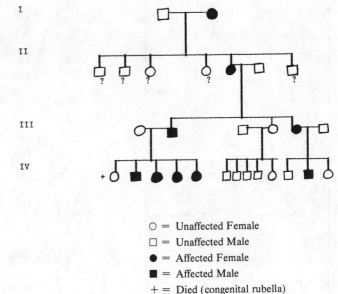

O = Unaffected Female
□ = Unaffected Male
● = Affected Female
■ = Affected Male
+ = Died (congenital rubella)

Figure 1

PHYSICAL EXAMINATION: Joint swelling was not noted. There was no palpable organomegaly.

Laboratory Results

A. Screening Procedures

	Patient	Normal
Prothrombin time	12 seconds	10–12 seconds
APTT	35 seconds	<42 seconds
Platelet count	86,500/μl	130,000–400,000/μl
Bleeding time	>15 minutes	1–8 minutes

Questions

1. Does the history of thrombocytopenia in the paternal grandmother have clinical implications?
2. What pattern of inheritance does the family tree suggest?
3. What additional laboratory procedures are indicated?

STORAGE POOL DISEASE IN ASSOCIATION WITH AUTOSOMAL DOMINANT THROMBOCYTOPENIA

CLINICAL PICTURE

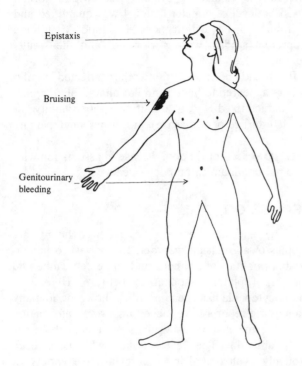

Epistaxis

Bruising

Genitourinary bleeding

PATHOPHYSIOLOGIC BASIS

Alpha granules

Transmission em-equatorial section (schematic)

No dense bodies were demonstrated

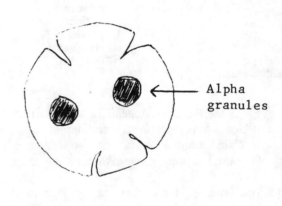

Alpha granules

LABORATORY FINDINGS

A. Screening Procedures

Test	Patient's Result	Normal Range
Prothrombin time	Normal	10–12 seconds
APTT	Normal	<42 seconds
Platelet count	Abnormal	130,000–400,000/μl
Bleeding time	Abnormal	1–8 minutes

B. Confirmatory Procedures

Factor VIII R:RCo	Normal	50% to 150%
Platelet aggregation	See tracings	
Platelet ATP	Abnormal	
Bone marrow	Increased number of megakaryocytes	

TREATMENT

Judicious use of platelet concentrates
Cryoprecipitate (?)
Avoidance of aspirin containing compounds

Laboratory Results

B. Confirmatory Procedures

	Patient	Normal
Factor VIII:C	104%	50% to 150%
Factor VIII R:Ag	90%	50% to 150%
Factor VIII R:RCo	85%	50% to 150%

Platelet Aggregation Studies (see platelet aggregation tracings, Figure 2)

	Patient	Normal
Adenosine diphosphate	Primary wave	Biphasic aggregation
Collagen	Prolonged lag phase with minimal aggregation	Full-range monophasic aggregation
Epinephrine	No response	Biphasic aggregation
Ristocetin	Full-range agglutination	Full-range monophasic agglutination or biphasic agglutination
Platelet retention (glass-bed column)	25%	40% to 90%

To evaluate the thrombocytopenia, a bone marrow aspirate and biopsy was performed. Examination of the sample was within normal limits, with an adequate number of normal-appearing megakaryocytes being found.

Additional special studies were undertaken; they included arachidonic acid-induced platelet aggregation (see tracing). There was a normal response to arachidonic acid-induced aggregation, indicating that the platelets contained an adequate amount of cyclooxygenase. Platelet nucleotide levels were quantified. The total platelet content of adenosine triphosphate was decreased and was subsequently found to be decreased in other family members with a bleeding history.

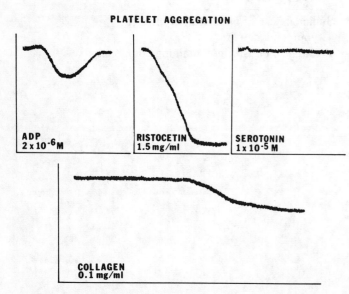

PLATELET AGGREGATION

ADP 2 x 10⁻⁶ M — RISTOCETIN 1.5 mg/ml — SEROTONIN 1 x 10⁻⁵ M — COLLAGEN 0.1 mg/ml

Figure 2

Further studies included transmission electron microscopy, which showed an absence of dense granules in thin sections, thus substantiating the biochemical evidence of a decreased level of adenosine diphosphate. Results of studies of other cell organelles, such as microtubules, mitochondria, alpha granules and elements of the surface connecting system, were within normal limits. The level of platelet factor 4 was quantified and also found to be within normal limits. Membrane glycoprotein studies were performed, and the results were normal.

It should be noted that other affected family members appeared to have a similar abnormality, which was characterized by a qualitative abnormality of platelets (storage pool disease) and thrombocytopenia.

DIAGNOSIS: Storage pool disease in association with autosomal dominant thrombocytopenia

Discussion

This case and members of the patient's family are examples of an unusual disorder. In contrast to hereditary abnormalities of red cells and white cells, inherited disorders of platelets appear to be rare. Hereditary thrombocytopenia has been described; however, in many instances the reports have lacked important information concerning the history as well as pertinent laboratory data (Table 1). The few families who have been thoroughly evaluated display a remarkable variety of clinical features and genetic patterns. A few well-

Table 1
Classification of Hereditary Thrombocytopenia

Sex-Linked Recessive
  Wiskott-Aldrich syndrome and variants
  "Isolated" thrombocytopenia
  Thrombocytopenia with increased IgA and renal disease

Autosomal Dominant
  Thrombopathic thrombocytopenia
    Storage pool disease
    "Aspirin-like" defect
  Isolated thrombocytopenia
  Associated with a generalized disorder
    May-Hegglin anomaly
    Hemoglobin Köln

Autosomal Recessive
  Bernard-Soulier syndrome
  Associated with a generalized disease
    Chédiak-Higashi syndrome
    Thrombocytopenia-absent radius syndrome
    Inborn errors of metabolism

Unclassified Forms
  Associated with some other heritable disorder of hemostasis
    von Willebrand's disease
    Christmas disease

Table 2

Platelet Kinetics in Thrombocytopenic States*

	Amegakaryocytic	Megakaryocytic			
	Bone Marrow Hypoplasia	Ineffective Thrombopoiesis	Altered Distribution	Platelet Destruction	Immune System-Mediated Thrombocytopenia
Platelet number	↓	↓	↓	↓	↓
Megakaryocyte mass	↓	↑	↑	↑	↑
Effective platelet production	↓	↓	↑	↑	↑
Percentage recovery (^{51}Cr tagging)	↔	↔	↓	↔	↔
Survival (^{51}Cr tagging)	(graph: % Recovery, 65→10, Days)	(graph: 65→10, Days)	(graph: 65/30→10, Postoperative, Preoperative, % Recovery, Days)	↓ (graph: 65, Hours)	(graph: 65, Postoperative, Preoperative, Hours, Days)

*From Triplett DA: Platelet Disorders in Murano G, Bick RL: Basic Concepts of Hemostasis and Thrombosis. Boca Raton, Florida: CRC Press, 1980, p 126.

defined syndromes have been characterized; they include Wiskott-Aldrich syndrome, May-Hegglin anomaly and Bernard-Soulier syndrome. A number of cases of hereditary thrombocytopenia in association with intrinsic abnormalities of platelet function also have been described. In most instances, the nature of the abnormality of platelet function has not been characterized.

Pathophysiologic Basis. The combination of hereditary thrombocytopenia and a qualitative abnormality of platelet function has been sporadically reported. Because of the rarity of cases and because many cases were reported before specialized tests of platelet function became available, the pathophysiologic basis of the thrombocytopenia and the qualitative abnormality of platelet function has in most instances been classified inadequately. In the past, the terms thrombocytopathy and thrombopathy were used to identify bleeding disorders in which the defects in platelet function were unlike the defects seen in Glanzmann's thrombasthenia. Most qualitative abnormalities have been described and characterized by demonstrating decreased availability of platelet factor 3. Since the introduction of the aggregometer for measuring platelet function and various other procedures for evaluating platelets, such as electron microscopy, qualitative abnormalities have been classified more thoroughly. Therefore, the terms thrombocytopathy and thrombopathy should probably be discarded because of their past association and identification with platelet factor 3. Isolated deficiency of platelet coagulant activity has rarely been reported.

This family showed an autosomal dominant pattern of inheritance for the thrombocytopenia and storage pool

disease. The thrombocytopenia was mild, with the platelet count ranging from 86,000 to 165,000/μl. Examination of bone marrow biopsy specimens from affected family members revealed hyperplasia of the megakaryocytes. Thus, the thrombocytopenia would fall into the megakaryocytic subgroup of hereditary thrombocytopenia. This subgroup includes ineffective thrombopoiesis and intrinsic defects of platelets that shorten their life span. Platelet kinetic studies in this family demonstrated a normal life span, suggesting that the underlying mechanism was ineffective thrombopoiesis (Table 2). Despite these findings, however, the platelet count in the paternal grandmother returned to normal after splenectomy. This observation suggests that the spleen was the primary site of destruction of the intrinsically abnormal platelets.

Most patients with hereditary thrombocytopenia do not respond to splenectomy. An exception is a family that has been described by Murphy and colleagues. In that family, thrombocytopenia was inherited as a sex-linked recessive trait and was associated with reduction of platelet size and life span. The platelet defect was similar to that seen in Wiskott-Aldrich syndrome; however, those patients showed only mild eczema, and recurrent infection or other immunologic abnormalities were absent. It was thought that those patients had a variant of Wiskott-Aldrich syndrome with a minimal immunologic defect.

In the case being discussed, the platelet contents of adenosine diphosphate and triphosphate were decreased, and the ratio of the level of the triphosphate to the level of the diphosphate was increased. This finding is typical of storage pool disease. Also, the level of platelet factor 4

Table 3
Classification of Storage Pool Disease

Congenital Disease*
  Autosomal dominant form
  With small platelets
  Associated with autosomal dominant form of thrombocytopenia
  Chédiak-Higashi syndrome
  Thrombocytopenia-absent radius syndrome
  Hermansky-Pudlak syndrome
  Wiskott-Aldrich syndrome
  With absence of alpha granules

Acquired Disease
  Disseminated intravascular coagulation
  Immune system mediated (i.e., systemic lupus erythematosus)
  After cardiopulmonary bypass

*May also be classified according to granular defects: δ-dense bodies absent, α-alpha granules absent. δα-combined alpha granules and dense body deficiencies, hysosomes may also be absent.

was within normal limits. Thus, the abnormality in this family would appear to be a storage pool defect involving dense bodies but not affecting alpha granules.

Storage pool disease has been described in association with a number of clinical conditions, including Hermansky-Pudlak syndrome, Chédiak-Higashi syndrome, Wiskott-Aldrich syndrome and thrombocytopenia-absent radius (TAR) syndrome, all of which are hereditary (Table 3). When storage pool disease is not associated with these syndromes, it often is inherited as an autosomal dominant disorder and is characterized by easy bruising and prolonged bleeding from minor wounds. Patients with storage pool disease represent a heterogeneous group. They may have a deficiency only of dense bodies, deficiencies of dense bodies and alpha granules or a deficiency only of alpha granules (gray platelet syndrome).

Other qualitative abnormalities have been described in patients with hereditary thrombocytopenia. In one family, it was believed that thrombocytopenia was coexisting with von Willebrand's disease, and in another, an isolated deficiency of platelet factor 3 and a disturbance of aggregation with collagen accompanied thrombocytopenia.

Clinical Picture. Patients with qualitative abnormalities of platelets often have a mild bleeding syndrome. Chief complaints include "easy bruising" together with mucous membrane bleeding, such as epistaxis, gastrointestinal bleeding or genitourinary bleeding.

Treatment. The treatment of choice for a bleeding episode in this family would include platelet concentrates. However, they should be used judiciously to prevent isoimmunization to platelet antigens. Splenectomy might be considered if bleeding became a serious problem.

Interestingly, several patients with storage pool disease have been reported to respond to cryoprecipitate. The physiologic basis of this response is unknown.

Bibliography

Bigler C, Gasser C, Gugler E: A family with X-linked hereditary thrombocytopenia. *Schweiz Med Wochenschr* 109:321–327, 1979.

Bithell TC, Parakh SJ, Strong RR: Platelet function studies in the Bernard-Soulier syndrome. *Ann NY Acad Sci* 201:145–160, 1972.

Cohn J, Hague M, Anderson V, et al: Sex linked hereditary thrombocytopenia with immunologic defects. *Hum Hered* 25:309–317, 1975.

Epstein CJ, Sahud MA, Piel CF, et al: Hereditary macrothrombocytopathia, nephritis and deafness. *Amer J Med* 52:299–310, 1972.

Falcao L, Libanska J, Gautier A: Hereditary hypogranular thrombopathic thrombocytopenia with deficient thrombopoiesis. (Abstract) *Clin Stud* 2:258, 1971.

Holmsen H, Storm E, Day HG: Determination of ATP and ADP in blood platelets: A modification of the firefly luciferase assay for plasma. *Anal Biochem* 46:489–501, 1972.

Moore JR: X-linked idiopathic thrombocytopenia. *Clin Genet* 5:344–346, 1974.

Murphy S: Hereditary thrombocytopenia. *Clin Haematol* 1:359–366, 1972.

Murphy S: Intrinsic platelet defects in hereditary thrombocytopenia. *Ann NY Acad Sci* 201:421–428, 1972.

Murphy S, Oski FA, Gardiner FH: Hereditary thrombocytopenia with an intrinsic platelet defect. *N Engl J Med* 281:857–862, 1969.

Murphy S, Oski FA, Naiman JL, et al: Platelet size and kinetics in hereditary and acquired thrombocytopenia. *N Engl J Med* 286:499–504, 1972.

Myllyla G, Pelkonen R, Ikkala E, et al: Hereditary thrombocytopenia: Report of three families. *Scand J Haematol* 4:421–425, 1967.

Parsa KP, Lee DBN, Zamboni L, et al: Hereditary nephritis, deafness and abnormal thrombopoiesis. *Amer J Med* 60:665–672, 1976.

Quick AJ, Hussey CV: Hereditary thrombopathic thrombocytopenia. *Amer J Med Sci* 245:643–653, 1963.

Smith TP, Dodds WJ, Tartaglia AP: Thromboasthenic-thrombopathic thrombocytopenia with giant, "Swiss-cheese" platelets. A case report. *Ann Intern Med* 79:828–834, 1973.

Spitler LE, Levin AS, Stites DP, et al: The Wiskott-Aldrich syndrome: Results of transfer factor therapy. *J Clin Invest* 51:3216–3219, 1972.

CASE
51

PATIENT: 27-year-old woman

CHIEF COMPLAINT: This patient presented with a petechial rash over the legs and epistaxis.

MEDICAL HISTORY: The patient had been hospitalized only for delivery of two children. Approximately 3 weeks before presentation, an influenza-like illness developed, and the patient became fatigued. Approximately 4 days before this evaluation, she noticed a "rash" over the legs.

FAMILY HISTORY: Noncontributory

DRUG HISTORY: No medication

PHYSICAL EXAMINATION: Petechiae were noted over the legs and upper portion of the chest. In addition, several large ecchymotic areas were noted over the thighs. There was no palpable organomegaly.

Laboratory Results

A. Screening Procedures

	Patient	Normal
Prothrombin time	12 seconds	10–12 seconds
APTT	35 seconds	<42 seconds
Platelet count	6000/μl	130,000–400,000/μl
Bleeding time	Not performed	1–8 minutes

Questions

1. What is the most likely diagnosis?
2. What additional laboratory procedures are indicated?

Laboratory Results

B. Confirmatory Procedures

	Patient	Normal
Antinuclear antibody	Negative	Negative
Coombs' test	Negative	Negative

BONE MARROW EXAMINATION: A bone marrow aspirate and biopsy showed approximately 60% cellularity, with normal numbers of erythroid and mye-loid elements. There appeared to be an increase in the number of megakaryocytes, and many megakaryocytes were thought to be immature, having vacuolated cytoplasm.

DIAGNOSIS: Acute autoimmune thrombocytopenia*

Discussion

This case is an example of acute autoimmune thrombocytopenia. This disorder is relatively common during childhood, but it occasionally occurs during adulthood as well. There is no apparent predilection for either sex, and the maximal incidence is in children between 2 and 5 years of age. There appears to be some correlation with prior viral infection, and most cases occur in the winter and spring. Thrombocytopenia in this disorder characteristically develops 1 to 3 weeks after viral infection has occurred. The offending organism is frequently unknown. Acute autoimmune thrombocytopenia may follow many episodes of a viral infection such as influenza, pharyngitis or gastroenteritis. In the differential diagnosis a number of possibilities must be considered. These include various collagen vascular diseases such as systemic lupus erythemistosis (SLE). Consequently an antinuclear antibody study was obtained. It is important to remember that autoimmune thrombocytopenia is a diagnosis of exclusion.

Clinical Course. Acute autoimmune thrombocytopenia is characteristically fulminant, with the initial platelet count often ranging from zero to 20,000/μl. Kinetic studies demonstrate reduction of the platelet life span. Typically, the bone marrow has an increased number of megakaryocytes, which frequently have an immature appearance.

Acute autoimmune thrombocytopenia usually subsides without treatment within 3 weeks (range, within several days to 6 months). Patients who do not recover within 6 months are diagnosed as having chronic autoimmune thrombocytopenia. Patients whose thrombocytopenia ultimately proves to be chronic often present with a higher platelet count (i.e., 20,000 to 75,000/μl).

Treatment. There is no firm evidence that corticosteroid therapy is beneficial in patients with acute autoimmune thrombocytopenia. In a patient with severe autoimmune

*also caused idiopathic thrombocytopenic purpura (ITP)

ACUTE AUTOIMMUNE THROMBOCYTOPENIA

CLINICAL PICTURE

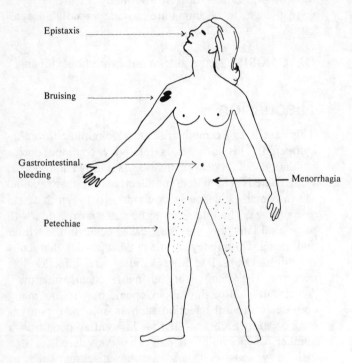

Epistaxis

Bruising

Gastrointestinal bleeding

Menorrhagia

Petechiae

PATHOPHYSIOLOGIC BASIS

Immune system-mediated destruction of platelets

LABORATORY FINDINGS

A. Screening Procedures

Test	Patient's Result	Normal Range
Prothrombin time	Normal	10–12 seconds
APTT	Normal	<42 seconds
Platelet count	Abnormal	130,000–400,000/μl
Bleeding time	Abnormal	1–8 minutes

B. Confirmatory Procedures

Antinuclear antibody	Negative	Negative
Coombs' test	Negative	Negative
Bone marrow	Increased number of megakaryocytes	
Platelet antibodies	Positive	Negative

TREATMENT

Corticosteroids in some cases
Platelet transfusions in cases of life-threatening bleeding

thrombocytopenia, a short course of corticosteroids is appropriate during the first few days of the disease, when hemorrhagic symptoms are prominent. Platelet transfusions may be effective in patients with life-threatening hemorrhage, such as intracranial bleeding. However, platelet transfusion should not be used except in the above circumstance. The mortality of acute autoimmune thrombocytopenia is approximately 1 to 2%.

Bibliography

Pathophysiologic Basis

Cines DB, Dusak B, Tomaski A, et al: Immune thrombocytopenic purpura and pregnancy. *N Engl J Med* 306:826–831, 1982.

McMillan R: The pathogenesis of immune thrombocytopenic purpura. *CRC Crit Rev Clin Lab Sci* 8(4):303–331, November 1977.

McMillan R: Immune thrombocytopenia. *Clin Haematol* 12:69–88, 1983.

Antibody Detection

Dixon R, Rosse W, Ebbert L: Quantitative determination of antibody in idiopathic thrombocytopenic purpura—Correlation of serum and platelet bound antibody with clinical response. *N Engl J Med* 292:230–236, 1975.

Harmon JA, Miller WV: Platelet antibodies: Their detection and significance. *Amer J Med Technol* 47:797–802, 1981.

Saleem A, Banez EI, Siters B: Enzyme labeled immunosorbant assay (ELISA) for detection of platelet antibodies. *Ann Clin Lab Sci* 12:68–72, 1982.

Treatment

Ahn YS, Harrington WJ, Seelman RC, et al: Vincristine therapy of idiopathic and secondary thrombocytopenias. *N Engl J Med* 291:376–380, 1974.

Caplan SN, Berkman EM: Immunosuppressive therapy of idiopathic thrombocytopenic purpura. *Med Clin North Amer* 60:971–986, 1976.

Fehr J, Hofmann V, Kappeler U: Transient reversal of thrombocytopenia in idiopathic thrombocytopenic purpura by high dose intravenous gamma globulin. *N Engl J Med* 306:1254–1258, 1982.

Lacey JV, Penner JA: Management of idiopathic thrombocytopenic purpura in the adult. *Semin Thromb Haemostasis* 3:160–174, 1977.

CASE
52

PATIENT: 22-year-old woman

CHIEF COMPLAINT: This patient was referred for evaluation of "easy bruising." This problem had first appeared while the patient was in nursing school approximately 4 years before this evaluation. At that time, she had been seen by an internist and was found to have a platelet count of 60,000/μl. A bone marrow aspirate and biopsy were performed, and an adequate number of megakaryocytes was seen in the biopsy specimen. Because of the minor symptoms, a decision was made to follow up the patient without prescribing medication.

The patient had not seen her physician since the initial episode until 8 months before this admission, when she was found to have a platelet count of 40,000/μl. She was placed on prednisone at a dosage of 60 mg per day, and her platelet count increased to 180,000/μl. For the last 6 months, the dosage of prednisone had been decreased, and the medication was eventually discontinued before this admission.

FAMILY HISTORY: Noncontributory

DRUG HISTORY: No medication

PHYSICAL EXAMINATION: A number of ecchymotic areas were noted over the legs and trunk.

Laboratory Results

A. Screening Procedures

	Patient	Normal
Prothrombin time	12 seconds	10–12 seconds
APTT	37 seconds	<42 seconds
Platelet count	50,000/μl	130,000–400,000/μl
Bleeding time	7 minutes and 30 seconds	1–8 minutes

Questions

1. What is the most likely diagnosis?
2. What is the treatment of choice?

Laboratory Results

B. Confirmatory Procedures

	Patient	Normal
Antinuclear antibody	Negative	Negative
Platelet-associated IgG	35 fg/platelet	<10 fg/platelet

A bone marrow biopsy was performed. Examination of the biopsy specimen revealed an increased number of megakaryocytes. Some of them appeared to be immature.

DIAGNOSIS: Chronic autoimmune thrombocytopenia

Discussion

This case is an example of chronic autoimmune thrombocytopenia. Most patients with this disorder are between 20 and 50 years of age. There is a predilection for females, the sex ratio being approximately 3:1. Chronic autoimmune thrombocytopenia often has an insidious onset, and the platelet count at the time of presentation is variable. Spontaneous remission is relatively rare.

Biochemical Aspects. Plasma from patients with chronic autoimmune thrombocytopenia contains an IgG fraction that is adsorbed by platelets. This immunoglobulin is species specific and reacts in vivo in all respects like antiplatelet antibodies, which may be seen in patients with isoimmune antibody formation or drug-induced antibodies (Table 1).

A number of laboratory procedures have been used to quantify or semiquantify the amount of immunoglobulin on surfaces of platelets or in plasma. One group of tests makes use of the availability or release of a platelet constituent as a means of evaluating platelet antibodies in plasma or serum. The two most frequently used tests in this category are availability of platelet factor 3 and release of ^{14}C-labeled serotonin. These tests are semiquantitative and are not recommended.

One semiquantitative test that provides useful clinical information is quantification of solubilized platelet-associated IgG by immunodiffusion. This procedure is relatively easy and may be performed in laboratory settings where more sophisticated procedures are not available.

CHRONIC AUTOIMMUNE THROMBOCYTOPENIA

CLINICAL PICTURE

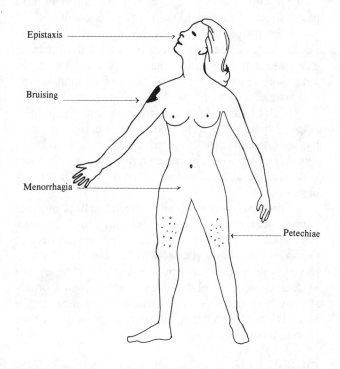

Epistaxis

Bruising

Menorrhagia

Petechiae

PATHOPHYSIOLOGIC BASIS

Immune system-mediated destruction of platelets

LABORATORY FINDINGS

A. Screening Procedures

Test	Patient's Result	Normal Range
Prothrombin time	Normal	10–12 seconds
APTT	Normal	<42 seconds
Platelet count	Abnormal	130,000–400,000/μl
Bleeding time	Normal or abnormal	1–8 minutes

B. Confirmatory Procedures

Platelet IgG	Abnormal	<10 fg/platelet
Bone marrow	Increased number of megakaryocytes	

TREATMENT

Corticosteroids
Splenectomy
Vincristine-loaded platelets (refractory cases)
Immunosuppressive agents (refractory cases)
Intravenous immunoglobulin (refractory cases)
Plasmapheresis

Table 1
Classification of Immune System-Mediated Thrombocytopenia

Idiopathic Thrombocytopenic Purpura
    Acute
    Chronic
    Relapsing

Alloantibodies
    Neonatal
    Post Transfusion Purpura

Other Clinical States
    Collagen vascular disease
    Lymphoproliferative disorders
    Solid tumor
    Infection
        Viral
        Bacterial
        Parasitic
    Drug reaction

Quantitative tests for platelet-associated immunoglobulin include Coombs' consumption test, direct measurement of ^{125}I-labeled antihuman immunoglobulin bound by platelet-associated immunoglobulin, solid-phase radioimmunoassay and enzyme-linked immunosorbent assay. All these procedures have been used in patients with chronic autoimmune thrombocytopenia. Platelets from healthy persons contain from 1 to 11 fg of immunoglobulins. When these sensitive procedures have been used, from 69% to 100% of patients with autoimmune thrombocytopenia have been found to have elevated levels of platelet-associated immunoglobulins. In general, levels of immunoglobulins on surfaces of platelets are inversely correlated with the platelet count in patients with autoimmune thrombocytopenia. There also appears to be an inverse relationship between platelet life span and levels of platelet-associated immunoglobulins. Patients who respond to treatment often show decreases in or a return to normal of levels of platelet-associated immunoglobulins.

Most patients in whom thrombocytopenia is due to mechanisms that are clearly nonimmune have normal levels of platelet-associated immunoglobulins. Patients in whom thrombocytopenia is associated with infection may have elevated levels of platelet-associated immunoglobulins.

Also, it should be noted that approximately 50% of patients with systemic lupus erythematosus have elevated levels of platelet-associated immunoglobulins and that approximately 30% to 40% of patients who are in remission from chronic autoimmune thrombocytopenia have elevated levels of platelet-associated immunoglobulins. In these instances, the elevation of levels of platelet-associated immunoglobulins is believed to be

evidence of a compensated thrombocytolytic state. Platelets of patients with autoimmune thrombocytopenia have a shortened life span; however, circulating platelets are hemostatically effective. In fact, there may be surprisingly few bleeding symptoms despite the marked depression of the platelet count. Platelet survival in patients with autoimmune thrombocytopenia is in most cases directly proportional to the platelet count.

Once the platelets have been sensitized by immunoglobulins, they are apparently destroyed by extravascular sequestration rather than by direct lysis in the circulation. Patients with low titers of antiplatelet immunoglobulin respond well to splenectomy or corticosteroid therapy; however, patients with high titers respond poorly to either form of therapy. In such patients, the liver is the primary site of destruction of sensitized platelets. The bone marrow and lymph nodes may also be sites of sequestration and destruction of platelets.

Corticosteroids have an immediate effect in many patients with mild cases of chronic autoimmune thrombocytopenia. There is evidence that corticosteroids suppress the phagocytic activity of the reticuloendothelial system and that such agents inhibit phagocytosis of antibody-coated platelets by granulocytes. Corticosteroids may also prevent adsorption of immunoglobulins by platelets; in high doses, they may decrease production of immunoglobulins.

Clinical Picture. Autoimmune thrombocytopenia is the most common diagnosis in patients who present with an isolated finding of thrombocytopenia. In most cases of chronic autoimmune thrombocytopenia, the onset is insidious and the patient's only complaints may be of menorrhagia, recurrent epistaxis or, occasionally, easy bruising. In some instances, the disorder is an unexpected finding during routine blood examination. A diagnosis of autoimmune thrombocytopenia is one of exclusion.

In the differential diagnosis, other causes of isolated thrombocytopenia, including drug-induced thrombocytopenia must be considered (Table 2). Also, if a patient has recently received a transfusion, the possibility of post-transfusion purpura should be considered. Other causes of thrombocytopenia, such as disseminated intravascular coagulation, infection, thrombotic thrombocytopenia purpura and decreased bone marrow production, usually are readily identified on the basis of associated clinical and laboratory findings.

Treatment. Corticosteroid therapy and splenectomy are the only established treatments for autoimmune thrombocytopenia. Typically, patients with mild cases of autoimmune thrombocytopenia (platelet count above 20,000/μl) respond readily to corticosteroid therapy. Patients who show an immediate response to corti-

Table 2
Classification of Thrombocytopenia

Decreased Production of Platelets
  Constitutional anemia (Fanconi's syndrome)
  Thrombocytopenia-absent radius baby syndrome (absence of megakaryocytes)
  Deficiency of thrombopoietin (two published cases)
  Rubella and other viral illnesses
  Neonatal thrombocytopenia (maternal drug ingestion, i.e., thiazides)
  Hereditary thrombocytopenia
    May-Hegglin anomaly
    Thrombocytopenia with giant platelets
  Infiltrative diseases of bone marrow
    Carcinoma, leukemia, lymphoma
    Myelofibrosis
    Osteopetrosis
    Miliary tuberculosis
  Radiation therapy and myelosuppressive drug therapy
  Drug administration (thiazides, alcohol, estrogens)
  Cyclic thrombocytopenia
  Megaloblastic anemia
  Paroxysmal nocturnal hemoglobinuria
  Tidal platelet dysgenesis

Increased Destruction of Platelets
  Acute hemolytic reaction (i.e., erythroblastosis)
  Disseminated intravascular coagulation
  Infection
  Drug sensitivity (quinine, quinidine)
  Isoimmune thrombocytopenia
  Idiopathic thrombocytopenic purpura
  Thrombotic thrombocytopenic purpura
  Hemolytic-uremic syndrome
  Posttransfusion purpura
  Kasabach-Merritt syndrome
  Drug administration (e.g., ristocetin)
  Malaria

Increased Sequestration of Platelets
  Hypersplenism
  Hypothermia

Loss of Platelets
  Hemorrhage and multiple blood transfusions
  Extracorporeal circulation

costeroid therapy have a much more favorable prognosis than do those who are initially refractory to such therapy. The dosage of corticosteroids is variable, but in many instances, approximately 1 to 1.2 mg of prednisone per kilogram of body weight per day is used as the starting dosage. Once the platelet count has responded favorably

(usually within 5 to 10 days), the dosage may be tapered. By tapering the dosage, a minimal effective dosage may be identified. In patients who continue to have symptoms or in whom recurrence occurs after corticosteroid therapy has been discontinued, splenectomy is the treatment of choice.

Splenectomy results in major improvement in 70% to 90% of patients and in complete and permanent remission in 45% to 60% of patients. After splenectomy has been performed, the platelet count increases rapidly, often as much as 20,000/μl per day. Within 7 to 12 days, the platelet count typically exceeds 500,000/μl in patients who show a favorable response to splenectomy.

Various other forms of therapy have been tried in patients with chronic autoimmune thrombocytopenia. Such therapies include plasmapheresis, platelet transfusion, intravenous administration of immunoglobulins, and immunosuppressive therapy. These therapies have not yielded satisfactory results.

Bibliography

Cines DB, Dusak B, Tomaski A, et al: Immune thrombocytopenia. *N Engl J Med* 306:826–830, 1982.

McMillan R: Chronic idiopathic thrombocytopenic purpura. *N Engl J Med* 304:1135–1137, 1981.

McMillan R: Immune Thrombocytopenia *Clin Haematol* 12:69–88, 1983.

Moake JL, Rudy CK, Troll JH, et al: Unusually large plasma factor VIII: von Willebrand factor multimers in chronic relapsing thrombotic thrombocytopenic purpura. *N Engl J Med* 307:1432–1435, 1982.

Morse BS, Giuliani D, Nussbaum M: Quantitation of platelet-associated IgG by radial immunodiffusion. *Blood* 57:809–811, 1981.

Rosse WF: Management of chronic immune thrombocytopenia. *Clin Haematol* 12:267–284, 1983.

Shulman NR, Jordan JN Jr: Platelet Immunology. In Colman RW, Hirsh J, Marder VJ, Salzman EW (eds): *Hemostasis and Thrombosis*. Philadelphia: J. B. Lippincott Company, 1982, pp 274–342.

Stuart MJ, Kelton JG, Allen JB: Abnormal platelet function and arachidonate metabolism in chronic idiopathic thrombocytopenic purpura. *Blood* 58:326–329, 1981.

CASE
53

PATIENT: 61-year-old man

CHIEF COMPLAINT: This patient presented to the emergency room because of copious rectal bleeding of 3 hours' duration.

MEDICAL HISTORY: The patient had a history of peptic ulcer disease, which was quiescent. He also had a mild case of adult-onset diabetes, which was controlled by dietary measures.

FAMILY HISTORY: Noncontributory

DRUG HISTORY: The patient had taken cimetidine for peptic ulcer disease. He had avoided aspirin, substituting Tylenol (acetaminophen) for routine analgesic needs.

PHYSICAL EXAMINATION: No mass was palpable on rectal examination. Because of the profuse bleeding, sigmoidoscopy was difficult to perform.

Laboratory Results

A. Screening Procedures

	Patient	Normal
Prothrombin time	12 seconds	10–12 seconds
APTT	39 seconds	<42 seconds
Platelet count	1,480,000/μl	130,000–400,000/μl
Bleeding time	>15 minutes	1–8 minutes

Questions

1. What is the most likely diagnosis?
2. What additional laboratory procedures are indicated?
3. Would correction of the platelet count affect the bleeding time?

Laboratory Results

B. Confirmatory Procedures

A complete blood count showed the following results:

	Patient	Normal
Hemoglobin level	14.9 g/dl	14–18 g/dl
Red cell count	7×10^6/μl	$4.7–6.1 \times 10^6$/μl

	Patient	Normal
White cell count	15,400/μl	4900–10,800/μl
Hematocrit	44.7%	42% to 52%

Bone marrow aspirate and biopsy were essentially 100% cellular. All three cell lines (myeloid, erythroid, megakaryocytic) were increased, however, the erythroid series was proportionately increased more than the myeloid and megakaryocytic series. Special stains for iron (Prussian Blue) revealed no iron stores.

Platelet aggregation studies were performed after platelet-rich plasma had been prepared and after the platelet count had been lowered to 300,000/ml by dilution. When the diluted platelet-rich plasma was used, normal aggregation was found with adenosine diphosphate, collagen and epinephrine, and normal agglutination with ristocetin was observed.

DIAGNOSIS: Polycythemia vera in association with iron deficiency anemia

Discussion

This case is an example of a myeloproliferative disease that presented wtih gastrointestinal bleeding of apparently sudden onset. The hematocrit was, however, within normal limits; nevertheless, it was assumed that the hematocrit had been much higher before the onset of the massive gastrointestinal bleeding. This assumption was supported by the red cell count of 7,000,000/μl.

The platelet count was elevated so markedly that the possibility of hemorrhagic thrombocythemia also had to be considered (Table 1). The distinction between polycythemia vera and hemorrhagic thrombocythemia is often a difficult one because of the many similarities among the various myeloproliferative disorders.

Patients with myeloproliferative disorders may have qualitative abnormalities of platelet function. Such an abnormality is illustrated by this case. The bleeding time was greater than 15 minutes; however, the results of platelet aggregation studies performed on platelet-rich plasma adjusted to a count of 300,000/μl by dilution were within normal limits. Various abnormalities of platelets have been described in patients with myeloproliferative disorders. They include abnormalities of receptor sites on platelet membranes as well as abnormalities of the lipoxygenase pathway.

POLYCYTHEMIA VERA WITH SECONDARY
IRON DEFICIENCY

CLINICAL PICTURE

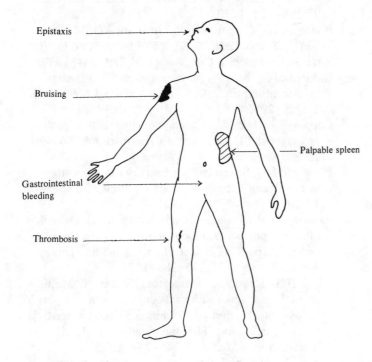

Epistaxis

Bruising

Gastrointestinal
bleeding

Thrombosis

Palpable spleen

PATHOPHYSIOLOGIC BASIS OF BLEEDING IN POLYCYTHEMIA VERA

Abnormalities of membrane receptor sites (decreased numbers of alpha-adrenergic receptors and prostaglandin D_2 receptors)
Deficiency of lipoxygenase activity
Decreased numbers of dense bodies and alpha granules

LABORATORY FINDINGS

A. Screening Procedures

Test	Patient's Result	Normal Range
Prothrombin time	Normal*	10–12 seconds
APTT	Normal*	<42 seconds
Platelet count	Abnormal	130,000–400,000/μl
Bleeding time	Abnormal	1–8 minutes

B. Confirmatory Procedures

Bone marrow	Hypercellular
Unadjusted platelet aggregation	Abnormal

May be abnormal if citrate volume is not adjusted.

TREATMENT

Chemotherapy (alkylating agents)
^{32}P lowers platelet count rapidly
Plateletpheresis
Antiplatelet agents if thrombosis is a presenting sign

Table 1
Classification of Causes of an Elevated Platelet Count

Thrombocytosis
  Secondary or reactive (transient)
    Acute blood loss
    Postpartum
    Infection
    Posttraumatic
    After splenectomy
    Exercise
    Postoperative state
    Drug administration (epinephrine)
    After thrombocytopenia
      Pernicious anemia (after treatment)
      Acute thrombocytopenic purpura
      Alcohol-induced thrombocytopenia
      Drug-induced thrombocytopenia
    Ovulation
    Sarcoidosis
    Adrenal hyperplasia
    Osteoporosis
    Hemophilia A
  Chronic
    Inflammatory bowel disease
      Ulcerative colitis
      Granulomatous colitis
    Rheumatoid arthritis
    Neoplasm
      Hodgkin's disease
      Carcinoma
      Osteogenic sarcoma
      Retinoblastoma
      Mesothelioma
    Iron deficiency (late in iron deficiency may see thrombocytopenia)
    Chronic hemolytic anemia with splenectomy
    Splenic atrophy

Thrombocythemia
  As a predominant feature
    Essential thrombocythemia
  As an accompanying feature of myeloproliferative disorder
    Polycythemia vera
    Myeloid metaplasia
    Chronic myelocytic leukemia

Bibliography

Berger S, Aledort LM, Gilbert HS, et al: Abnormalities of platelet function in patients with polycythemia vera. *Cancer Res* 33:2683–2687, 1973.

Boneu B, Nouvel C, Sie P, et al: Platelets in myeloproliferative disorders. I. A comparative evaluation with certain platelet function tests. *Scand J Haematol* 25:214–220, 1980.

Boughton BJ, Corbett WEN, Ginsburg AD: Myeloproliferative disorders: A paradox of in vivo and in vitro platelet function. *J Clin Pathol* 30:228–234, 1977.

Caranobe C, Sie P, Nouvel C, et al: Platelets in myeloproliferative disorders. *Scand J Haematol* 25:289–295, 1980.

Cooper B, Ahern D: Characterization of the platelet prostaglandin D_2 receptor. *J Clin Invest* 64:586–590, 1979.

Hoagland HC, Silverstein M: Primary thrombocythemia in the young patient. *Mayo Clin Proc* 53:578–580, 1978.

Keenan JP, Wharton J, Shephard AJN, et al: Defective platelet lipid peroxidation in myeloproliferative disorders: A possible defect of prostaglandin synthesis. *Brit J Haematol* 35:275–283, 1977.

Klein HG, Kessler C, Anderson KC, et al: Multiple arterial and venous thromboemboli in a man with chronic myelogenous leukemia and occult metastatic breast carcinoma: The significance of thrombocythemia. *South Med J* 75:745–747, 1982.

Okuma M, Uchino H: Altered arachidonate metabolism by platelets in patients with myeloproliferative disorders. *Blood* 54:1258–1271, 1979.

Schafer AL: Deficiency of platelet lipoxygenase activity in myeloproliferative disorders. *N Engl J Med* 306:381–386, 1982.

Wasserman LR, Gilbert HS: Surgery in polycythemia vera. *N Engl J Med* 269:1226–1230, 1963.

CASE
54

PATIENT: 96-year-old woman

CHIEF COMPLAINT: This patient was transferred from a nursing home after her body temperature rose to 103°F and a diminished sensorium developed. At the time of admission, x-ray film of the chest revealed an infiltrate of the right lower lobe consistent with pneumonia.

MEDICAL HISTORY: The patient's medical history was complicated. She had adult-onset diabetes, hypertension and arteriosclerotic heart disease.

FAMILY HISTORY: Noncontributory

DRUG HSITORY: After admission, the patient was placed on various antibiotics, including ticarcillin.

PHYSICAL EXAMINATION: At the time of admission, physical findings were consistent with right lower lobe pneumonia. In addition, there was edema of the legs.

HOSPITAL COURSE: Three days after ticarcillin therapy had been instituted, serious oral pharyngeal hemorrhage developed. The volume of blood loss was so large that transfusion of 2 units of packed red cells was necessary.

Laboratory Results

A. Screening Procedures

	Patient	Normal
Prothrombin time	12 seconds	10–12 seconds
APTT	32 seconds	<42 seconds
Platelet count	463,000/μl	130,000–400,000/μl
Bleeding time	15 minutes	1–8 minutes

Questions

1. What is the most likely diagnosis?
2. What additional laboratory procedures are indicated?

Laboratory Results

B. Confirmatory Procedures

	Patient	Normal
Fibrinogen	500 mg/dl	170–410 mg/dl
Antithrombin III activity	90%	85% to 115%
Fibrin split products	>10 μg/ml but <40 μg/ml	<10 μg/ml
Protamine sulfate	Negative	Negative

Platelet Aggregation Studies (see platelet aggregation tracings, Figure 1)

	Patient	Normal
Adenosine diphosphate	Primary wave with disaggregation	Biphasic aggregation
Epinephrine	Primary wave with disaggregation	Biphasic aggregation
Collagen	Decreased response	Full-range monophasic aggregation
Ristocetin	Full-range monophasic response	Full-range monophasic agglutination or biphasic agglutination

DIAGNOSIS: Qualitative abnormality of platelets (secondary to ticarcillin)

Discussion

Penicillin and its derivatives have been associated with acquired abnormalities of platelets (Table 1). Such abnormalities are thought to be due to alteration of membrane charge or permeability.

Treatment of this patient involved discontinuation of ticarcillin and substitution of an alternate antibiotic.

QUALITATIVE ABNORMALITY OF PLATELETS
(SECONDARY TO TICARCILLIN)

CLINICAL PICTURE

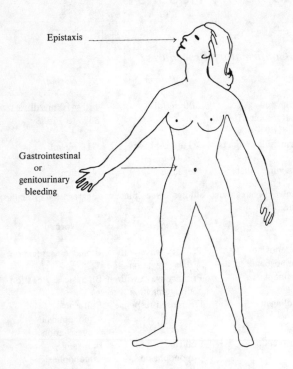

Epistaxis

Gastrointestinal
or
genitourinary
bleeding

PATHOPHYSIOLOGIC BASIS OF DRUG-INDUCED PLATELET DYSFUNCTION

Altered membrane characteristics
Altered metabolism of prostaglandins
Altered metabolism of 3',5'-cyclic adenosine monophosphate

LABORATORY FINDINGS

A. Screening Procedures

Test	Patient's Result	Normal Range
Prothrombin time	Normal	10–12 seconds
APTT	Normal	<42 seconds
Platelet count	Normal	130,000–400,000/μl
Bleeding time	Abnormal	1–8 minutes

B. Confirmatory Procedures

Fibrinogen	Normal	170–410 mg/dl
AT III activity	Normal	85–115%
Fibrin split products	Normal	<10 μg/ml
Protamine sulfate	Normal	Negative
Platelet aggregation	See tracings	

TREATMENT

Discontinue offending drug

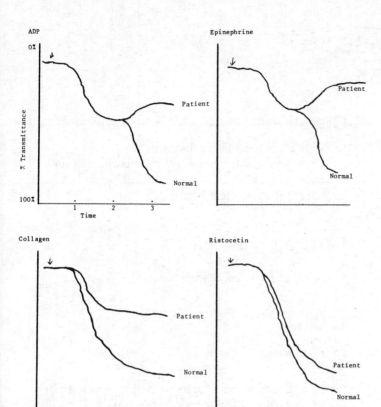

Figure 1

Bibliography

Brown CH III, Bradshaw MW, Natelson EA, et al: Defective platelet function following the administration of penicillin compound. *Blood* 47:949, 1976.

Brown CH III, Natelson EA, Bradshaw MW, et al: Study of the effects of ticarcillin on blood coagulation and platelet function. *Antimicrob Agents Chemother* 7:652–657, 1975.

McClure P, Caserly J, Monsier GH, et al: Carbenicillin-induced bleeding disorder. *Lancet* 2:1307–1308, 1970.

Table 1
Drugs that Alter Platelet Function

Drugs Not Containing Aspirin That Inhibit Platelet Aggregation

Acetaminophen		
Aminopyrine	Heparin	(Furadantin)
(Pyramidon)	Ibufenac (Dytransin)	Phenothiazines
Clofibrate	Ibuprofen (Motrin)	Phenylbutazone
(Atromid-S)	Indomethacin	Penicillins and
Dextran	(Indocin)	cephalothins
Dextropropoxy-	Imipramine	Sulfinpyrazone
phene (Doloxene)	hydrochloride	(Anturane)
Dipyridamole	(tricyclic	Volatile general
(Persantine)	antidepressants)	anesthetics
Ethanol	Meclofenamic acid	
Furosemide	Mefenamic acid	
(Lasix)	(Ponstel)	

Drugs That Affect Retention
Clofibrate
(Atromid-S)
Local anesthetics
Glycerol
guaiacolate
Sodium warfarin
(Coumadin) (?)

CASE
55

PATIENT: 62-year-old woman

CHIEF COMPLAINT: This patient was admitted in a confused state and was unable to give a coherent history. According to friends, her confusion was of recent onset and somewhat episodic. It had increased substantially during the several days that immediately preceded hospitalization. The admitting physician had thought that a toxic psychosis might account for the bizarre mental confusion.

MEDICAL HISTORY: Not obtainable

FAMILY HISTORY: Not obtainable

DRUG HISTORY: It was known that the patient had adult-onset diabetes, which had been controlled with oral hypoglycemic agents and dietary measures.

PHYSICAL EXAMINATION: In addition to the neurologic findings described above, several large bruises were noted over the legs.

Laboratory Results

A. Screening Procedures

	Patient	Normal
Prothrombin time	12 seconds	10–12 seconds
APTT	40 seconds	<42 seconds
Platelet count	48,000/μl	130,000–400,000/μl
Bleeding time	8 minutes and 30 seconds	1–8 minutes

Other admitting laboratory test results were as follows:

Hemoglobin level	6.9 g/dl	12–16 g/dl
Hematocrit	20.7%	37% to 47%
Reticulocyte count	4.5%	0.5% to 1.5%
Bilirubin	3 mg/dl	0.2–1 mg/dl
Blood urea nitrogen	30 mg/dl	<25 mg/dl

Examination of a peripheral blood smear revealed nucleation of numerous red cells together with basophilic stippling. Marked anisocytosis and poikilocytosis were observed. Schistocytes and helmet cells were identified.

Questions

1. What is the most likely diagnosis?
2. What additional laboratory procedures are indicated?
3. What is the treatment of choice?

Laboratory Results

B. Confirmatory Procedures

	Patient	Normal
Antithrombin III activity	90%	85% to 115%
Fibrin split products	<10 μg/ml	<10 μg/ml
Protamine sulfate	Negative	Negative

Examination of a bone marrow biopsy specimen revealed marked megakaryocytic hyperplasia.

DIAGNOSIS: Thrombotic thrombocytopenic purpura

Discussion

This case is a classical example of thrombotic thrombocytopenic purpura. After the patient had entered the hospital, her mental state continued to deteriorate, and on the fourth hospital day, she died. At autopsy, a enlarged spleen, weighing 420 g, was found, as were marked pulmonary congestion and edema and adrenal atrophy. Microscopic examination of tissues at autopsy revealed subintimal fibrinous deposits in the capillaries.

Moschcowitz first described thrombotic thrombocytopenic purpura in 1925. It continues to be a perplexing, frequently fatal disorder. Many cases have now been reported in the literature; however, there is a great difference of opinion regarding clinical features, laboratory findings, diagnostic criteria, pathogenesis and treatment.

Pathophysiologic Basis and Biochemical Aspects. The thrombocytopenia seen in this disorder varies in severity, with the platelet count ranging from 10,000 to 120,000/μl. It is often accompanied by hemolytic anemia, with a hemoglobin level of less than 11 g/dl, and an elevated reticulocyte count.

Examination of a peripheral blood smear typically shows evidence of red cell fragmentation, which is

THROMBOTIC THROMBOCYTOPENIC PURPURA

CLINICAL PICTURE

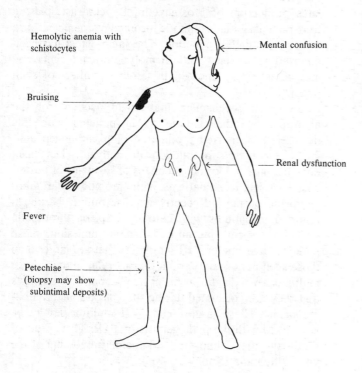

Hemolytic anemia with schistocytes

Bruising

Fever

Petechiae
(biopsy may show
subintimal deposits)

Mental confusion

Renal dysfunction

PATHOPHYSIOLOGIC BASIS

Platelet thrombi with endothelial proliferation
Platelet aggregating factor??
Decreased production of prostacyclin (prostaglandin I_2)
Decreased production of plasminogen activator by endothelial cells
Presence of large von Willebrand factor multimers in plasma

LABORATORY FINDINGS

A. Screening Procedures

Test	Patient's Result	Normal Range
Prothrombin time	Normal	10–12 seconds
APTT	Normal	<42 seconds
Platelet count	Abnormal	130,000–400,000/μl
Bleeding time	Abnormal	1–8 minutes
Peripheral blood	Schistocytes	Normal morphologic features

B. Confirmatory Procedures

Bone marrow	Megakaryocytic hyperplasia	
Fibrin split products	<10 μg/ml	<10 μg/ml
Protamine sulfate	Negative	Negative
Coombs' test	Negative	Negative

TREATMENT

Antiplatelet agents (of doubtful usefulness)
Splenectomy (of doubtful usefulness)
Plasmapheresis and exchange transfusion
Infusion of prostacyclin

thought to occur intravascularly when the red cells are sliced as they pass over fibrin strands. Nucleated red cells are also frequently seen. Coombs' test gives a negative result.

The renal disease that occurs in thrombotic thrombocytopenic purpura usually is mild and manifested by proteinuria, hematuria, azotemia and urinary casts. The degree of involvement varies from series to series, and the distinction between the disorder and hemolytic-uremia syndrome is not always clear. Hemolytic-uremia syndrome occurs most frequently in children and is characterized by more severe renal involvement and a better overall prognosis than are the case for thrombotic thrombocytopenic purpura.

With the exception of the thrombocytopenia, the results of coagulation laboratory tests usually are normal, whereas the results of such tests usually are abnormal in patients with disseminated intravascular coagulation.

Gingival or petechial lesion biopsy has been suggested as a means of confirming the clinical diagnosis. However, such biopsy specimens must be examined carefully and the findings interpreted with caution. Published experience with gingival biopsy suggests that such specimens are positive in approximately one-half of cases. A negative biopsy specimen is not adequate evidence for ruling out the diagnosis nor is a positive biopsy specimen a firm basis for establishing the diagnosis.

The pathogenesis of thrombotic thrombocytopenic purpura remains a subject of controversy. Despite the lack of laboratory evidence of intravascular coagulation, there is undisputed morphologic evidence of vascular wall damage and widespread thrombus formation in the microvasculature. The thrombi consist of fibrin and platelets with variable degrees of endothelial cell proliferation. It has been suggested that the thrombi in this disorder derive almost exclusively from platelets and that the fibrin is derived from platelet fibrinogen. The process would appear to be mediated primarily by platelets and not by generation of thrombin. This assumption is supported by several observations, including decreased platelet life span and normal fibrinogen life span in patients with thrombotic thrombocytopenic purpura.

Current belief is that endothelial cells are the site of the initial injury in patients with this disorder. The type of injury is unknown, although it may be immunologic, either cell mediated or IgG mediated. One theory is that there is a platelet-aggregating factor in plasma of patients with thrombotic thrombocytopenic purpura. This factor is thought to stimulate platelet aggregation directly. It has not been demonstrated in plasma of patients with other types of thrombocytopenia, and some authors believe that normal plasma may contain an inhibitor of this factor. These two observations would explain the therapeutic benefit of plasmapheresis, or plasma infusion, that has recently been described.

Another suggested mechanism is decreased production of prostacyclin (prostaglandin I_2). Recently, it has been demonstrated that when normal plasma is incubated with normal endothelial cell cultures, it stimulates production of prostacyclin. By contrast, plasma from patients with thrombotic thrombocytopenic purpura fails to stimulate production. The same defect has been reported in patients with hemolytic-uremic syndrome and, interestingly enough, in family members of such patients.

Another mechanism that might account for the abnormal endothelial function in patients with this disorder is decreased production of plasminogen activator. Decreased production of activator has been demonstrated in biopsy specimens of segments of thrombosed vessels from patients with thrombotic thrombocytopenic purpura. Recently another finding has been reported in patients with chronic relapsing thrombotic thrombocytopenic purpura. When in remission, these patients have Factor VIII multimers that are larger than those seen in normal plasma. During relapse these large multimers will disappear from the plasma. This suggests that they are consumed during the episode of thrombocytopenia. These large factor VIII multimers may be associated with the pathogenesis of TTP. Their production may reflect abnormal endothelial processing of the von Willebrand factor.

Clinical Picture. The diagnosis of this disorder is based on a pentad of findings. The three of major importance are thrombocytopenia (with or without purpura), fragmentation hemolytic anemia and fluctuating neurologic signs. Mild renal disease and fever are of lesser importance. Laboratory findings of disseminated intravascular coagulation are absent.

Thus, it is clear that thrombotic thrombocytopenic purpura is a syndrome rather than a single disease. It may occur in a fulminating form or in a chronic form punctuated by periods of remission and relapse.

Treatment. A number of therapies have been tried; they include administration of antiplatelet agents, splenectomy and immunosuppressive therapy. However, the greatest advance in the field is the use of exchange transfusion and plasmapheresis. One suggested treatment regimen involves plasma exchange daily for 5 to 7 days and replacement with 2 to 4 liters of fresh-frozen plasma per day. Another possible therapy is infusion of prostacyclin.

Bibliography

Amir J, Krauss S: Treatment of thrombotic thrombocytopenic purpura with antiplatelet drugs. *Blood* 42:27–33, 1973.

Brain MC, Neame PB: Thrombotic thrombocytopenic purpura and the hemolytic uremic syndrome. *Semin Thromb Haemostasis* 8:186–197, 1982.

Bukowski RM, King JW, Hewlett JS: Plasmapheresis in the treatment of thrombotic thrombocytopenic purpura. *Blood* 50:413–417, 1977.

Chen YC, McLeod B, Hall ER, et al: Accelerated prostacyclin degradation in thrombotic thrombocytopenic purpura. *Lancet* 2:267–269, 1981.

Crain SM, Choudhury AM: Thrombotic thrombocytopenic purpura. *J Amer Med Ass* 246:1243–1246, 1981.

Fitzgerald GA, Maas RL, Stein R, et al: Intravenous prostacyclin in thrombotic thrombocytopenic purpura. *Ann Intern Med* 95:319–322, 1981.

Gutterman LA, Stevenson TD: Treatment of thrombotic thrombocytopenic purpura with vincristine. *J Amer Med Ass* 247:1433–1436, 1982.

Machin SJ, McVerry BA, Parry H, et al: A plasma factor inhibiting prostacyclin-like activity in thrombotic thrombocytopenic purpura. *Acta Haematol* 67:8–12, 1982.

Moake JL, Rudy CK, Troll J, et al: Unusually large factor VIII: von Willebrand factor multimers in chronic relapsing thrombotic thrombocytopenic purpura. *N Engl J Med* 307:1432, 1982.

Moake JL, Rudy C, Troll J, et al: Unusually large plasma factor: von Willebrand factor multimers during acute episodes of thrombotic thrombocytopenic purpura: their persistance following recovery predicts subsequent recurrence. (Abstract) *Blood* 60:281, 1982.

Marcus AJ: Moschowitz revisited. *N Engl J Med* 307:1447–1448, 1982.

Nalbandian RM, Henry RL: A proposed comprehensive pathophysiology of thrombotic thrombocytopenic purpura with implicit novel tests and therapies. *Semin Thromb Haemostasis* 6:356–390, 1980.

Pini M, Manotti C, Megha A, et al: Normal prostacyclin-like activity and response to plasma exchange in thrombotic thrombocytopenic purpura. *Acta Haematol* 67:198–205, 1982.

Rosove MH, Ho WG, Goldfinger D: Ineffectiveness of aspirin and dipyridamole in the treatment of thrombotic thrombocytopenic purpura. *Ann Intern Med* 96:27–33, 1982.

Wu KK, Hall ER, Papp A: Prostacyclin stabilizing factor deficiency in thrombotic thrombocytopenic purpura. (Letter to the editor) *Lancet* 1:460–461, 1982.

CASE
56

PATIENT: 67-year-old man

CHIEF COMPLAINT: This patient was admitted with a provisional diagnosis of deep-vein thrombosis and pulmonary embolus. When he was seen in the emergency room, he reported shortness of breath and chest pain. He also described a bout of coughing, during which fresh blood was expectorated, immediately before his hospital visit.

MEDICAL HISTORY: Noncontributory

FAMILY HISTORY: Noncontributory

DRUG HISTORY: The patient had taken cimetidine for peptic ulcer disease.

PHYSICAL EXAMINATION: The pulse was rapid and somewhat thready at 110 pulsations per minute, and the respiratory rate was also increased at 35 inspirations per minute. Blood pressure was 100/60 mm Hg. There was slight splinting of the right hemithorax. In addition, the legs revealed a trace of pitting edema, with localized tenderness being noted in the upper portion of the right thigh.

Laboratory Results

A. Screening Procedures (admitting)

	Patient	Normal
Prothrombin time	12 seconds	10–12 seconds
APTT	30 seconds	<42 seconds
Platelet count	380,000/μl	130,000–400,000/μl
Bleeding time	6 minutes	1–8 minutes

HOSPITAL COURSE: The admitting complete blood count and platelet count were within normal limits. The patient was evaluated with a ventilation perfusion scan together with a pulmonary arteriogram, and a diagnosis of pulmonary embolism was established. The patient was started on heparin, 6000 units every four hours, after a loading dose of 20,000 units. He was continued on heparin for 9 days, at which time oozing from venipuncture sites was noted. The following laboratory results were obtained:

Laboratory Results

B. Screening Procedures (follow-up)

	Patient	Normal
Prothrombin time	14 seconds	10–12 seconds
APTT	80 seconds	<42 seconds
Platelet count	10,500/μl	130,000–400,000/μl
Bleeding time	Not performed	

Questions

1. What is the cause of the thrombocytopenia?
2. What additional laboratory procedures are indicated?
3. What is the treatment of choice?

Laboratory Results

C. Confirmatory Procedures

	Patient	Normal
Thrombin time	150 seconds	20–24 seconds
Fibrinogen	740 mg/dl	170–410 mg/dl
Protamine sulfate	Negative	Negative

It was believed that the results of the confirmatory laboratory tests ruled out a diagnosis of disseminated intravascular coagulation. Results of studies undertaken to demonstrate heparin-induced platelet antibodies were positive.

DIAGNOSIS: Heparin-induced thrombocytopenia

Discussion

Thrombocytopenia has recently been recognized as an increasingly common complication of heparin administration. The frequency of this complication has not been clearly established but has been reported as occurring in less than 1% to more than 20% of patients receiving heparin. This wide variation may be attributable to differences in heparin preparations. It appears that this complication occurs more frequently in patients who have received bovine lung heparin than in those who have received porcine mucosal preparations of heparin.

HEPARIN-INDUCED THROMBOCYTOPENIA

CLINICAL PICTURE

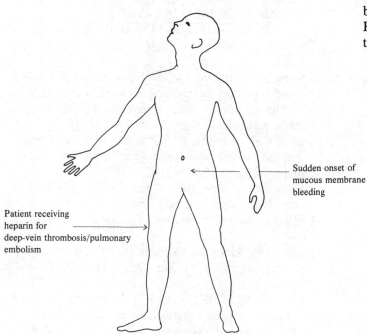

Sudden onset of mucous membrane bleeding

Patient receiving heparin for deep-vein thrombosis/pulmonary embolism

PATHOPHYSIOLOGIC BASIS

Heparin-induced antibody formation
Heparin-induced platelet aggregation and sequestration by the spleen
Heparin-induced disseminated intravascular coagulation

LABORATORY FINDINGS

A. Screening Procedures

Test	Patient's Result	Normal Range
Prothrombin time	Abnormal	10–12 seconds
APTT	Abnormal	<42 seconds
Platelet count	Abnormal	130,000–400,000/μl
Bleeding time	Abnormal	1–8 minutes

B. Confirmatory Procedures

Heparin-dependent antibody	Present

TREATMENT

Discontinue heparin (may switch to heparin of different tissue origin)
Start oral anticoagulant therapy
Dextran therapy

Biochemical Aspects. The pathophysiologic mechanism for heparin-induced thrombocytopenia has been widely debated in the literature. At least three different mechanisms may be involved: platelet aggregation with sequestration in the spleen, heparin-induced antibody formation and heparin-induced thrombosis with disseminated intravascular coagulation. Of these phenomena, heparin-induced antibody formation appears to be the most frequent cause of the thrombocytopenia.

Clinical Picture. Almost all patients who receive heparin show a transient decrease in the platelet count after administration of heparin. This transient decrease may be due to platelet aggregation and sequestration by the spleen.

More striking decreases in the platelet count, as occurred in this case, are often seen after several days of heparin administration. Two possible mechanisms are involved: heparin-induced antibody formation and heparin-induced thrombosis with disseminated intravascular coagulation. In this case, antibodies were demonstrated.

Treatment. In severe thrombocytopenia, heparin should be discontinued. Occasionally, it is possible to switch to another preparation of heparin and not have severe thrombocytopenia. However, in most cases, this approach is not recommended. This patient was treated with oral anticoagulant therapy. The platelet count quickly rebounded to within the normal range, and the patient was discharged with no further complications.

Bibliography

Chong BH, Grace CS, Rozenberg MC: Heparin-induced thrombocytopenia: Effect of heparin platelet antibody on platelets. *Brit J Haematol* 49:531–540, 1981.

Chong BH, Pitney WR, Castaldi PA: Heparin induced thrombocytopenia: Association of thrombotic complications with heparin-dependent IgG antibody that induces thromboxane synthesis and platelet aggregation. *Lancet* 2:1246–1248, 1982.

Cimes DB, Kaywin P, Bina M, et al: Heparin associated thrombocytopenia. *N Engl J Med* 303:788–795, 1980.

Hussey CV, Bernhard VM, McLean MR, et al: Heparin induced platelet aggregation. In vitro confirmation of thrombotic complications associated with heparin therapy. *Ann Clin Lab Sci* 9:487–492, 1979.

Kapsch CN, Adelstein EH, Rhodes GR, et al: Heparin induced thrombocytopenia, thrombosis and hemorrhage. *Surgery* 86:148–155, 1979.

Rhodes GR, Dixon RH, Silver D: Heparin induced thrombocytopenia: Eight cases with thrombotic hemorrhagic complications. *Ann Surg* 186:752–758, 1977.

Triplett DA: Heparin: Biochemistry, therapy, and laboratory monitoring. *Ther Drug Mon* 1:173–197, 1979.

White PW, Sadd JR, Nensel RE: Thrombotic complications of heparin therapy—Including 6 cases of heparin-induced skin necrosis. *Ann Surg* 190:595–598, 1979.

CASE
57

PATIENT: 57-year-old man

CHIEF COMPLAINT: This patient presented to the emergency room after a fall that resulted in laceration of the left hip with formation of a large hematoma.

MEDICAL HISTORY: The patient had been hospitalized on a number of occasions for problems associated with ethanol abuse. He had several episodes of delirium tremens and was known to have cirrhosis, which had been documented by liver biopsy, together with portal hypertension and splenomegaly. On at least one occasion, he had been diagnosed and treated for bleeding esophageal varices.

FAMILY HISTORY: Noncontributory

DRUG HISTORY: In addition to ethanol abuse, the patient had a history of drug abuse.

PHYSICAL EXAMINATION: There was a large laceration and hematoma over the left hip. The abdomen was slightly distended, although a fluid wave was not elicited. The liver was palpable approximately 10 fingerbreadths below the right costal margin, and the spleen was palpable approximately three fingerbreadths below the left costal margin. Spider angiomas were noted over the distribution of the superior vena cava. There was palmar erythema with clubbing. There also was muscle atrophy of the arms and legs (spider habitus).

Laboratory Results

A. Screening Procedures (admitting)

	Patient	Normal
Prothrombin time	14 seconds	10–12 seconds
APTT	39 seconds	<42 seconds
Platelet count	90,000/μl	130,000–400,000/μl
Bleeding time	8 minutes	1–8 minutes

HOSPITAL COURSE: After the patient had been admitted to the medicine service, a fever developed, and blood cultures grew coagulase-positive Staphylococcus aureus. The patient was placed on antibiotics. Shortly thereafter, oozing was noted from venipuncture sites and the wound over the left hip.

Laboratory Results

B. Screening Procedures (follow-up)

	Patient	Normal
Prothrombin time	17 seconds	10–12 seconds
APTT	43 seconds	<42 seconds
Platelet count	35,000/μl	130,000–400,000/μl
Bleeding time	10 minutes and 30 seconds	1–8 minutes

Questions

1. What is the most likely diagnosis?
2. What additional laboratory procedures are indicated?
3. What are the possible causes of thrombocytopenia?
4. Why was the prothrombin time on admission slightly prolonged?

Laboratory Results

C. Confirmatory Procedures

	Patient	Normal
Factor VIII:C	40%	50% to 150%
Fibrinogen	100 mg/dl	170–410 mg/dl
Antithrombin III (activity)	55%	85% to 115%
Fibrin split products	>100 μg/ml	<10 μg/ml
Protamine sulfate	Positive	Negative

DIAGNOSIS: Disseminated intravascular coagulation complicating chronic liver disease and staphylococcal septicemia

Discussion

This patient was placed on antibiotics, and heparin was administered to manage the disseminated intravascular coagulation. In addition, the local wound was debrided. After heparinization had been achieved, coagulation parameters improved. Levels of fibrin split products decreased, and the platelet count increased to approximately 90,000/μl, which was similar to the admitting value.

Although coagulation parameters improved, local bleeding at the site of wound debridement was exa-

DISSEMINATED INTRAVASCULAR COAGULATION COMPLICATING CHRONIC LIVER DISEASE AND STAPHYLOCOCCAL SEPTICEMIA

CLINICAL PICTURE

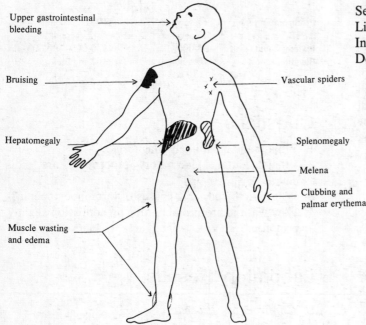

Upper gastrointestinal bleeding

Bruising

Hepatomegaly

Muscle wasting and edema

Vascular spiders

Splenomegaly

Melena

Clubbing and palmar erythema

PATHOPHYSIOLOGIC BASIS OF DISSEMINATED INTRAVASCULAR COAGULATION

Septicemia and associated endothelial injury
Liver unable to clear activated coagulation factors
Increased fibrinolysis
Decreased production of coagulation factors

LABORATORY FINDINGS

A. Screening Procedures

Test	Patient's Result	Normal Range
Prothrombin time	Abnormal	10–12 seconds
APTT	Abnormal	<42 seconds
Platelet count	Abnormal	130,000–400,000/μl
Bleeding time	Abnormal	1–8 minutes

B. Confirmatory Procedures

Test	Patient's Result	Normal Range
Factor VIII:C	Abnormal	50% to 150%
Antithrombin III	Abnormal	85% to 115%
Fibrin split products	Abnormal	<10 μg/ml

TREATMENT

Manage septicemia
Replace coagulation factors (fresh-frozen plasma)
Heparin (rarely)

cerbated by heparin therapy. This consequence was, however, anticipated, and heparin administration was not decreased because of local bleeding.

This case illustrates the use of heparin in the management of disseminated intravascular coagulation. In patients with an open wound or an injured mucosal surface, bleeding may be worsened by administration of heparin. This consequence is expected, even though the systemic disseminated intravascular coagulation is abat-

ing. Therefore, it is more important to monitor laboratory values to follow the course of the coagulation disturbance. It should not be assumed that increased local bleeding indicates a lack of response to heparin.

Bibliography

(See Bibliography for Case 31)

CASE
58

PATIENT: 36-year-old man

CHIEF COMPLAINT: This patient was admitted with pain in the right leg. He had first noticed the pain approximately 4 days before admission; however, he had not sought medical attention until the pain became intolerable.

MEDICAL HISTORY: The patient had previously been hospitalized on two occasions, for tonsillectomy with adenoidectomy at 9 years of age and for hernia repair at 21 years of age. There were no bleeding problems with either surgical procedure.

FAMILY HISTORY: Noncontributory

DRUG HISTORY: No medication

PHYSICAL EXAMINATION: The right leg was swollen from the middle of the thigh to the ankle. The circumference of the right thigh was approximately 1½ inches greater than the circumference of the left thigh. In addition, there was tenderness over the upper aspect of the right leg.

Laboratory Results

A. Screening Procedures

	Patient	Normal
Prothrombin time	12 seconds	10–12 seconds
APTT	26 seconds	<42 seconds
Platelet count	350,000/μl	130,000–400,000/μl
Bleeding time	7 minutes and 30 seconds	1–8 minutes

HOSPITAL COURSE: Doppler and impedance studies were ordered and, on the basis of the results of these studies, a diagnosis of right femoral vein thrombosis was made. The patient was started on 1000 units of heparin per hour, given by continuous intravenous infusion. The activated partial thromboplastin time (APTT) was monitored to follow the course of the heparin therapy. After 24 hours of intravenous administration of heparin (second hospital day), the APTT was measured. It was greater than 200 seconds, and the prothrombin time was 70 seconds.

Questions

1. Is the patient's APTT appropriate for this dosage of heparin?
2. Is his prolonged prothrombin time appropriate for this dosage of heparin?
3. What is the treatment of choice?

Laboratory Results

B. Confirmatory Procedures

The patient was given protamine sulfate. Six hours later, repeat tests were performed, and the following results were obtained:

	Patient	Normal
Prothrombin time	20 seconds	10–12 seconds
APTT	150 seconds	<42 seconds

DIAGNOSIS: Overdose of heparin

Discussion

This patient obviously had received too much heparin. An APTT of greater than 200 seconds together with a prothrombin time of 70 seconds would indicate an overdose of heparin. Heparin given at a dosage of 1000 units per hour would not prolong the prothrombin time to 70 seconds, nor would it be expected to prolong the APTT to greater than 200 seconds. The key in making the diagnosis of overdose of heparin in this patient was the markedly prolonged prothrombin time.

Subsequently, careful evaluation revealed that the patient had received 10,000 units of heparin per hour rather than 1000 units of heparin per hour. This error occurred because the label on the heparin bottle had been misread.

Bibliography

Triplett DA: Heparin: Clinical use and laboratory monitoring: In Triplett DA (ed): *Laboratory Evaluation of Coagulation*. Chicago: American Society of Clinical Pathologists, 1982, pp 271–313.

CASE
59

PATIENT: 22-year-old man

CHIEF COMPLAINT: This patient was admitted with a swollen right leg. Doppler and impedance studies indicated thrombosis of the proximal portion of the saphenous vein. .

MEDICAL HISTORY: Noncontributory

FAMILY HISTORY: A maternal great-grandfather had died of myocardial infarction.

DRUG HISTORY: No medication

PHYSICAL EXAMINATION: The right leg was swollen, and there was tenderness over the proximal portion of the right thigh.

Laboratory Results

A. Screening Procedures (admitting)

	Patient	Normal
Prothrombin time	12 seconds	10–12 seconds
APTT	27 seconds	<42 seconds
Platelet count	300,000/μl	130,000–400,000/μl
Bleeding time	6 minutes	1–8 minutes

HOSPITAL COURSE: The patient was placed on intermittent intravenous infusion of heparin (6000 units every 4 hours). However, the clinician thought that the response to heparin was insufficient, as judged by the activated partial thromboplastin time (APTT).

Laboratory Results (obtained while receiving heparin on sixth day of therapy)

B. Screening Procedures (follow-up)

	Patient	Normal
Prothrombin time	12 seconds	10–12 seconds
APTT	70 seconds	<42 seconds
Platelet count	210,000/μl	130,000–400,000/μl
Bleeding time	8 minutes	1–8 minutes

Questions

1. Is this APTT adequate for anticoagulation?
2. What additional laboratory procedures are indicated?

Laboratory Results

C. Confirmatory Procedures

	Patient	Normal
Antithrombin III (activity)	65%	85% to 115%
Antithrombin III (immunologic)	16 mg/dl	23–40 mg/dl

Because of the possibility of hereditary deficiency of antithrombin III, family members were evaluated:

	Patient	Normal
Brother (20 years old)		
Antithrombin III (activity)	92.5%	85% to 115%
Anithrombin III (immunologic)	37.2 mg/dl	23–40 mg/dl
Father (49 years old)		
Antithrombin III (activity)	90%	85% to 115%
Antithrombin III (immunologic)	35.2 mg/dl	23–40 mg/dl
Mother (46 years old)		
Antithrombin III (activity)	103%	85% to 115%
Antithrombin III (immunologic)	41.4 mg/dl	23–40 mg/dl

DIAGNOSIS: Decreased antithrombin III (due to infusion of heparin)

Discussion

This case illustrates the importance of knowing that heparin depresses the level of antithrombin III (Table 1). The antithrombin III level in this patient was monitored while he was receiving heparin. Follow-up studies done after heparin therapy had been discontinued revealed normal antithrombin III activity and antigenic content in the plasma.

It is important in assessing the response to heparin to have a baseline APTT for each patient. In this patient, the baseline APTT was short; the APTT noted above may well represent adequate anticoagulation. Many

Table 1
Classification of Causes of an Altered Antithrombin III Level

Decreased Antithrombin III	Increased Antithrombin III
Acquired	Acquired
Diminished synthesis	Acute hepatitis
Cirrhosis	Renal transplantation
Chronic hepatitis	Inherited
Cardiovascular disease	Hemophilias A and B
Arteriosclerosis	Combined deficiency of
Adult-onset diabetes	factors VIII and V
mellitus	Drug Therapy
Fatty liver of pregnancy	Courmarin
Increased utilization	17α-Alkylated
Disseminated	corticosteroids
intravascular coagulation	
Postoperative states	
Pulmonary embolism	
Myocardial infarction	
Protein-losing enteropathy	
Nephrotic syndrome	
Drugs	
Oral contraceptive use	
Heparin therapy	
L-Asparaginase therapy	
Fibrinolytic therapy	
(streptokinase)	

investigators advocate using the patients baseline APTT as a reference point in determining adequate heparinization.

Bibliography

Marciniak E, Gockerman JP: Heparin induced decrease in circulating antithrombin III. *Lancet* 2:581–584, 1977.

McGann MA, Triplett DA: Interpretation of antithrombin III activity. *Lab Med* 13:742–749, 1982.

Rao AK, Guzzo J, Niewiarowski S, et al: Antithrombin III levels during heparin therapy. *Thromb Res* 24:181–186, 1981.

CASE
60

PATIENT: 68-year-old woman

CHIEF COMPLAINT: This patient presented to the emergency room because of chest pain of sudden onset. In addition, there was hemoptysis.

MEDICAL HISTORY: The patient had been hospitalized on several occasions for various medical and surgical problems. Her surgical history included hysterectomy and cholecystectomy. In addition, she had been hospitalized on several occasions for complications of diabetes.

FAMILY HISTORY: There was a history of diabetes on the maternal side of the family.

DRUG HISTORY: The patient had taken insulin, thiazide diuretics and Valium (diazepam).

PHYSICAL EXAMINATION: Splinting of the left hemithorax and a pleural friction rub were noted. There also were physical findings of consolidation on the left side, including increased tactile fremitus, dullness to percussion and tubular breath sounds.

Laboratory Results

A. Screening Procedures (admitting)

	Patient	Normal
Prothrombin time	12 seconds	10–12 seconds
APTT	30 seconds	<42 seconds
Platelet count	280,000/μl	130,000–400,000/μl
Bleeding time	6 minutes	1–8 minutes

HOSPITAL COURSE: On the basis of these findings, a presumptive diagnosis of pulmonary embolism was made. A ventilation perfusion scan was also consistent with pulmonary embolism and an arteriogram confirmed the diagnosis.

The patient was placed on a loading dose of 10,000 units of heparin, which was followed by a dosage of approximately 1000 units per hour by continuous intravenous infusion. On the second hospital day, the following test results were obtained:

Laboratory Results

B. Screening Procedures (follow-up)

	Patient	Normal
Prothrombin time	15 seconds	10–12 seconds
APTT	82 seconds	<42 seconds
Platelet count	190,000/μl	130,000–400,000/μl
Bleeding time	7 minutes	1–8 minutes

The patient did well until the sixth hospital day, when she was feeling anxious and restless and had an increased pulse and backache. The following laboratory results were obtained:

	Patient	Normal
Prothrombin time	21 seconds	10–12 seconds
APTT	>150 seconds	<42 seconds

Questions

1. What is the most likely diagnosis?
2. What additional laboratory procedures are indicated?

Laboratory Results

C. Confirmatory Procedures

A CAT scan of the abdomen revealed a large retroperitoneal hematoma.

DIAGNOSIS: Retroperitoneal hemorrhage (due to overdose of heparin)

Discussion

This patient had received an overdose of heparin. Early on the fifth hospital day, an intern had noted that the activated partial thromboplastin time (APTT) was 40 seconds. As a result, he had increased the dosage of heparin from 1000 units to 1600 units per hour. When the patient was found to be feeling anxious and was somewhat hypotensive and complaining of backache, a CAT scan was ordered; it revealed a large retroperitoneal hematoma.

This case points out the need for careful follow-up of patients who are receiving heparin. A dose of heparin should never be modified on the basis of the result of a single laboratory test. In addition, it should be remembered that patients who are receiving heparin rarely bleed during the first 2 or 3 days of therapy. Presumably at this point in the thrombotic process, there is a need for a relatively high level of heparin to diminish the generation of thrombin and to control extension of the thrombus. However, after this initial period, the need for heparin decreases. Patients who bleed during heparin therapy typically do so on the fourth, fifth and sixth hospital days. Also, postmenopausal women appear to have an increased risk for bleeding during heparin therapy.

This patient was treated by reducing the dosage of heparin and shifting to Coumadin (sodium warfarin).

Bibliography

Triplett DA: Heparin: Clinical use and laboratory monitoring. In Triplett DA (ed): *Laboratory Evaluation of Coagulation*. Chicago: American Society of Clinical Pathologists, 1982, pp 271–313.

CASE
61

PATIENT: 55-year-old man

CHIEF COMPLAINT: This patient presented to the emergency room because of severe chest pain and shortness of breath. Complete evaluation indicated pulmonary embolism, as established on the basis of a mismatch between a ventilation perfusion scan and positive pulmonary arteriograms.

MEDICAL HISTORY: Noncontributory

FAMILY HISTORY: There was a maternal family history of arteriosclerosis and diabetes.

DRUG HISTORY: The patient was taking no medication at the time of admission.

PHYSICAL EXAMINATION: Physical findings were consistent with pulmonary embolism of the right lung. A friction rub was heard, and there was dullness to percussion.

Laboratory Results

A. Screening Procedures (admitting)

	Patient	Normal
Prothrombin time	11 seconds	10–12 seconds
APTT	29 seconds	<42 seconds
Platelet count	380,000/μl	130,000–400,000/μl
Bleeding time	7 minutes	1–8 minutes

HOSPITAL COURSE: The patient was placed on heparin, for 10 days. During the last 5 days of heparin therapy, the patient was started on oral anticoagulants. He was discharged receiving 10 mg of Coumadin (sodium warfarin) per day. Because of insomnia during his hospital stay, the patient also received Seconal (secobarbital) nightly.

Laboratory Results

B. Discharge Values

	Patient	Normal
Prothrombin time	19 seconds	10–12 seconds
APTT	40 seconds	<42 seconds
Platelet count	200,000/μl	130,000–400,000/μl
Bleeding time	Not performed	

POSTHOSPITAL COURSE: The patient was instructed to return to his physician's office on a weekly

basis for follow-up measurements of the prothrombin time. Approximately 8 days after discharge, he was seen in the physician's office.

Laboratory Results

C. Postdischarge Values

	Patient	Normal
Prothrombin time	54 seconds	10–12 seconds
APTT	49 seconds	<42 seconds

Table 1
Drugs That Alter the Response to Oral Anticoagulants

Anticoagulant Effect Enhanced	Anticoagulant Effect Reduced
Most predictable offenders	Barbiturates
Phenylbutazone (Butazolidin)	Glutethimide (Doriden)
Oxyphenbutazone (Tandearil)	Ethchlorvynol (Placidyl)
Phenyramidol hydrochloride (Analexin)	Halperidol (Haldol)
Norethandrolone (Nilevar)	Oral contraceptives, estrogens
Methandrostenolone (Dianabol)	Corticosteroids, corticotropin
Dextrothyroxine sodium (Choloxin)	Griseofulvin (Fulvicin)
Glucagon	Meprobamate (Miltown)
Clofibrate (Atromid-S)	Antacids
Less predictable offenders	Cholestyramine
Disulfiram (Antabuse)	
Methylphenidate hydrochloride (Ritalin)	
Aspirin	
p-Aminosalicylic acid	
Methylsalicylic acid	
Quinidine	
Quinine	
Acetaminophen (Tylenol)	
Antibiotics	
Other offenders	
Levothyroxine sodium	
Thiouracils	
Phenytoin (Dilantin)	
Indomethacin (Indocin)	
Tolbutamide (Orinase)	
Chloral hydrate	
Monamine oxidase inhibitors	
Diazoxide	
Mefanamic acid	
Ethacrynic acid	
Nalidixic acid	

Questions

1. What is the most likely diagnosis?

DIAGNOSIS: Overdose of Coumadin (due to interaction with Seconal)

Discussion

This case illustrates a relatively common problem. A number of drugs potentiate the action of oral anticoagulants, but many other drugs diminish the effectiveness of oral anticoagulants (Table 1). This patient had been taking Coumadin and Seconal at the time of discharge. He had been on maintenance therapy with Coumadin at a dosage of 10 mg per day, which had proved to be an effective anticoagulant dosage during his hospital stay. After the patient had returned to his home, he discontinued the Seconal but continued to take Coumadin at a dosage of 10 mg per day. Seconal is known to diminish the effectiveness of oral anticoagulants by increasing the rate of metabolism of Coumadin in the liver. Therefore, once the Seconal had been discontinued, the dosage of Coumadin was in excess of that needed to maintain proper anticoagulation. Consequently, when the patient returned to the physician for a follow-up measurement of the prothrombin time 8 days later, it was found to be markedly abnormal.

The dosage of Coumadin was decreased to approximately 5 mg per day, which proved to be effective in this patient.

Bibliography

Breckenridger A: Oral anticoagulant drugs: Pharmacokinetic aspects. *Semin Hematol* 15:19–26, 1978.

Deykin D: Warfarin therapy. *N Engl J Med* 283:691–694, 801, 1970.

CASE
62

PATIENT: 60-year-old man

CHIEF COMPLAINT: This patient had traveled from London to Chicago on a business trip. He had been instructed by his physician in London to consult a cardiologist in Chicago to monitor his oral anticoagulant therapy.

MEDICAL HISTORY: The patient had a documented episode of thrombophlebitis with pulmonary embolism 4 months before he made the trip. He had been hospitalized and treated with heparin and oral anticoagulants and was undergoing maintenance therapy with oral anticoagulants at the time of his visit to the United States.

FAMILY HISTORY: Noncontributory

DRUG HISTORY: The patient had been taking Coumadin (sodium warfarin) at a dosage of 5 mg per day.

PHYSICAL EXAMINATION: Noncontributory

Laboratory Results

A. London Screening Procedures

	Patient	Normal
Prothrombin time	45 seconds	<18 seconds
APTT	48 seconds	<50 seconds

B. Chicago Results

Prothrombin time	20 seconds	10–12 seconds
APTT	41 seconds	<42 seconds

Questions

1. Should this patient's dosage of Coumadin be changed on the basis of the results obtained in Chicago?
2. What is the most likely explanation for the difference between the two prothrombin time measurements?

DIAGNOSIS: Adequate anticoagulation

Discussion

This case illustrates the problems in a highly mobile society of patients who are receiving oral anticoagulant therapy. The sensitivity of various thromboplastins to the action of oral anticoagulants differs markedly according to the source of a thromboplastin. In this case, the prothrombin time was measured in London, where human brain thromboplastin is used as the standard reagent (British comparative thromboplastin). The therapeutic range for human brain thromboplastin is much different from those of thromboplastins from other animal sources. The thromboplastin used in Chicago was of rabbit origin and therefore had a different normal range as well as a different therapeutic range.

In this instance, the two results are comparable and, accordingly, the dosage of Coumadin was not altered. Currently, efforts are under way to standardize measurement of the prothrombin time so that this type of situation can be readily recognized and appreciated by physicians who are consulted by patients taking oral anticoagulants. Several reference thromboplastins have been prepared through the efforts of a program sponsored by the European Economic Community. These reference prothromboplastins may be used by manufacturers to calibrate their batches of commercial thromboplastin. Using these reference thromboplastins International Normalized Ratios (INRs) may be calculated. Thus results between two different thromboplastins can be readily compared.

Bibliography

Duxbury BMCD: Therapeutic control of oral anticoagulant treatment. *Brit Med J* 284:702–704, 1982.

Poller L: Oral anticoagulant therapy. In Bloom AL, Thomas DP (eds): *Haemostasis and Thrombosis*. Edinburgh: Churchill Livingstone, 1981.

Shinton NK: Therapeutic control of anticoagulant treatment. *Brit MEd J* 284:1871–1874, 1982.

Triplett DA: Anticoagulant therapy: Monitoring techniques. *Lab Man* 20:31–42, 1982.

Triplett DA (ed): *Standardization of Coagulation Assays: An Overview*. Skokie, Illinois: College of American Pathologists, 1982.

Index

Page numbers followed by an "f" refer to figures and those followed by a "t" indicate tabular material.

A

Acquired immune deficiency syndrome (AIDS), 95
    as a complication of hemophilia, 109
Activated partial thromboplastin time (APTT), 66t, 67f, 68
    normal value, 76
    prolonged, 88
        in case report, 81
Adenocarcinoma, metastatic
    chronic disseminated intravascular coagulation, 220
Afibrinogenemia, 63t
    congenital, case report, 167-170
    and deficiency of Factor XIII, 182
Alcoholism, 208-210
Allergic reactions,
    and fibrinolytic therapy, 38
trans-p-aminomethylcyclohexane carboxylic acid
        (AMCA), 39-40
    pharmacologic aspects, 40
Amyloidosis, primary systemic, 249-251
Angiokeratoma, 64t
Anticoagulants
    development of, 4
    following fibrinolytic therapy, 37
    oral, 5, 188
    therapy, complications of, 80
Antifibrinolytic agents, mechanisms of action, 39-40
Antifibrinolytic therapy, clinical use of, 39, 40
α_2 antiplasmin, and hemorrhage, 36
Antiplasmin levels, clinical states with altered, 192
Antiplatelet medication, 37
Antithrombin III, 22-23
    activity test, 76
    altered level, classification of causes, 308t
    antigen test, 76
    decreased, due to infusion of heparin, 307-308
    deficiency
        acquired, case report, 230-232
        similarity to Protein C deficiency, 198
        variants of, 189
    hereditary deficiency of, case report, 186-189
Aprotinin, 39
Arachidonic acid
    and platelet membrane, 48
    and synthesis of prostaglandin, 50
Arterial spiders, 64t
Arterial thromboembolic disease,
    role of platelets in, 45

Aspirin, 51
    frequent ingestion of, 201
    and hemostatic disorders, 63
    medications containing (list), 77-79t
    and platelet abnormality, 201-204
    qualitative abnormality of platelets, secondary to,
        106
    and streptokinase therapy, 37
Atherosclerosis,
    role of platelets in, 45, 46f

B

Bernard-Soulier syndrome, 48
    case report, 268-270
Bethesda assay, 76
Bleeding
    disorders, congenital, 63t
    early childhood, 190
    and family history, 62-63
    in first week of life, 207
    gastrointestinal, 210, 290
    infant, 98
    lifelong history of, 163
    and liver disease, 209
    localized, and antifibrinolytic therapy, 39
    at multiple sites, 215
    neonatal, 161
    and patient history, 61-62
    postoperative
        and Factor XI deficiency, 90
        history of, 62
    severe, 146
        and hereditary deficiency of α_2-antiplasmin, 192
    and trauma, 192
    upper respiratory, 210
    uterine, 171
Bleeding time
    for evaluating primary hemostasis, 65-66
    template, 66t
Bone marrow examination, 65-66
Breast feeding, and risk of hemorrhage, 203
Bruising, and Hemophilia B, 94
Burn injury, and coagulopathy, case report, 211-216

C

Calcium, 49
Campbell-deMorgan spot, 64t
Capillary hemostasis, 61
γ-carboxyglutamic acid, 5f
    and discovery of other Vitamin-K dependent
        plasma proteins, 13-14